Yearbook of Diabetes 2025

Yearbook of Diabetes 2025

Editor-in-Chief
Sujoy Ghosh
Professor
Department of Endocrinology
Institute of Post Graduate Medical Education and Research
Kolkata, West Bengal, India

Assistant Editor
Anjan Roy
Field Based Medical Affairs/Medical Science Liaison Expert
Kolkata, West Bengal, India

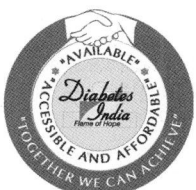

Under the Aegis of Diabetes India

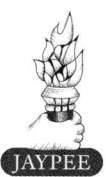

JAYPEE BROTHERS MEDICAL PUBLISHERS
The Health Sciences Publisher
New Delhi | London

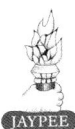

Jaypee Brothers Medical Publishers (P) Ltd

Headquarters
EMCA House
23/23-B, Ansari Road, Daryaganj
New Delhi 110 002, India
Landline: +91-11-23272143, +91-11-23272703
+91-11-23282021, +91-11-23245672
E-mail: jaypee@jaypeebrothers.com

Corporate Office
Jaypee Brothers Medical Publishers (P) Ltd.
4838/24, Ansari Road, Daryaganj
New Delhi 110 002, India
Phone: +91-11-43574357
Fax: +91-11-43574314
E-mail: jaypee@jaypeebrothers.com

Overseas Office
JP Medical Ltd.
83, Victoria Street, London
SW1H 0HW (UK)
Phone: +44-20 3170 8910
Fax: +44(0)20 3008 6180
E-mail: info@jpmedpub.com

Website: www.jaypeebrothers.com
Website: www.jaypeedigital.com

© 2025, Jaypee Brothers Medical Publishers

The views and opinions expressed in this book are solely those of the original contributor(s)/author(s) and do not necessarily represent those of editor(s) or publisher of the book.

All rights reserved. No part of this publication may be reproduced, stored or transmitted in any form or by any means, electronic, mechanical, photocopying, recording or otherwise, without the prior permission in writing of the publishers.

All brand names and product names used in this book are trade names, service marks, trademarks or registered trademarks of their respective owners. The publisher is not associated with any product or vendor mentioned in this book.

Medical knowledge and practice change constantly. This book is designed to provide accurate, authoritative information about the subject matter in question. However, readers are advised to check the most current information available on procedures included and check information from the manufacturer of each product to be administered, to verify the recommended dose, formula, method and duration of administration, adverse effects and contraindications. It is the responsibility of the practitioner to take all appropriate safety precautions. Neither the publisher nor the author(s)/editor(s) assume any liability for any injury and/or damage to persons or property arising from or related to use of material in this book.

This book is sold on the understanding that the publisher is not engaged in providing professional medical services. If such advice or services are required, the services of a competent medical professional should be sought.

Every effort has been made where necessary to contact holders of copyright to obtain permission to reproduce copyright material. If any have been inadvertently overlooked, the publisher will be pleased to make the necessary arrangements at the first opportunity.

Inquiries for bulk sales may be solicited at: jaypee@jaypeebrothers.com

Yearbook of Diabetes 2025 / Sujoy Ghosh

First Edition: **2025**

ISBN: 978-93-6616-193-8

Printed at: Samrat Offset Pvt. Ltd.

Contributors

SECTION EDITORS

Abhranil Dhar
Postdoctoral Trainee
Department of Endocrinology
Institute of Post Graduate
Medical Education and Research
Kolkata, West Bengal, India

Anirban Sinha
Associate Professor
Department of Endocrinology
Calcutta Medical College and
Hospital
Kolkata, West Bengal, India

Arijit Singha
Assistant Professor
Department of Endocrinology
Institute of Post Graduate
Medical Education and Research
Kolkata, West Bengal, India

Indira Maisnam
Assistant Professor
Department of Endocrinology
Institute of Post Graduate
Medical Education and Research
Kolkata, West Bengal, India

Mainak Banerjee
Consultant Endocrinologist
Narayan Health Rabindranath
Tagore International Institute of
Cardiac Sciences
Kolkata, West Bengal, India

Nisha Batra
Postdoctoral Trainee
Department of Endocrinology
Institute of Post Graduate
Medical Education and Research
Kolkata, West Bengal, India

Pritam Biswas
Postdoctoral Trainee
Department of Endocrinology
Institute of Post Graduate
Medical Education and Research
Kolkata, West Bengal, India

Soham Tarafdar
Consultant Endocrinologist
Manipal Hospitals, Dhakuria
Kolkata, West Bengal, India

Sunetra Mondal
Assistant Professor
Department of Endocrinology
Nil Ratan Sircar Medical College
and Hospital
Kolkata, West Bengal, India

Editorial Board

- Peter Schwarz, Germany
- SR Arvind, India
- Abdul Basit, Pakistan
- Shashank Joshi, India
- Nadima Shegen, Jordan
- Sanjeev Phatak, India
- Rajeev Chawla, India
- Sanjay Agarwal, India
- Jothydev Kesavadev, India
- Sanjay Karla, India
- Azad Khan, Bangladesh
- Banshi Saboo, India
- Biswajeet Bhomik, Bangladesh
- Manoj Chawla, India
- Partha Kar, United Kingdom
- Kamlesh Kunthi, United Kingdom
- Brij Mohan Makkar, India
- Atul Kalhaan, United Kingdom
- Rakesh Parikh, India
- Anuj Maheswari, India

Foreword

It is indeed a matter of great pride that DiabetesIndia is publishing *"Yearbook of Diabetes 2025"* which will be released at the World Congress of Diabetes at Ahmedabad, India, on 13th to 16th February 2025 and also at IDF World Diabetes Congress at Bangkok, Thailand on 7th to 10th April 2025. One of the key endeavors of DiabetesIndia has been to promote research and education in the field of diabetes in India. A *"yearbook,"* a compilation of assorted research papers in diabetes and allied subjects published during the preceding 1 year, will be an important source of all the recent developments in understanding of diabetes and provide a great knowledge tool for physicians, postgraduates, and researchers. Hopefully this will ultimately translate into motivation for more research in diabetes and better patient care. Personally, I am more than pleased to be part of this great educational venture. My compliments go to Dr Sujoy Ghosh and the editorial team and my best wishes for the *"Yearbook of Diabetes 2025"*.

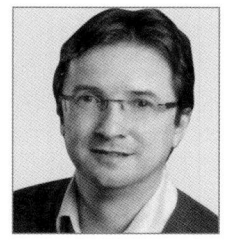

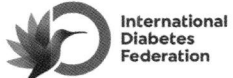 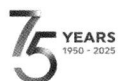

Peter Schwarz
President
International Diabetes Federation

Message from the DiabetesIndia

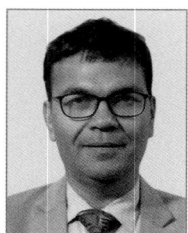

Banshi Saboo
Secretary, DiabetesIndia
Consultant Diabetologist
Dia Care – Diabetes Care and
Hormone Clinic
Ahmedabad, Gujarat, India

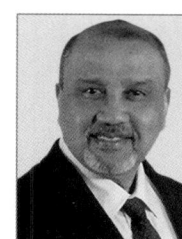

SR Aravind
President
DiabetesIndia
Chairman and
Managing Director
Diacon Hospital (Diabetes
Care and Research Centre)
Bengaluru, Karnataka, India

The *"Yearbook of Diabetes 2025"* brings you the abstracts of the articles that reported recent and breakthrough developments in diabetes during 1st January 2024 to 31st December 2024, carefully selected from many journals worldwide. Expert commentaries evaluate the clinical importance of each article.

This book allows the reader to quickly identify and understand topics of interest which translate into practical application. The goals of the book are to be current, be compact, make the information accessible, and be understandable by students of medicine of all ages.

The book is divided into nine sections arranging closely related subjects into clusters. The sections span the spectrum of diabetes from basic science to futuristic.

Together, we salute and thank the Editor-in-Chief Dr Sujoy Ghosh for his expertise in the shaping and collation and for showing extraordinary commitment to maintaining the excellent standard. We are especially grateful to the editorial team comprising Drs Peter Schwarz, Abdul Bashit, Atul Kalhaan, Biswajeet Bhowmik, Kamlesh Kunthi, Nadima Shegen, Patha Kar, Abhay Sahoo, Amit Gupta, Anoop Mishra, Anup Maheswari, Banshi Saboo, Bharat Saboo, Brij Mohan Makkar, G Vijay Kumar, Jayant Panda, Kamalakar Tripathi, Manoj Chawla, Rajeev Chawla, Rutul Goklani, Sadhasiv Rao, Sanjay Agarwal, Sanjay Kalra, Sanjay Reddy, Sanjeev Phatak, Shashank Joshi, and SR Arvind who have provided endless support. We thank Drs Arijit Singha, Soham Tarafdar, Indira Maisnam, Mainak Banerjee, Pritam Biswas, Abhranil Dhar, Sunetra Mondal, Anirban Sinha, and Nisha Batra for their extremely valuable contribution. We would also like to thank Assistant Editor Dr Anjan Roy who has been instrumental in compiling this extensive work.

We all take immense pride in producing an outstanding book and hope that the reader will agree that the excellence of the writing and scholarly rigor displayed by the authors make a strong argument for its endurance as an outstanding resource for education and teaching in diabetes.

Preface

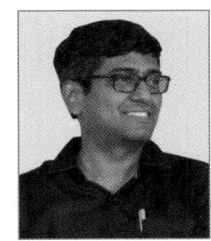

Given the fact that 63,773 articles related to diabetes have been published on PubMed in 2024 itself, it is not surprising that no one has embarked upon taking the herculean task of writing a yearbook on diabetes.

Being a teacher, I have been often asked by students which studies to read and how to interpret them. Clinicians, both primary care and specialists, often attend conferences and clinical meetings with the expectation to update their understanding of diabetology. Clinical service delivery makes it difficult for most to keep abreast with all the new studies published. Others have at various points expressed their inability to interpret clinical studies and at other times physicians have been swayed by deliberate or inadvertent biased interpretation of clinical studies by both pharmaceutical companies and "key opinion leaders."

Hence, it is imperative that a yearbook be published that contains the most important publications which are summarized in an easy-to-read format for the physician. DiabetesIndia is one of the biggest organizations in the field of diabetology worldwide and is, therefore, the apt organization to take up the responsibility.

But why did I agree upon taking this challenge? As I took up this challenge with our editorial team/authors, I was reminded of the words of author Conan Doyle (The Hound of the Baskervilles), "the boldest, or it may be the most drunken, rode forward."

We decided to screen all diabetes-related articles (major publications, from major journals) published between January 1, 2024 and December 31, 2024. We screened almost 15,000 original research articles and then divided up the selected articles into nine subsections and wrote up a critical appraisal of all the selected ones. The unstructured writeups tried to provide background information on what was already known about the issue prior to the particular publication, what the study added in terms of medical knowledge, and what the take home for the physician is as well as highlights the possible strengths and limitations of the study and the scope of future research.

I was fortunate to be working with an outstanding team of doctors, including a dynamic editorial team consisting of a mix of doctors (including specialists in pharmacology), physicians, diabetologists, and endocrinologists. I would like to put on record my thanks to my Assistant Editor Dr Anjan Roy and also Dr Ranjini Sen for her scientific support. The entire writing team of doctors for the book has done a splendid job, that too at such a short notice.

The book would never have seen the day of light without the persistence, help, support, and guidance that I received from Mr Sabyasachi Hazra (Associate Director, Publishing) of Jaypee Brothers Medical Publishers (P) Ltd, New Delhi, India.

Finally, I would like to thank all my colleagues at work and my family who have been a constant source of encouragement and support.

I dedicate this book to all those involved in the management of patients with diabetes and hope this helps in improvement of patient care and outcome.

Sujoy Ghosh

Contents

Section 1: BASIC SCIENCE
Section Editor: Arijit Singha

1. Large-scale Proteomics Improve Prediction of Chronic Kidney Disease in People with Diabetes 1
2. tRNA-derived Fragments are Altered in Diabetes 2
3. Islet Autoantibody Frequency in Relatives of Children with Type 1 Diabetes Who have a Type 2 Diabetes Diagnosis 3
4. Bone Marrow Mesenchymal Stem Cell-derived Exosomal miR-221-3p Promotes Angiogenesis and Wound Healing in Diabetes via the Downregulation of Forkhead Box P1 5
5. The Metabolomic Signature of Weight Loss and Remission in the Diabetes Remission Clinical Trial (DiRECT) 6
6. Multi-omic Prediction of Incident Type 2 Diabetes 8
7. HOMA-IR and the Matsuda Index as Predictors of Progression to Type 1 Diabetes in Autoantibody-positive Relatives 10
8. Zinc Finger BED-type Containing 3 Promotes Hepatic Steatosis by Interacting with Polypyrimidine Tract-binding Protein 1 11
9. Week-long Normoglycemia in Diabetic Mice and Minipigs via a Subcutaneous Dose of a Glucose-responsive Insulin Complex 13

Section 2: EPIDEMIOLOGY
Section Editor: Soham Tarafdar

1. Association between Age at Diabetes Diagnosis and Subsequent Incidence of Cancer: A Longitudinal Population-based Cohort 15
2. Natural History of Type 2 Diabetes in Indians: Time to Progression 17
3. Association of Baseline Factors with Glycemic Outcomes in GRADE: A Comparative Effectiveness Randomized Clinical Trial 19
4. The Difference between Cystatin C- and Creatinine-based Estimated Glomerular Filtration Rate and Risk of Diabetic Microvascular Complications Among Adults With Diabetes: A Population-based Cohort Study 22
5. The Effect of City-level Sugar-sweetened Beverage Taxes on Longitudinal HbA1c and Incident Diabetes in Adults with Prediabetes 24

6. Association of Glucagon-like Peptide-1 Receptor Agonists with Suicidal Ideation and Self-injury in Individuals with Diabetes and Obesity: A Propensity-weighted, Population-based Cohort Study — 26

7. Associations between Diabetes and Cancer: A 10-year National Population-based Retrospective Cohort Study — 28

8. 5-year Follow-up of the Randomised Diabetes Remission Clinical Trial (DiRECT) of Continued Support for Weight Loss Maintenance in the UK: An Extension Study — 31

9. Adiposity and Metabolic Health in Asian Populations: An Epidemiological Study Using Dual-energy X-ray Absorptiometry in Singapore — 33

10. Association of Glycaemic Index and Glycaemic Load with Type 2 Diabetes, Cardiovascular Disease, Cancer, and All-cause Mortality: A Meta-analysis of Mega Cohorts of more than 100,000 Participants — 36

11. Associations of the Glycaemic Index and the Glycaemic Load with Risk of Type 2 Diabetes in 127,594 People from 20 Countries (PURE): A Prospective Cohort Study — 38

12. Daily Low-dose Aspirin and Incident Type 2 Diabetes in Community-dwelling Healthy Older Adults: A Post-hoc Analysis of Efficacy and Safety in the ASPREE Randomised Placebo-controlled Trial — 41

13. Early Findings from the NHS Type 2 Diabetes Path to Remission Programme: A Prospective Evaluation of Real-world Implementation — 43

14. Food Additive Emulsifiers and the Risk of Type 2 Diabetes: Analysis of Data from the NutriNet-Santé Prospective Cohort Study — 46

15. Meat Consumption and Incident Type 2 Diabetes: An Individual-participant Federated Meta-analysis of 1.97 Million Adults with 100,000 Incident Cases from 31 Cohorts in 20 Countries — 48

Section 3: COMORBIDITIES
Section Editor: Pritam Biswas

1. Comparative Effectiveness of Aspirin Dosing in Cardiovascular Disease and Diabetes Mellitus: A Subgroup Analysis of the ADAPTABLE Trial — 51

2. A Methodological Framework for Meta-analysis and Clinical Interpretation of Subgroup Data: The Case of Major Adverse Cardiovascular Events With GLP-1 Receptor Agonists and SGLT-2 Inhibitors in Type 2 Diabetes — 52

3. Effect of Semaglutide on Regression and Progression of Glycemia in People with Overweight or Obesity but without Diabetes in the SELECT Trial — 54

4. Semaglutide and Cardiovascular Outcomes by Baseline HbA1c and Change in HbA1c in People with Overweight or Obesity but without Diabetes in SELECT — 55

5. Metabolomic Fingerprints of Medical Therapy versus Bariatric Surgery in Patients with Obesity and Type 2 Diabetes: The STAMPEDE Trial — 57

6. Cardiovascular and Mortality Outcomes with GLP-1 Receptor Agonists versus Other Glucose-lowering Drugs in Individuals with NAFLD and Type 2 Diabetes: A Large Population-based Matched Cohort Study — 58

7. Circulating Metabolomic Markers Linking Diabetic Kidney Disease and Incident Cardiovascular Disease in Type 2 Diabetes: Analyses from the Hong Kong Diabetes Biobank — 60
8. Effect of Sodium-glucose Cotransporter-2 Inhibitors on Myocardial Infarction Incidence: A Systematic Review and Meta-analysis of Randomized Controlled Trials and Cohort Studies — 61
9. Prediction of New-onset Heart Failure in Patients with Type 2 Diabetes Derived from ALTITUDE and CANVAS — 63
10. Impact of Glycaemic Status on the Cardiac Effects of Empagliflozin when Initiated Immediately after Myocardial Infarction: A Post-hoc Analysis of the EMMY Trial — 64
11. Impact of Empagliflozin on Insulin Needs in Patients with Heart Failure and Diabetes: An EMPEROR-Pooled Analysis — 65
12. Diabetes and Risk of Heart Failure in People with and without Cardiovascular Disease: Systematic Review and Meta-analysis — 67
13. Semaglutide in Patients with Obesity-related Heart Failure and Type 2 Diabetes — 68
14. Effects of Empagliflozin on Progression of Chronic Kidney Disease: A Prespecified Secondary Analysis from the EMPA-KIDNEY Trial — 69
15. Efficacy and Safety of Once-weekly Semaglutide 2.4 mg versus Placebo in People with Obesity and Prediabetes (STEP 10): A Randomised, Double-blind, Placebo-controlled, Multicentre Phase 3 Trial — 71
16. Impact of Primary Kidney Disease on the Effects of Empagliflozin in Patients with Chronic Kidney Disease: Secondary Analyses of the EMPA-KIDNEY Trial — 73

Section 4: COMPLICATIONS
Section Editor: Abhranil Dhar

1. Mortality in the Glycemia Reduction Approaches in Diabetes: A Comparative Effectiveness Study (GRADE) — 76
2. Risk of Diabetic Retinopathy and Diabetic Macular Oedema with Sodium-glucose Cotransporter-2 Inhibitors and Glucagon-like Peptide 1 Receptor Agonists in Type 2 Diabetes: A Real-world Data Study from a Global Federated Database — 78
3. Effect of Preceding Drug Therapy on the Renal and Cardiovascular Outcomes of Combined Sodium-glucose Cotransporter-2 Inhibitor and Glucagon-like Peptide-1 Receptor Agonist Treatment in Patients with Type 2 Diabetes and Chronic Kidney Disease — 80
4. Comparing Clinical Outcomes in Patients with Type 2 Diabetes Mellitus after Ischaemic Stroke: Sodium-glucose Cotransporter-2 Inhibitors Users versus Non-users. A Propensity Score Matching National Cohort Study — 82
5. Uric Acid-lowering Effects of Sodium-glucose Cotransporter 2 Inhibitors for Preventing Cardiovascular Events and Mortality: A Systematic Review and Meta-analysis — 84
6. A Meta-analysis of Randomized Controlled Studies Examining the Effects of Sodium-glucose Cotransporter-2 Inhibitors on Peripheral Artery Disease and Risk of Amputations — 85

7. Efficacy of Aspirin for Primary Prevention among Adults with High-risk Type 2 Diabetes in the ACCORD Trial — 87
8. Glycaemic Control and Macrovascular and Microvascular Outcomes: A Systematic Review and Meta-analysis of Trials Investigating Intensive Glucose-lowering Strategies in People with Type 2 Diabetes — 88
9. Incidence and Progression of Diabetic Retinopathy in Patients Treated with Glucagon-like Peptide-1 Receptor Agonists versus Sodium-glucose Cotransporter 2 Inhibitors: A Population-based Cohort Study — 90
10. Normoalbuminuria—Is It Normal? The Association of Urinary Albumin within the 'Normoalbuminuric' Range with Adverse Cardiovascular and Mortality Outcomes: A Systematic Review and Meta-analysis — 93
11. Comparison of Estimated Glomerular Filtration Rate Change with Sodium-glucose Cotransporter-2 Inhibitors versus Glucagon-like Peptide-1 Receptor Agonists among People with Diabetes: A Propensity-score Matching Study — 95
12. Major Adverse Events in Youth-onset Type 1 and Type 2 Diabetes: The SEARCH and TODAY Studies — 96
13. Effect of Proteinuria on the Rapid Kidney Function Decline in Chronic Kidney Disease Depends on the Underlying Disease: A Post Hoc Analysis of the BRIGHTEN Study — 98
14. Editorials: Diabetic Kidney Disease—Semaglutide Flows into the Mainstream — 100
15. A Phase 2 Randomized Trial of Survodutide in MASH and Fibrosis — 102
16. Tirzepatide for Metabolic Dysfunction–associated Steatohepatitis with Liver Fibrosis — 103
17. Effects of Semaglutide on Chronic Kidney Disease in Patients with Type 2 Diabetes — 105
18. Effect of SGLT2 Inhibitors on Heart Failure Outcomes and Cardiovascular Death Across the Cardiometabolic Disease Spectrum: A Systematic Review and Meta-analysis — 107

Section 5: TYPE 1 DIABETES MELLITUS
Section Editor: Mainak Banerjee

1. Disparities in Continuous Glucose Monitor Use between Children with Type 1 Diabetes Living in Urban and Rural Areas — 113
2. Longitudinal Assessment of Pancreas Volume by MRI Predicts Progression to Stage 3 Type 1 Diabetes — 114
3. Low-dose Antithymocyte Globulin: A Pragmatic Approach to Treating Stage 2 Type 1 Diabetes — 116
4. Exploring Factors that Influence Postexercise Glycemia in Youth with Type 1 Diabetes in the Real World: The Type 1 Diabetes Exercise Initiative Pediatric (T1DEXIP) Study — 118
5. A Randomized Comparison of Postprandial Glucose Excursion Using Inhaled Insulin versus Rapid-acting Analog Insulin in Adults with Type 1 Diabetes Using Multiple Daily Injections of Insulin or Automated Insulin Delivery — 120
6. Comparing the Glycaemic Outcomes between Real-time Continuous Glucose Monitoring (rt-CGM) and Intermittently Scanned Continuous Glucose Monitoring (isCGM) among Adults and Children with Type 1 Diabetes: A Systematic Review and Meta-analysis of Randomised Controlled Trials — 121

7. A First-in-Human, Open-label Phase 1b and a Randomised, Double-blind Phase 2a Clinical Trial in Recent-onset Type 1 Diabetes with AG019 as Monotherapy and in Combination with Teplizumab 123

8. Progression of Type 1 Diabetes is Associated with High Levels of Soluble PD-1 in Islet Autoantibody-positive Children 125

9. Autoimmune Comorbidity in Type 1 Diabetes and its Association with Metabolic Control and Mortality Risk in Young People: A Population-based Study 126

10. The Association of Chronic Complications with Time in Tight Range and Time in Range in People with Type 1 Diabetes: A Retrospective Cross-sectional Real-world Study 128

11. Safety and Efficacy of Teplizumab in the Treatment of Type 1 Diabetes Mellitus: An Updated Systematic Review and Meta-analysis of Randomized Controlled Trials 130

12. Mortality in Type 1 Diabetes Mellitus: A Single Centre Experience from the ICMR–Youth Onset Diabetes Registry in India 132

13. Islet-after-kidney Transplantation versus Kidney Alone in Kidney Transplant Recipients with Type 1 Diabetes (KAIAK): A Population-based Target Trial Emulation in France 134

14. Prediction of Progression to Type 1 Diabetes with Dynamic Biomarkers and Risk Scores 136

Section 6: GESTATIONAL DIABETES MELLITUS AND PREGNANCY IN DIABETES MELLITUS
Section Editor: Indira Maisnam

1. Perinatal Outcomes Associated with Metformin Use during Pregnancy in Women with Pregestational Type 2 Diabetes Mellitus 138

2. Earlier Detection of Gestational Diabetes Impacts on Medication Requirements, Neonatal and Maternal Outcomes 139

3. Prevalence of Gestational Diabetes Mellitus Risk Factors in Singleton Pregnancies Obtained by Assisted Reproductive Technology: An Observational, Retrospective, Real-world Study from a Pregnancy Registry 141

4. Comparing the Different Phenotypes of Diabetes in Pregnancy: Are Outcomes Worse for Women with Young-onset Type 2 Diabetes Mellitus Compared to Type 1 Diabetes? 142

5. Comparing Advanced Hybrid Closed Loop Therapy and Standard Insulin Therapy in Pregnant Women with Type 1 Diabetes (Cristal): A Parallel-group, Open-label, Randomised Controlled Trial 144

6. Early Pregnancy HbA1c as the First Screening Test for Gestational Diabetes: Results from Three Prospective Cohorts 145

Section 7: DRUGS AND THERAPEUTICS
Section Editor: Sunetra Mondal

1. Comparative Effects of Randomized Second-line Therapy for Type 2 Diabetes on a Composite Outcome Incorporating Glycemic Control, Body Weight, and Hypoglycemia: An Analysis of the Glycemia Reduction Approaches in Diabetes: A Comparative Effectiveness Study (GRADE) 148

2. Impact of Canagliflozin on Kidney and Cardiovascular Outcomes by Type 2 Diabetes Duration: A Pooled Analysis of the CANVAS Program and CREDENCE Trials — 150

3. Occurrence of Gastrointestinal Adverse Events Upon GLP-1 Receptor Agonist Initiation with Concomitant Metformin Use: A Post Hoc Analysis of LEADER, STEP 2, SUSTAIN-6, and PIONEER 6 — 151

4. Early-onset Type 2 Diabetes and Tirzepatide Treatment: A Post Hoc Analysis from the SURPASS Clinical Trial Program — 153

5. Efficacy and Safety of LX9211 for Relief of Diabetic Peripheral Neuropathic Pain (RELIEF-DPN 1): Results of a Double-blind, Randomized, Placebo-controlled, Proof-of-concept Study — 155

6. Glucose-lowering Drugs and Liver-related Outcomes Among Individuals with Type 2 Diabetes: A Systematic Review of Longitudinal Population-based Studies — 156

7. Dose-response Effects on HbA1c and Bodyweight Reduction of Survodutide, a Dual Glucagon/GLP-1 Receptor Agonist, Compared with Placebo and Open-label Semaglutide in People with Type 2 Diabetes: A Randomised Clinical Trial — 158

8. Subcutaneously Administered Tirzepatide vs Semaglutide for Adults with Type 2 Diabetes: A Systematic Review and Network Meta-analysis of Randomised Controlled Trials — 160

9. Ultra-rapid Lispro Improved Postprandial Glucose Control Compared to Insulin Lispro in Predominantly Chinese Patients with Type 1 Diabetes: A Prospective, Randomized, Double-blind Phase 3 Study — 162

10. Once-daily Oral Small-molecule Glucagon-like Peptide-1 Receptor Agonist Lotiglipron (PF-07081532) for Type 2 Diabetes and Obesity: Two Randomized, Placebo-controlled, Multiple-ascending-dose Phase 1 Studies — 164

11. Effect of Tirzepatide on Body Fat Distribution Pattern in People with Type 2 Diabetes — 166

12. Glucagon-like Peptide-1 Receptor Agonist-based Agents and Weight Loss Composition: Filling the Gaps — 168

13. Oral or Injectable Semaglutide for the Management of Type 2 Diabetes in Routine Care: A Multicentre Observational Study Comparing Matched Cohorts — 169

14. Effectiveness of Switching from Dipeptidyl Peptidase-4 Inhibitor to Oral Glucagon-like Peptide-1 Receptor Agonist in Japanese Participants with Type 2 Diabetes Mellitus: Prospective Observational Study Using Propensity Score Matching — 171

15. Inclisiran in Individuals with Diabetes or Obesity: Post Hoc Pooled Analyses of the ORION-9, ORION-10 and ORION-11 Phase 3 Randomized Trials — 173

16. Pioglitazone Reduces Serum Ketone Bodies in Sodium-glucose Cotransporter-2 Inhibitor-treated Non-obese Type 2 Diabetes: A Single-centre, Randomized, Crossover Trial — 175

17. Are the Cardiovascular Properties of GLP-1 Receptor Agonists Differentially Modulated by Sulfonylureas? Insights from Post-hoc Analysis of EXSCEL — 177

18. Tirzepatide 5, 10 and 15 mg versus Injectable Semaglutide 0.5 mg for the Treatment of Type 2 Diabetes: An Adjusted Indirect Treatment Comparison — 179

19. Continuous Glucose Monitoring-based Metrics and the Duration of Hypoglycaemia Events with Once-weekly Insulin Icodec versus Once-daily Insulin Glargine U100 in Insulin-naive Type 2 Diabetes: An Exploratory Analysis of ONWARDS 1 — 181

20. Efficacy and Safety of SGLT2 Inhibitors with and without Glucagon-like Peptide 1 Receptor Agonists: A SMART-C Collaborative Meta-analysis of Randomised Controlled Trials — 183
21. Once-weekly Insulin Icodec as Compared to Once-daily Basal Insulins: A Meta-analysis — 185
22. Insulin Efsitora versus Degludec in Type 2 Diabetes without Previous Insulin Treatment — 186

Section 8: NEWER TECHNOLOGIES
Section Editor: Anirban Sinha

1. Efficacy and Safety of Continuous Glucose Monitoring and Intermittently Scanned Continuous Glucose Monitoring in Patients with Type 2 Diabetes: A Systematic Review and Meta-analysis of Interventional Evidence — 189
2. Estimating Glycemia from HbA1c and CGM: Analysis of Accuracy and Sources of Discrepancy — 190
3. Relationship between Sensor-detected Hypoglycemia and Patient-reported Hypoglycemia in People with Type 1 and Insulin-treated Type 2 Diabetes: The Hypo-METRICS Study — 192
4. Does Fully Closed-loop Automated Insulin Delivery Improve Glycemic Control in Patients with Type 2 Diabetes? A Meta-analysis of Randomized Controlled Trials — 193
5. Real Time Continuous Glucose Monitoring in High-risk People with Insulin-requiring Type 2 Diabetes: A Randomised Controlled Trial — 195
6. Continuous Glucose Monitoring with Structured Education in Adults with Type 2 Diabetes Managed by Multiple Daily Insulin Injections: A Multicentre Randomised Controlled Trial — 196
7. Comparison between a Tubeless, On-body Automated Insulin Delivery System and a Tubeless, On-body Sensor-augmented Pump in Type 1 Diabetes: A Multicentre Randomised Controlled Trial — 198
8. Performance of the MiniMed 780G System on Mitigating Menstrual Cycle-dependent Glycaemic Variability — 199

Section 9: OTHERS
Section Editor: Nisha Batra

1. Optimal Dose and Type of Physical Activity to Improve Glycemic Control in People Diagnosed With Type 2 Diabetes: A Systematic Review and Meta-analysis — 201
2. Suicidal Ideation, Suicide Attempts, and Suicide Deaths in Adolescents and Young Adults with Type 1 Diabetes: A Systematic Review and Meta-analysis — 203
3. Individualizing Treatment of Type 2 Diabetes after Metformin: More Insights from GRADE — 205
4. Diabetes Management in Detention Facilities: A Statement of the American Diabetes Association — 207

5. Dapagliflozin Improves Erectile Dysfunction in Patients with Type 2 Diabetes Mellitus: An Open-label, Non-randomized Pilot Study 209
6. Footwear Fit as a Causal Factor in Diabetes-related Foot Ulceration: A Systematic Review 211
7. Effectiveness and Safety of Empagliflozin: Final Results from the EMPRISE Study 213
8. Impact of the Timing of Metformin Administration on Glycaemic and Glucagon-like Peptide-1 Responses to Intraduodenal Glucose Infusion in Type 2 Diabetes: A Double-blind, Randomised, Placebo-controlled, Crossover Study 215
9. Efficacy and Safety of Oral Semaglutide Monotherapy versus Placebo in a Predominantly Chinese Population with Type 2 Diabetes (PIONEER 11): A Double-blind, Phase IIIa, Randomised Trial 217
10. Comparative Renal Outcomes of Matched Cohorts of Patients with Type 2 Diabetes Receiving SGLT2 Inhibitors or GLP-1 Receptor Agonists Under Routine Care 219
11. Glucagon-like Peptide-1 Receptor Agonists and Risk of Thyroid Cancer: A systematic Review and Meta-analysis of Randomized Controlled Trials 221
12. Beneficial Effect of Oral Semaglutide for Type 2 Diabetes Mellitus in Patients with Metabolic Dysfunction-associated Steatotic Liver Disease: A Prospective, Multicentre, Observational Study 223
13. Fluoroquinolones and the Risk of Severe Hypoglycaemia Among Sulphonylurea Users: Population-based Cohort Study 225
14. Denosumab, for Osteoporosis, Reduces the Incidence of Type 2 Diabetes, Risk of Foot Ulceration and All-cause Mortality in Adults, Compared with Bisphosphonates: An Analysis of Real-world, Cohort Data, with a Systematic Review and Meta-analysis 227
15. The Use of Composite Endpoints in Cardiovascular Outcome Trials for Diabetes: A Review of 22 Randomized Clinical Trials Published Since 2008 229
16. Efficacy, Adherence and Persistence of Various Glucagon-like Peptide-1 Agonists: Nationwide Real-life Data 231
17. Association of Iron Status with All-cause and Cause-specific Mortality in Individuals with Diabetes 233
18. Fair Allocation of GLP-1 and Dual GLP-1–GIP Receptor Agonists 235
19. Intensive Blood-pressure Control in Patients with Type 2 Diabetes 237
20. Type 2 Diabetes in Patients with G6PD Deficiency 239

Index **247**

Section 1: BASIC SCIENCE

Section Editor: Arijit Singha

1. Large-scale Proteomics Improve Prediction of Chronic Kidney Disease in People with Diabetes

Ref: Ye Z, Zhang Y, Zhang Y, Yang S, He P, Liu M, et al. Large-Scale Proteomics Improve Prediction of Chronic Kidney Disease in People With Diabetes. Diabetes Care. 2024;47(10):1757-63.

ABSTRACT

Objective: Chronic kidney disease (CKD) polygenic risk score and a validated clinical risk model [CKD Prediction Consortium (CKD-PC)] will be compared with the predictive ability of a protein risk score for CKD prediction in diabetic patients.

Research design and methods: 2,094 diabetic patients having proteomics and genetic data from the UK Biobank Pharma Proteomics Project who had no prior history of CKD were included in this cohort analysis. A CKD protein risk score comprising 11 proteins was created in the training set (which included 1,047 participants and 117 CKD occurrences) based on almost 3,000 plasma proteins.

Results: 12.1 years was the median follow-up period. The CKD protein risk score was positively correlated with incident CKD [per standard deviation (SD) increment; hazard ratio 1.78; 95% confidence interval (CI) 1.44, 2.20] in the test sample, which included 1,047 patients and 112 CKD incidents. The prediction performance of incident CKD was significantly improved by the CKD protein risk score (C-index increase 0.122; 95% CI 0.071, 0.177) and the CKD-PC risk factors (C-index increase 0.175; 95% CI 0.126, 0.217) when compared to the basic model (age + sex + race, C-index, 0.627; 95% CI 0.578, 0.675). However, there was no significant improvement in the CKD polygenic risk score (C-index increase 0.007; 95% CI 20.016, 0.025).

The continuous 10-year net reclassification (0.199; 95% CI 0.059, 0.299) and 10-year integrated discrimination index (0.041; 95% CI 0.007, 0.083) were both markedly improved by adding the CKD protein risk score to the CKD-PC risk factors. This resulted in the largest C-index of 0.825 (C-index from 0.802 to 0.825; difference 0.023; 95% CI 0.006, 0.044).

Conclusion: The discrimination and reclassification of CKD risk in diabetic individuals was much enhanced by the addition of the CKD protein risk score to a validated clinical risk model.

CRITICAL APPRAISAL

What was Known Prior to this Study?

Chronic kidney disease (CKD) is a significant and increasingly prevalent global health issue, affecting 10% of adults worldwide. Polygenic risk scores, which include sequence variants, have the potential to improve screening and prevention efforts for CKD. However, the clinical applicability of these polygenic risk scores in assessing CKD risk in patients with diabetes requires validation through prospective studies. The potential of proteomic profiling lies in its ability to identify novel biomarkers that may indicate the onset of CKD before it occurs. Some studies have investigated the relationship between various circulating proteins and the risk of CKD progression in individuals with diabetic kidney disease. However, there is a notable lack of research regarding the predictive value of circulating proteins in assessing CKD risk among people with diabetes. The Chronic Kidney Disease Prediction Consortium (CKD-PC) has developed an equation to predict the incidence of CKD in individuals with diabetes. Enhancing the validated CKD-PC model by incorporating a panel of multiple protein biomarkers and addressing various pathophysiological pathways of CKD may significantly improve the accuracy of CKD risk prediction—a hypothesis that has not yet been explored.

What this Study Adds?

The study developed and validated a protein risk score for CKD derived from large-scale proteomics. This score serves as a robust and independent predictor of incident CKD in individuals with diabetes. It significantly enhances the ability to discriminate and reclassify CKD risk in diabetic patients, whether used in conjunction with age and sex or when added to an established clinical risk model for CKD.

Limitations of the Study

The UK Biobank is composed primarily of individuals with European ancestry, warranting future investigations to assess the translation of the protein risk score across diverse populations and ethnicities. These proteins are not easily measured in routine clinical chemistry. Further validations outside this cohort would be good to be able to use these as risk protein markers.

Impact on Clinical Practice

Incorporating the CKD protein risk score into clinical practice leads to better risk stratification and earlier prevention for patients with diabetes at risk for developing CKD.

2. tRNA-derived Fragments are Altered in Diabetes

Ref: Ng N, Gibriel HAY, Halang L, Jirström E, Ioana JA, Burke M, et al. tRNA-derived fragments are altered in diabetes. Diabet Med. 2024;41(2):e15258.

ABSTRACT

Aim: Due to its diverse clinical presentation, maternally inherited diabetes and deafness (MIDD), an uncommon form of adult-onset diabetes, can be challenging to diagnose. A new and developing class of small noncoding RNAs (sncRNAs) transfers RNA-derived tiny fragments and shows great potential as serum biomarkers because of their abundance, stability, simplicity of detection, and stress-induced production.

Methods: We examined the amounts of tiRNA 5'ValCAC (both alone and in conjunction with miR-23b-3p) found in serum samples from MIDD, type 1 diabetes, type 2 diabetes, and healthy controls based on small RNA sequencing investigations.

Results: Subjects with MIDD and type 2 diabetes had lower serum levels of 5'ValCAC than controls. Serum levels of miR-23b-3p were higher in individuals with type 2 diabetes than in any other group. The potential of 5'ValCAC and miR-23b-3p as MIDD indicators was demonstrated by Receiver operating characteristic analysis; the combination demonstrated good separation from people with type 2 diabetes.

Conclusion: This is the first study demonstrating that individuals with diabetes had changed tiRNA levels in their serum. Serum biomarkers 5'ValCAC and miR-23b-3p together may be able to distinguish between individuals with MIDD and those with type 2 diabetes.

CRITICAL APPRAISAL

What was Known Prior to this Study?
Maternally inherited diabetes and deafness (MIDD) is a rare form of adult-onset diabetes (0.5–2.8% of cases) caused by mutations in mitochondrial DNA (mtDNA). The diagnosis of MIDD can be difficult due to phenotypic variability, and diabetes can often be misdiagnosed as type 1 or type 2 diabetes. High-pitched sensorineural hearing loss may not be detected until an audiogram is performed. Therefore, early accessible biomarkers may aid to guide subsequent genetic testing for MIDD. Small noncoding RNAs (sncRNAs) have been identified as potential biomarkers for MIDD, with several studies highlighting miRNAs to be differentially abundant in blood and muscle compared to controls. Transfer RNA-derived small fragments (tsRNAs) are a novel class of sncRNAs derived from transfer RNAs. A subclass of tsRNAs, the so-called tRNA-derived stress-induced RNAs (tiRNAs), is produced by cleavage of tRNAs in their anticodon loop in response to metabolic, hypoxic, or oxidative stress. In the pancreas, tiRNAs 5'HIS-GTG and 5'GLU-GTC have been found to control mitochondrial respiration, β-cell proliferation and insulin secretion. In this study, small RNA-seq analysis of pooled serum samples from MIDD, type 1 diabetes and type 2 diabetes subjects, as well as healthy controls was performed to identify sncRNAs with altered expression.

What this Study Adds?
Serum levels of 5'ValCAC were found to be reduced in subjects with MIDD (mitochondrial diabetes) and type 2 diabetes when compared to control groups. In contrast, individuals with type 2 diabetes had higher serum levels of miR-23b-3p compared to all other subjects. Receiver operating characteristic (ROC) analysis indicated that both 5'ValCAC and miR-23b-3p have potential as biomarkers for MIDD, and their combination shows excellent differentiation from subjects with type 2 diabetes.

Strength of the Study
This report is the first to show altered serum levels of tiRNAs in subjects with diabetes.

Limitations of the Study
Absence of functional studies to determine the biological role of tiRNA in diabetes and small sample size are significant limitations of the study. Presence of hypertension, dyslipidemia, and medications could potentially alter the expression of tiRNA.

Impact on Clinical Practice/Future Scope of Research
Levels of tiRNAs 5'ValCAC and 5'GlyGCC in the serum of MIDD and type 2 diabetes subjects and suggest that the differing expression levels seen here may be associated with reduced skeletal muscle insulin sensitivity. Combined use of 5'ValCAC and miR-23b-3p as serum biomarkers may help differentiate MIDD from type 2 diabetes patients and possibly type 1 diabetes patients.

3. Islet Autoantibody Frequency in Relatives of Children with Type 1 Diabetes Who have a Type 2 Diabetes Diagnosis

Ref: Lewis SJ, Williams CL, Mortimer GL, Oram RA, Hagopian WA, Gillespie KM, et al.; AWAF; BOX Study Group. Islet autoantibody frequency in relatives of children with type 1 diabetes who have a type 2 diabetes diagnosis. Diabet Med. 2024;41(9):e15394.

ABSTRACT

Aim: The purpose of this study was to assess autoimmune traits in people with a type 2 diagnosis who are related to children with type 1 diabetes.

Methods: The type 1 diabetes genetic risk score (GRS2) and autoantibodies to glutamate decarboxylase 65 (GADA), islet antigen-2 (IA-2A), zinc transporter 8 (ZnT8A), and insulin (IAA) were measured in prediagnosis samples (median 17 months prior to onset) from relatives who were subsequently diagnosed with type 2 diabetes. Fisher's exact and t-tests were used to examine relationships between islet autoantibodies, insulin therapy, and GRS2.

Results: 32 (14%) of the 226 relatives (64% male; mean age at sampling 41 years; mean age at diagnosis 54 years) tested positive for at least one islet autoantibody >10 years prior to diagnosis. Insulin was used to treat around half of them ($n = 15$). Relatives receiving insulin had higher GADA-positivity than relatives not receiving insulin [12/18 (67%) vs. 6/18 (33%), $p < 0.001$]. 13 out of 32 (41%) relatives with autoantibodies had IAA-positivity. Autoantibody-positive relatives had higher GRS2 scores ($p = 0.032$), but there was no conclusive evidence of a treatment-related difference ($p = 0.072$).

Conclusion: This study emphasizes how crucial it is to measure islet autoantibodies, such as IAA, in family members of individuals with type 1 diabetes in order to prevent misdiagnosis.

CRITICAL APPRAISAL

What was Known Prior to this Study?

Earlier study found that children who were newly diagnosed with type 1 diabetes and had a family history of type 2 diabetes exhibited certain phenotypic characteristics typical of type 2 diabetes. However, genome-wide association studies indicate that the underlying causes of these conditions are different. This study focuses on first-degree relatives of individuals with type 1 diabetes who were later diagnosed with type 2 diabetes. The aim of the study was to determine whether these relatives possess immunogenetic features associated with type 1 diabetes.

What this Study Adds?

Distinguishing between type 1 and type 2 diabetes in adults is complex, as clinical features alone cannot accurately classify the type of diabetes. There is ongoing debate among some clinicians about whether all new diabetes cases in individuals under 30 years of age should be referred to secondary care. Recent studies on postdiagnosis type 2 diabetes have identified islet autoantibodies. Notably, there has been a first report documenting prediagnosis islet autoimmunity and genetic risk score (GRS) in samples from relatives who were later diagnosed with type 2 diabetes. The presence of islet autoantibodies, along with a high GRS, can support a diagnosis of adult-onset type 1 diabetes. Testing for islet autoantibodies in family members of individuals with type 1 diabetes could help reduce misclassification in primary diabetes care and inform future testing guidelines.

Strength of the Study

Detection of islet autoantibodies before diabetes onset in relatives of probands with type 1 diabetes.

Limitations of the Study

The sample size for this study is relatively small when compared to other population studies. Additionally, it did not include analyses of C-peptide, hemoglobin A1c (HbA1c), or body mass index (BMI). Previous research has indicated that BMI may influence islet autoimmunity in individuals with type 2 diabetes, noting that individuals who are GADA-positive tend to have a lower BMI than those who are GADA-negative. Our sample population was predominantly of White European descent. The study also examined the use of GRS in relatives of individuals with type 1 diabetes. By definition, these relatives are expected to have a higher type 1 diabetes GRS compared to the general population.

Impact on Clinical Practice/Future Research

This study has revealed that some individuals may have been misdiagnosed with type 2 diabetes, even though they are relatives of children with type 1 diabetes. These individuals were clearly positive for autoantibodies and/or had a high GRS prior to their type 2 diabetes diagnosis. Further research is necessary to develop a more specific and sensitive method for clinicians to accurately identify type 1 diabetes in adults.

4. Bone Marrow Mesenchymal Stem Cell-derived Exosomal miR-221-3p Promotes Angiogenesis and Wound Healing in Diabetes via the Downregulation of Forkhead Box P1

Ref: Qiu ZY, Xu WC, Liang ZH. Bone marrow mesenchymal stem cell-derived exosomal miR-221-3p promotes angiogenesis and wound healing in diabetes via the downregulation of forkhead box P1. Diabet Med. 2024;41(9):e15386.

ABSTRACT

Aim: Diabetes patients may develop nonhealing ulcers as a result of impaired wound healing. This work is to explore the mechanism of bone marrow mesenchymal stem cells (BMSCs)-isolated exosomal miR-221-3p in angiogenesis and diabetic wound healing since BMSC exosomes can aid in wound healing.

Methods: Human umbilical vein endothelial cells (HUVECs) were exposed to high glucose (HG) in order to simulate diabetes in vitro. Transmission electron microscopy (TEM), western blot analysis, and dynamic light scattering (DLS) were used to identify the exosomes that were isolated from BMSCs. Alizarin red, alkaline phosphatase (ALP), and oil red O staining were used to evaluate the capacity to distinguish BMSCs. Using confocal microscopy, the capacity to internalize exosomes labeled with PKH26 was evaluated. Scratch, MTT, and tube formation tests were used independently to assess migration, cell viability, and angiogenesis. Western blotting or quantitative reverse transcriptase polymerase chain reaction (qRT-PCR) were used to analyze the amounts of miRNA and protein. The dual-luciferase reporter, ChIP, and RIP assays were used to ascertain the connection between miR-221-3p, FOXP1, and SPRY1.

Results: After being successfully extracted from BMSCs, exosomal miR-221-3p was introduced into HUVECs. Exosomal miR-221-3p isolated from BMSCs decreased the angiogenesis, cell survival, and migration of HUVECs, which were reported to be suppressed by HG. FOXP1 has the potential to transcriptionally upregulate SPRY1, and by downregulating SPRY1, FOXP1 silencing reversed the inhibition of HG-stimulated angiogenesis, cell survival, and migration in HUVECs. Conversely, miR-221-3p specifically targeted FOXP1, and the beneficial effect of exosomal miR-221-3p on HUVEC angiogenesis was counteracted by FOXP1 overexpression.

Conclusion: Through the FOXP1/SPRY1 axis, exosomal miR-221-3p that was isolated from BMSCs stimulated angiogenesis in diabetic wounds. Additionally, the results of this study can offer fresh perspectives on diabetes prevention techniques.

CRITICAL APPRAISAL

What was Known Prior to this Study?
Diabetic foot ulcer (DFU) is a debilitating complication of chronic hyperglycemia and often leads to significant morbidity and mortality. Though some interventions can slow the progression of diabetic wound healing, the persistent nature of these wounds presents a significant clinical challenge. A key factor in impaired healing is the inhibition of angiogenesis, which is often observed in diabetic patients. Surgical interventions may restore peripheral blood flow, but their effectiveness can be limited. Therefore, promoting angiogenesis is essential for advancing the treatment of diabetic wounds. Bone marrow mesenchymal stem cells (BMSCs) are multipotent stem cells capable of self-renewal and differentiation into various cell types. A recent study highlighted the therapeutic benefits of using BMSCs for tissue repair and regeneration. Although BMSC-based wound healing therapies have shown promising results in preclinical studies, they are still in the early stages of clinical trials. Furthermore, the molecular mechanisms underlying the role of BMSCs in diabetic wound healing require further investigation. Exosomes are extracellular vehicles (EVs) with a diameter of 30–150 nm that can transport RNAs to target cells, where they exert various effects. Additionally, BMSC-derived exosomes have demonstrated beneficial effects on diabetic wounds by delivering RNAs. Moreover, miR-221-3p is present in exosomes secreted by BMSCs and BMSC-derived exosomal miR-221-3p has been shown to alleviate asthma; however, it remains to be determined whether BMSC-derived exosomes can promote wound healing in diabetes by containing miR-221-3p. In this study, the role of BMSC-derived exosome on angiogenesis was evaluated.

What this Study Adds?
Exosomes containing miR-221-3p isolated from BMSCs alleviated HG-mediated inhibition of angiogenesis in human umbilical vein endothelial cells (HUVECs). miR-221-3p could directly sponge FOXP1 and downregulates SPRY1. BMSCs-isolated exosomal miR-221-3p promoted wound healing in diabetic mice by targeting FOXP1/SPRY1 axis.

Limitations of the Study
The clinical samples were not included in this study, which may limit the applicability of the findings to real-world scenarios. Furthermore, additional mechanisms underlying exosomal miR-221-3p in diabetic wounds have not yet been investigated.

Impact on Clinical Practice/Future Scope
The significant findings of this study could facilitate the development of effective therapies for curing diabetic foot in the clinical setting.

---

5. The Metabolomic Signature of Weight Loss and Remission in the Diabetes Remission Clinical Trial (DiRECT)

Ref: Corbin LJ, Hughes DA, Bull CJ, Vincent EE, Smith ML, McConnachie A, et al. The metabolomic signature of weight loss and remission in the Diabetes Remission Clinical Trial (DiRECT). Diabetologia. 2024;67(1):74-87.

ABSTRACT

Aim/Hypothesis: A consistent metabolomic signature of type 2 diabetes and overweight has been shown using high-throughput metabolomics technologies in a range of experimental types. Little research has been done on how much weight loss and diabetes remission can reverse these metabolomic abnormalities. Our goal was to describe the metabolomic effects of a weight-loss program in people with type 2 diabetes.

Methods: 574 fasting serum samples ($n = 298$) obtained from an ongoing randomized controlled trial (RCT) [the Diabetes Remission Clinical Trial (DiRECT)] were analyzed. Participants in the trial were randomly allocated (1:1) to treat patients with type 2 diabetes with either a weight management program (intervention) or best-practice care according to guidelines (control). Here, samples obtained at baseline and after a year were subjected to metabolomics analysis using both untargeted mass spectrometry (MS) and targeted 1H-nuclear magnetic resonance (^{1}H-NMR) spectroscopy. To assess how the intervention affected metabolite levels, multivariable regression models were built.

Results: The intervention was linked to increases in sphingolipids, plasmalogens, and metabolites involved with fatty acid metabolism and decreases in sugars, low-density lipoprotein (LDL) triglycerides, and branched-chain amino acids (Holm-corrected $p < 0.05$). Those who achieved diabetic remission experienced higher reductions in glucose, fructose, and mannose than those who did not, among those who lost >9 kg between baseline and 12 months.

Conclusion/Interpretation: We have described the metabolomic impacts of a comprehensive weight-management program that has been demonstrated to result in both diabetes remission and weight loss. It seems that a significant amount of the metabolome is changeable. Change patterns were mostly and remarkably at odds with disturbances previously linked to the onset of type 2 diabetes.

CRITICAL APPRAISAL

What was Known Prior to this Study?

In the study of type 2 diabetes, the relationship among risk factors, intermediate metabolic phenotypes, and the disease has prompted interest in using metabolomics to clarify the biological mechanisms involved. Research has consistently identified a strong metabolomic signature related to both prevalent and newly diagnosed type 2 diabetes. Given the overlap in metabolomic profiles between type 2 diabetes and its precursors—overweight/obesity and insulin resistance—many changes observed in diagnosed individuals may also influence disease development. However, it remains unclear whether these changes are a systemic 'downstream' response to high glucose or an "upstream" response to excess adiposity.

To enhance the understanding, it is essential to assess the metabolomic response to disease remission following interventions. Weight loss has shown significant efficacy in managing type 2 diabetes, with sustained metabolic benefits lasting up to a decade. However, concerns about the reliability of existing metabolomics studies, often due to small sample sizes and single-arm designs, warrant further investigation. The study analyzed samples of the pivotal randomized controlled trial (RCT)—the Diabetes Remission Clinical Trial (DiRECT)—to characterize the metabolomic profile associated with this intensive weight management intervention.

What this Study Adds?

Baseline characteristics were similar when comparing the intervention group with the control group. Participants at intervention group lost ~10 kg weight at the end of 12 months. The intervention was associated with a decrease in branched-chain amino acids, sugars, and low-density lipoprotein (LDL) triglycerides, along with an increase in sphingolipids, plasmalogens, and metabolites related to fatty acid metabolism (Holm-corrected $p < 0.05$). Under a conservative correction for multiple testing, 26% of nuclear magnetic resonance (NMR)-derived metabolites and 12% of mass spectrometry (MS)-derived metabolites were altered by the intervention. This suggests that a sizeable proportion of metabolite changes in type 2 diabetes are modifiable. The changes were evident many weeks after the conclusion of the weight-loss phase of the intervention, indicating sustained benefits to health.

Major Strengths of the Study

The study utilized samples and clinical data from a relatively large cluster-randomized trial, which had a well-matched control group compared to existing literature. By measuring metabolites both at baseline and after 12 months, the analysis was strengthened. Additionally, the use of two complementary metabolomics platforms expanded the overall coverage of the metabolome beyond what has been previously evaluated.

Limitations of the Study

The MS data are semiquantitative meaning that these findings require further validation using targeted techniques to allow absolute quantification. It is a challenge to attribute those changes to specific elements of the intervention (e.g., to fat loss per se or "upstream" changes in diet). Effects of weight loss on metabolome should be interpreted cautiously and should be validated in larger cohort.

Impact on Clinical Practice/Future Research Scope

Findings suggest excess weight is upstream of many previously reported metabolomic changes connected with type diabetes mellitus and that energy restriction is an effective way of improving multiple metabolic health signals.

6. Multi-omic Prediction of Incident Type 2 Diabetes

Ref: Carrasco-Zanini J, Pietzner M, Wheeler E, Kerrison ND, Langenberg C, Wareham NJ. Multi-omic prediction of incident type 2 diabetes. Diabetologia. 2024;67(1):102-12.

ABSTRACT

Aim/Hypothesis: One important component of population-level prevention methods is the identification of individuals who are at high risk of developing type 2 diabetes. Prior research has assessed the predictive value of omics measures, including proteins, metabolites, and polygenic scores, but has done so in isolation. It is unknown how much better integrated omics biomarkers can be than the existing clinical standard models. Testing the predictive capabilities of the genome, proteome, metabolome, and clinical biomarkers in conjunction with well-established clinical prediction models for type 2 diabetes was the goal of this work.

Methods: In a prospective, nested type 2 diabetes case-cohort study ($n = 1,105$, incident type 2 diabetes cases = 375) with 10,792 person-years of follow-up, we created sparse interpretable prediction models. We used least absolute shrinkage and selection operator (LASSO) regression to select from 5,759 features across the genome, proteome, metabolome, and clinical biomarkers. We used a clinical model that included factors from the Cambridge Diabetes Risk Score and hemoglobin A1c (HbA1c) to examine the predictive ability of omics-derived predictors.

Results: The top 10 proteins by themselves performed the best among single omics prediction models that lacked clinical risk factors {concordance index (C index) = 0.82 [95% confidence interval (CI) 0.75, 0.88]}, indicating that the proteome is the most informative single omic layer when clinical data is lacking. Nonetheless, the top 10 variables across several omic layers produced the greatest increase in type 2 diabetes incidence prediction over and above the clinical model [C index = 0.87 (95% CI 0.82, 0.92), Δ C index = 0.05, $p = 0.045$].

The top 10 omic features also showed improvement in those with HbA1c < 42 mmol/mol (6.0%), the prediabetes threshold [C index = 0.84 (95% CI 0.77, 0.90), Δ C index = 0.07, $p = 0.03$], the group for which prediction would be most helpful because current clinical guidelines do not target them for preventative interventions. The primary factor in this subgroup's increase in prediction was the type 2 diabetes polygenic risk score, which also produced a similar improvement in performance when added to the clinical model alone [C index = 0.83 (95% CI 0.75, 0.90), Δ C index = 0.06, $p = 0.002$]. However, during a 20-year period, people with high polygenic risk in this group had only about half the absolute risk for type 2 diabetes compared to those with prediabetes.

Conclusion/Interpretation: Omic methods improved incident type 2 diabetes prediction by a small amount. Even those with a high polygenic burden in that cohort had a low absolute risk of type 2 diabetes, despite the fact that a polygenic risk score does improve prediction in those whose HbA1c falls within the normoglycemic range, the group in whom prediction would be most helpful. This implies that the implementation of targeted population-based genetic screening for preventative interventions may not be as feasible as it seems.

CRITICAL APPRAISAL

What was Known Prior to this Study?

Considering the burden of type 2 diabetes mellitus across the world, it is critically important to identify at risk people of development of diabetes. Several risk scores based on patient-derived data are available and they perform well to predict incident diabetes mellitus particularly in people with high-risk group. In addition, blood-based biomarkers [hemoglobin A1c (HbA1c), lipid profiles, uric acid] have been shown to improve the predictive model. Genome-wide association studies (GWAS) have identified hundreds of genetic risk variants; however, genome-wide polygenic risk sores (PRSs) have not shown clinically meaningful improvement over and above the simple clinical models. Integrating the multiomics (proteomics, metabolomics, clinical biomarkers, and genomics) may be helpful to improve the prediction of incident type 2 diabetes mellitus.

What this Study Adds?

It was a case-cohort prospective study which included 1,105 individuals without diabetes mellitus at baseline between 40 and 79 years of age and followed up for 10 years for development of diabetes mellitus. Genome-wide genotyping was performed using the Affymetrix UK Biobank Axiom Array. The Cambridge Diabetes Risk Score was used as clinical predictive score in addition to HbA1c. The study observed that combination of different omics layers achieved the largest improvement in predictive performance over a standard clinical score. Type 2 diabetes mellitus polygenic risk score accounted for the most of the improvement in in predictive performance in individuals without prediabetes. However, the absolute risk of type 2 diabetes mellitus without prediabetes with a high polygenic burden was low.

Major Strengths of the Study

Comprehensive case ascertainment and virtually complete follow-up among deeply phenotyped participants.

Limitations of the Study

The study included participants of European ancestry, limiting the generalizability of results across populations of different ethnic backgrounds. The technology used for proteomics profiling relies on preserved protein structure for recognition by the affinity reagents, meaning that protein-altering variants could lead to biased measurements. External replication of results is currently not possible due to the unique depth of information incorporated in these analyses.

Impact on Clinical Practice/Scope of Future Research

Whether society deems it acceptable to offer preventative interventions to individuals at half the risk of groups for whom interventions are now routinely offered is an economic and political decision.

7. HOMA-IR and the Matsuda Index as Predictors of Progression to Type 1 Diabetes in Autoantibody-positive Relatives

Ref: Petrelli A, Cugnata F, Carnovale D, Bosi E, Libman IM, Piemonti L, et al. HOMA-IR and the Matsuda Index as predictors of progression to type 1 diabetes in autoantibody-positive relatives. Diabetologia. 2024;67(2):290-300.

ABSTRACT

Aim/Hypothesis: We evaluated the potential correlation between type 1 diabetes stage transitions and the Matsuda Index and HOMA-IR.

Methods: Relatives of people with type 1 diabetes (n = 6,256) who tested positive for autoantibody (AAb) were examined. After adjusting for measures of insulin secretion, Index60, and insulinogenic index (IGI), associations between insulin resistance indicators (HOMA-IR) and insulin sensitivity indicators (Matsuda Index) and body mass index percentile (BMIp) and age were evaluated. To find out if tertiles of HOMA-IR and Matsuda Index predicted progression to Stage 3 [diabetes according to the World Health Organization/American Diabetes Association (WHO/ADA) criteria], from Stage 1 to Stage 2 (≥2 AAbs with dysglycemia), and from Not Staged (<2 AAbs) to Stage 1 (≥2 AAbs and normoglycemia), Cox regression was employed.

Results: The Matsuda Index (inverse) and HOMA-IR (positive) were strongly correlated with BMIp and baseline age ($p < 0.0001$). After controlling for Index60, moving from Stage 1 to Stage 2 was linked to lower Matsuda Index and higher HOMA-IR [HOMA-IR: hazard ratio (HR) 1.71, $p < 0.0001$; Matsuda Index, HR 0.40, $p < 0.0001$], just as moving from Stages 1 or 2 to Stage 3 was linked to lower Matsuda Index and higher HOMA-IR (HOMA-IR: HR 1.98, $p < 0.0001$; Matsuda Index: HR 0.46, $p < 0.0001$). In the absence of adjustments, the correlations between the progression to Stage 3 and the HOMA-IR were inverse, while the Matsuda Index was positive. However, the directionality changed when adjustments were made. The results were comparable when Index60 was substituted with IGI.

Conclusion/Interpretation: After accounting for insulin secretion, the Matsuda Index shows a decrease in progression to Stages 2 and 3 of type 1 diabetes, while the HOMA-IR shows an increase. Insulin secretion indicators seem useful for analyzing correlations between the Matsuda Index or HOMA-IR and the development of type 1 diabetes in families with AAb.

CRITICAL APPRAISAL

What was Known Prior to this Study?

Type 1 diabetes mellitus (DM) is a heterogeneous disorder characterized by auto-immune-mediated beta cell dysfunction leading to deficiency of insulin secretion. Depending upon the presence or absence of islet auto-antibody (Ab) and/or dysglycemia, type 1 DM has three stages, "Not staged"—Ab < 2 and normal glucose tolerance, "Stage 1"—Ab ≥ 2 and normal glucose tolerance, and "Stage 2"—Ab ≥ 2 and dysglycemia. The relative importance of the staging lies in the prevention of the disease. Notably, the rising incidence of obesity in children often poses significant difficulties in making the diagnosis. Furthermore, excess weight gain itself increases the risk of developing type 1 DM. It is important to know whether insulin resistance and insulin sensitivity are possible factors of type 1 DM development. HOMA-IR and Matsuda index are well-validated tool for insulin resistance and insulin sensitivity, respectively. However, deficient insulin secretion in Ab+ relatives of type 1 DM may be limiting factor to calculate the above two index. Having said that, adjustment of insulin secretion may be useful. Several studies have documented the insulinogenic index (IGI) and Index60 as surrogate markers of insulin secretion in Ab+ relatives. In this study the HOMA-IR and Matsuda Index, which were adjusted by IGI and Index60, were assessed to characterize the pathogenesis of type 1 DM.

What this Study Adds?

First- and second-degree relatives of individuals with type 1 diabetes were enrolled into the TrialNet Pathway to Prevention (TNPTP) study at the international clinical centers of the TrialNet network. All participants were screened for islet autoantibodies to glutamic acid decarboxylase (GAD) (GADA), insulin (microinsulin antibody assay, mIAA), and IA-2 (IA-2A). If any of these were positive in screening, ZnT8A and ICA were also tested. Participants identified as autoantibody positive, as well as a small subset of those autoantibody negative, were monitored with autoantibody testing, hemoglobin A1c (HbA1c) and an oral glucose tolerance test (OGTT) at 6- or 12-month intervals. A total of $n = 6,256$ relatives were included in this study, $n = 4,459$ < 18 years old and $n = 1,797 \geq 18$ years old. Estimation of insulin resistance with HOMA-IR and insulin sensitivity with the Matsuda Index was obtained from OGTT data. Beta cell function was measured from OGTTs using Index60, and the IGI. The study found that transitioning from Stage 1 to Stage 2 and progression to Stage 3 of type 1 diabetes was associated with increased levels of HOMA-IR and reduced levels of Matsuda Index, only when adjusted for insulin secretion. Importantly, adjustments with indicators of insulin secretion such as Index60 and IGI appear necessary. The association with HOMA-IR went from inverse to positive, while the association with Matsuda Index went from positive to inverse.

Major Strengths of the Study

This study used the novel approach of adjusting for insulin secretion in assessing whether insulin resistance and insulin sensitivity, indicated by HOMA-IR and the Matsuda Index, respectively, are factors involved in the progression toward type 1 diabetes.

Limitations of the Study

Participants were retrospectively selected in the study. HOMA-IR and Matsuda Index measurements used in this analysis have not been validated for AAb+ populations.

Implications of the Findings for the Clinicians

Insulin resistance play significant role in the progression of type 1 DM.

Scope of Future Research

Targeting insulin resistance to delay the progression of type 1 DM.

8. Zinc Finger BED-type Containing 3 Promotes Hepatic Steatosis by Interacting with Polypyrimidine Tract-binding Protein 1

Ref: Wu Y, Yang M, Wu SB, Luo PQ, Zhang C, Ruan CS, et al. Zinc finger BED-type containing 3 promotes hepatic steatosis by interacting with polypyrimidine tract-binding protein 1. Diabetologia. 2024;67(10):2346-66.

ABSTRACT

Aim/Hypothesis: It is generally known that type 2 diabetes mellitus, insulin resistance, and the metabolic syndrome are all related to metabolic dysfunction-associated steatotic liver disease (MASLD). Although type 2 diabetes mellitus and the metabolic syndrome have been associated with zinc finger BED-type containing 3 (ZBED3), its function in MASLD is yet unknown. Our goal in this study was to look at ZBED3's role in relation to MASLD.

Methods: ZBED3 expression levels were measured in cellular and animal models of MASLD as well as in MASLD patients. The function of ZBED3 in MASLD was examined in vitro and in vivo using a cellular model of MASLD produced by nonesterified fatty acid (NEFA) and an animal model of MASLD induced by a high-fat diet (HFD), respectively. Lentiviral infection or adeno-associated virus tail-vein injection enhanced ZBED3 expression. Bioinformatics analysis and RNA-seq were used to investigate the mechanisms by which ZBED3 regulates lipid accumulation.

Co-immunoprecipitation and LC-MS/MS were used to examine the molecular mechanisms by which ZBED3 regulates the sterol regulatory element binding-protein 1c (SREBP1c), as the results of these next-generation transcriptome sequencing studies showed that ZBED3 controls SREBP1c (also known as SREBF1; a gene involved in fatty acid de novo synthesis).

Results: In this investigation, we discovered that ZBED3 was markedly elevated in the livers of MASLD patients and MASLD animal models. In vitro, NEFA-induced triglyceride buildup in hepatocytes was facilitated by ZBED3 overexpression. Moreover, ZBED3 overexpression in hepatocytes accelerated hepatic steatosis. On the other hand, resistance to HFD-induced hepatic steatosis was the outcome of ZBED3 deletion specific to hepatocytes. In order to control SREBP1c mRNA stability and alternative splicing, ZBED3 mechanistically interacts directly with polypyrimidine tract-binding protein 1 (PTBP1) and influences its binding to the SREBP1c mRNA precursor.

Conclusion/Interpretation: According to this study, ZBED3 is a key regulator of the development of MASLD and encourages hepatic steatosis.

Data availability: RNA-seq data have been deposited in the NCBI Gene Expression Omnibus (www.ncbi.nlm.nih.gov/geo/query/acc.cgi?acc=GSE231875). MS proteomics data have been deposited to the ProteomeXchange Consortium via the iProX partner repository (https://proteomecentral.proteomexchange.org/cgi/GetDataset?ID=PXD041743).

CRITICAL APPRAISAL

What was Known Prior to this Study?

Currently metabolic dysfunction-associated steatotic liver disease (MASLD) is the most common liver disease affecting ~25% of adult population in the world. It is the second most common cause for liver transplantation in the United States. Overall, the pooled prevalence of MASLD in India is 38%. Notably, MASLD is a spectrum disorder ranging from simple steatosis to hepatocellular carcinoma, characterized by accumulation of triglyceride in liver. Hepatic de novo lipogenesis (DNL) is one of the predominant contributing factors of triglyceride accumulation in hepatocytes. Notably, DNL is upregulated in patients with MASLD, in addition, it is independent of adiposity, intrahepatic triglyceride and circulating lipids level. Sterol regulatory element-binding protein-1c (SREBP1c) is the main transcriptional regulator involved in DNL. While protein cleavage, phosphorylation and ubiquitination of *SREBP1c* are well documented, post-transcriptional regulation of alternative splicing of SREBP1c remains unexplored. The RNA-binding protein polypyrimidine tract-binding protein 1 (PTBP1) binds to mRNA sequence of *SREBP1c* and enhance the stability of *SREBP1c* mRNA. Zinc finger BED-type containing 3 (ZBED3) is a member of the zinc finger protein superfamily and studies have demonstrated ZBED3 level is significantly elevated in insulin resistance, type 2 diabetes mellitus and metabolic syndrome. Furthermore, ZBED3 level is correlated with HOMA, body mass index (BMI) and triglyceride levels, which implies that ZBED3 might be involved in the progression of MASLD. This study was done to explore the role of ZBED3 in hepatic steatosis as well as interaction of ZBED3 with the alternative splicing of *PTBP1* and *SREBP1c* mRNA.

What this Study Adds?

ZBED3 is upregulated in the livers of individuals with steatosis as compared to without steatosis. Similar observation was documented in three animal models. ZBED3 overexpression promoted nonesterified fatty acid (NEFA)-induced triglyceride accumulation in hepatocytes. Furthermore, ZBED3 directly interacts with PTBP1 and affects its binding with *SREBP1c* mRNA precursor to regulate *SREBP1c* mRNA stability and alternative splicing.

Limitations of the Study

The study found elevated ZBED3 levels in individuals with MASLD in only a small selection of human liver samples, and the clinical generalizability of this finding remains to be explored.

Impact on Clinical Practice/Future Research

Elucidating the mechanisms of aberrant RNA splicing could provide therapeutic *targets for diseases*. PTBP1 may provide a good therapeutic target for MASLD.

9. Week-long Normoglycemia in Diabetic Mice and Minipigs via a Subcutaneous Dose of a Glucose-responsive Insulin Complex

Ref: Zhang J, Wei X, Liu W, Wang Y, Kahkoska AR, Zhou X, et al. Week-long normoglycaemia in diabetic mice and minipigs via a subcutaneous dose of a glucose-responsive insulin complex. Nat Biomed Eng. 2024;8(10):1214-25.

ABSTRACT

Insulin formulations that respond to glucose levels can improve their therapeutic effectiveness and decrease the frequency of administration. However, developing single-dose formulations that provide both sustained and glucose-responsive insulin release has been difficult. This research introduces an innovative glucose-responsive formulation for subcutaneous injection that reduces fibrous capsule formation and sustains normal blood glucose levels with minimal risk of hypoglycemia in mice and minipigs with type 1 diabetes for up to seven days. The formulation consists of recombinant human insulin modified with gluconic acid, which strongly binds to poly-L-lysine that has been altered with 4-carboxy-3-fluorophenylboronic acid. This binding occurs through glucose-responsive phenylboronic acid-diol complexation and electrostatic attraction. In the presence of elevated glucose concentrations, the phenylboronic acid groups rapidly bind to glucose, disrupting the complex and reducing the positive charge density of the polymers, thus facilitating insulin release. The encouraging therapeutic performance of this long-acting single-dose formulation suggests the need for further evaluation and clinical translation studies.

CRITICAL APPRAISAL

What was Known Prior to this Study?

It has been over a century since the discovery of insulin, a pivotal advancement that has transformed diabetes from a condition characterized by significant morbidity and mortality into a manageable chronic illness. Currently, insulin therapy is advancing toward the objective of closely mimicking physiological endogenous insulin profiles, aided by the development of rapid and long-acting insulin formulations, continuous glucose monitoring systems, and hybrid closed-loop systems. Despite these advancements, many individuals living with diabetes continue to experience unmet insulin needs, resulting in prolonged periods of blood glucose levels that fall outside the recommended targets. Noteworthy innovations aimed at enhancing insulin therapy include the engineering of insulins that primarily target the liver, as well as the creation of glucose-responsive insulins (GRIs). These insulins activate when blood glucose levels increase and remain inactive when levels are within the normal range. By mimicking beta-cell function, GRIs release insulin as needed, thereby improving time spent within the target glucose range and decreasing the risks of hypoglycemia and hyperglycemia for those managing diabetes. Particularly relevant is the emergence of a new type of subcutaneously administered therapy.

What this Study Adds?

The authors conducted an evaluation of the GRI conjugate to determine its ability to meet both prandial and basal insulin needs through laboratory assessments and preclinical studies involving mouse and minipig models. The performance of this GRI was also tested in three diabetic minipigs, which closely resemble human physiological characteristics. The results indicated that the GRI maintained its effectiveness in controlling blood glucose levels for a week and showed improved efficacy compared to daily insulin glargine injections. Overall, these findings suggest that this GRI formulation may have clinical potential as a basal insulin. In both the mouse and minipig studies, minimal hypoglycemia was observed, and the insulin complex exhibited low toxicity with no significant formation of fibrous capsules.

Limitations of the Study

The Glucose Response Index must demonstrate responsiveness to a specific range of glucose levels, as this is necessary for effectively maintaining blood glucose in humans. However, the available in vivo studies do not clearly show that it meets this requirement. Additionally, it would be helpful to compare their Glucose Response Index formulation with the new weekly formulations currently in development, particularly regarding the burden of care on patients and the control of glucose levels. Long-term safety data is also needed.

Impact on Clinical Practice/Future Scope of Research

The study contributes to the expanding research on GRIs and presents a proof of concept for a biodegradable insulin complex formulation. This formulation releases insulin in a glucose-responsive manner, demonstrated long-term efficacy in vivo, and appeared to have minimal toxicity. However, further studies are necessary before this agent can be considered a viable option for human use.

Section 2: EPIDEMIOLOGY

Section Editor: Soham Tarafdar

1. Association between Age at Diabetes Diagnosis and Subsequent Incidence of Cancer: A Longitudinal Population-based Cohort

Ref: Li Y, Tian J, Hou T, Gu K, Yan Q, Sun S, et al. Association Between Age at Diabetes Diagnosis and Subsequent Incidence of Cancer: A Longitudinal Population-Based Cohort. Diabetes Care. 2024;47(3):353-61.

ABSTRACT

Objective: Diabetes is more aggressive when it manifests earlier in life. In a sizable Chinese population, we sought to investigate the relationship between the age at which type 2 diabetes mellitus (T2DM) was diagnosed and the prevalence of cancer later on.

Design and methods of research: There were 428,568 newly diagnosed T2DM patients in the prospective population-based longitudinal cohort between 2011 and 2018. Based on their age of diagnosis, participants were split into six groups: 20–54, 55–59, 60–64, 65–69, 70–74, and ≥75 years. The overall and 14 site-specific cancer incidences were compared to the 100,649,346 person-years of the Shanghai general population.

Results: The T2DM cohort and the general population had 18,853 and 582,643 total cancer cases, respectively. In people with type 2 diabetes, the standardized incidence ratio (SIR) was 1.10 (1.09, 1.12) and the age-standardized rate of total cancer was 501 [95% confidence interval (CI) 491, 511] per 100,000 person-years. A higher incidence of both general and site-specific malignancies was linked to a younger age at T2DM diagnosis. SIRs were 1.48 (1.41, 1.54), 1.30 (1.25, 1.35), 1.19 (1.15, 1.23), 1.06 (1.02, 1.10), and 0.86 (0.84, 0.89) for total cancer with T2DM diagnosis at ages 20–54, 55–59, 60–64, 65–69, 70–74, and ≥75 years, respectively. Site-specific malignancies, such as those of the lung, colorectum, stomach, liver, pancreas, bladder, central nervous system, kidney, gallbladder, and lymphoma, showed comparable patterns among both males and females.

Conclusion: Based on the age at diagnosis, our results emphasize the importance of stratifying T2DM treatment. Age-standardized cancer risks are higher in individuals with early onset T2DM than in those with later onset, as is the case with a variety of vascular events.

CRITICAL APPRAISAL

The study aimed to investigate the relationship between the age of onset of type 2 diabetes mellitus (T2DM) and the subsequent risk of developing various cancers in a large Chinese population. Prior research has established a general link between T2DM and cancer, with T2DM patients exhibiting an elevated risk of various cancers compared to the general population. Previously reported data in a Swedish cohort of T1DM has reported risk of cancer was mildly elevated in women with diabetes. Few studies have identified higher risks of site-specific cancers, including liver, pancreatic, and breast cancers, in T2DM patients. Diabetes onset at younger ages has been associated with a more aggressive disease progression, worse metabolic control, and higher complication rates, including cardiovascular diseases and nephropathy. However, the relationship between the age of diabetes diagnosis and cancer incidence across a broad-spectrum of malignancies remained insufficiently explored. While some earlier research had hinted at associations between early-onset diabetes and specific cancers such as pancreatic and colorectal cancers, prior studies were limited by small sample sizes, lack of comprehensive cancer type coverage, and short follow-up durations.

A large cohort 428,568 (51.98% female) with T2DM were enrolled during the study period with a median follow-up of 4.58 (0.99, 8.00) years. The younger cohort of <55 years had higher body mass index (BMI) and higher fasting blood glucose (FBG). A total of 18,853 cancer cases recorded in the T2DM cohort. Among Shanghai general population 2011–2018 there were 582,643 cancer cases. Comparing overall cancer in both the cohorts in 100,000 person-years the crude incidence rate and the age standardized rates (ASRs) were higher in T2DM (973, 501) compared to general population (579, 394). The relative risk was represented as a standardized incidence ratio (SIR) comparing the ratio of observed and expected cancer incidence in each year. The SIRs of overall cancer were 1.10 (1.09, 1.12) in all T2DM patients, 1.10 (1.07, 1.12) in males, and 1.11 (1.09, 1.13) in females. Patients diagnosed with T2DM between ages 20 and 54 exhibited the highest relative risk (SIR = 1.48) compared to the general population. In contrast, those diagnosed at 75 or older had a lower cancer risk (SIR = 0.86). Younger-onset T2DM was linked to a higher relative risk of several cancers, including pancreatic, bladder, thyroid, and breast cancers. Higher BMI exacerbated cancer risk in T2DM patients, with notable increases in hormone-related cancers such as breast and uterine cancers in women and prostate cancer in men. No significant increase in the incidence of respiratory and stomach cancers was observed among male patients with T2DM, while female patients did not exhibit an elevated risk of respiratory, stomach, central nervous system (CNS), or gallbladder cancers compared to the general population. This study demonstrated a 10% increased risk of all cause cancer in the T2DM cohort compared to general population.

The study utilized a very large dataset, which provided substantial statistical power to detect associations, including for site-specific cancers. This is a major strength, as it allows for more precise estimates and greater confidence in the findings. The use of age-standardized rates and SIRs allowed for comparisons across different age groups and with the general population, minimizing the confounding effect of age itself. The data collected from Shanghai Standardized Diabetes Management System (SSDMS) and the malignant tumor registry system operated by Shanghai Municipal Center for Disease Control and Prevention (SCDC) was quite comprehensive with regular follow-up for missing cases. The prevalence of missing reports was found to be only 0.5%. A sensitivity analysis was conducted for patients with multiple cancers, and the associations were similar regardless of whether only the first occurrence of cancer (sensitivity analysis) or all cancers (primary analysis) were included after the diagnosis of T2DM.

Few limitations to note include a possible selection bias as the registry used data selected from health checkup programs which may include people who were more health conscious or had better access to healthcare, which may not represent the actual general population. Information on smoking, alcohol consumption, and physical activity was available for only 60% of patients. Although sensitivity analyses accounted for this limitation, residual confounding cannot be excluded. The exclusion of individuals with pre-existing diabetes could result in a survivor bias, as the cohort may not be representative of a general diabetes population. Despite an 8-year follow-up, many younger patients had not yet reached the age range at which cancer becomes most prevalent, potentially leading to an underestimation of their lifetime cancer risk in early-onset T2DM. The risk of death from cancer cannot be ascertained from this study.

The study demonstrates a clear inverse relationship: The younger the age at T2DM diagnosis, the higher the subsequent risk of developing cancer. An early onset of type 2 diabetes may represent a distinct subgroup with significantly elevated cancer risk. By highlighting the importance of age at T2DM diagnosis, the study suggests the need for personalized prevention and management strategies. Younger individuals diagnosed with T2DM may benefit from more intensive cancer screening and prevention efforts. Diabetes prevention strategies should be highlighted, especially at younger age group by addressing obesity and insulin resistance.

Further research should investigate the mechanisms by which hyperglycemia, insulin resistance, and chronic inflammation contribute to the development of carcinogenesis in individuals with early-onset type 2 diabetes. Investigating the role of genetic predisposition and epigenetic modifications in mediating cancer risk in T2DM patients is critical. Given that this study is based on a Chinese cohort, replication in other ethnic and regional populations is necessary to ensure generalizability. Intervention studies are needed to determine whether targeted interventions, such as intensified screening or lifestyle modifications, can reduce cancer risk in individuals with early-onset T2DM. Long-term follow-up studies are needed to assess the long-term impact of early-onset T2DM on cancer risk and to identify critical periods for intervention.

2. Natural History of Type 2 Diabetes in Indians: Time to Progression

Ref: Narayan KMV, Kondal D, Chang HH, Mohan D, Gujral UP, Anjana RM, et al. Natural History of Type 2 Diabetes in Indians: Time to Progression. Diabetes Care. 2024;47(5):858-63.

ABSTRACT

Objective: The purpose of this study is to outline the natural course of diabetes among Indians.

Design and methods of research: Participants in the Centre for Cardiometabolic Risk Reduction in South Asia longitudinal research who are older than 20 years provide the data. The American Diabetes Association's definition of glycemic states was used. Annual transition probability and sojourn duration through states were estimated using Markov models.

Results: Of the 2,714 individuals without diabetes, 341 had impaired glucose tolerance (IGT) and 641 had isolated impaired fasting glucose (iIFG). Compared to 8.6% (7.3, 9.8) for iIFG, the yearly transition to diabetes was 13.9% [95% confidence interval (CI) 12.0, 15.9] for individuals with IGT.

In the normoglycemia ↔ iIFG → diabetes model, the average sojourn time was 9.7 (8.4, 11.4) years in iIFG and 40.3 (34.6, 48.2) years in normoglycemia. The mean sojourn time in the normoglycemia ↔ IGT → diabetes model was 34.5 (29.5, 40.8) years, while the sojourn time in IGT was 6.1 (5.3, 7.1) years.

Conclusion: Although people stay in normoglycemia for 35–40 years, prediabetes quickly turns into diabetes.

CRITICAL APPRAISAL

Previous studies have identified that South Asian populations, including Indians, are at higher risk of developing type 2 diabetes mellitus (T2DM) compared to other ethnic groups. This elevated risk is linked to factors such as genetics, urbanization, sedentary lifestyles, and dietary habits. Moreover, Indians tend to develop diabetes at a younger age and with lower body mass index (BMI), the "thin-fat" phenotype characterized by increased abdominal adiposity despite a lower BMI thresholds, which has been well-documented in previous cohort studies and cross-sectional analyses.

Prior research has also highlighted the existence of two prediabetic states: Isolated impaired fasting glucose (iIFG) and impaired glucose tolerance (IGT). These states differ in their underlying mechanisms and associated risk profiles. While iIFG is often associated with defective insulin secretion and fasting hyperglycemia, IGT is characterized by postprandial glucose dysregulation and insulin resistance. However, despite this understanding, the progression dynamics of glycemic states (normoglycemia → prediabetes → diabetes) in Indian populations remained poorly characterized. There was a lack of evidence on the duration individuals spend in normoglycemia or prediabetes and the annual probability of transitioning between states. This study has sought to provide much-needed data on the natural history and progression of diabetes in a specific population.

Data for this study was collected from the Chennai site of the longitudinal Centre for Cardiometabolic Risk Reduction in South Asia (CARRS) study (2010–2012) up to the fourth follow-up (2016–2017). The data was analyzed using a continuous-time Markov model. The study analyzed data from 2,714 diabetes-free participants in the CARRS study, categorizing them into normoglycemia, iIFG, and IGT. On average, individuals remain in normoglycemia for 35–40 years before progressing to pre-diabetes. Mean duration in iIFG is 9.7 (8.4, 11.4) years, while the duration in IGT is shorter, at 6.1 (5.3, 7.1) years before progression to diabetes, indicating faster progression to diabetes in IGT (13.9% vs. 8.6%). Key findings revealed that iIFG was nearly twice as prevalent as IGT, indicating elevated fasting glucose is more common than postmeal glucose elevation in this urban Indian population. The transition probabilities demonstrated a 7.5% (6.7%, 8.3%) annual progression from normoglycemia to iIFG and a 5.1% (4.4%, 5.7%) progression to IGT. Notably, there were substantial reversibility rates back to normoglycemia, with 22.8% (19.6%, 26.6%) for iIFG and 15.4% (11.9%, 19.4%) for IGT. Stratified analyses showed higher risks of prediabetes (iIFG and IGT) progression in individuals over 40 years, higher BMI (≥23 kg/m^2 for men) exhibited a higher risk of transitioning from IGT to diabetes, while women had a higher risk of transitioning from iIFG to diabetes. The study emphasizes the rapid progression of prediabetes to diabetes and underscores the reversibility of early dysglycemia. This knowledge is crucial for clinicians to identify high-risk individuals and promptly implement interventions to combat the diabetes epidemic in India.

This study's methodological strengths include its use of data from the CARRS study, a large longitudinal cohort, enabling observation of glycemic state transitions within individuals over time and minimizing interindividual variability. Standardized oral glucose tolerance tests (OGTTs), based on the American Diabetes Association (ADA) criteria, ensured objective and consistent classification of glycemic states, reducing misclassification bias. Markov models, specifically designed for analyzing transitions, accounts for bidirectional movement (progression and regression). These models facilitate the estimation of transition probabilities and sojourn times, offering a dynamic perspective on disease progression. Finally, the study population, drawn from Chennai, a major Indian urban center, offered a reasonably representative sample of this high-risk group.

The data collection was restricted to a single urban site (Chennai), potentially limiting the generalizability of the findings to rural populations or other regions in India. While the study presents annual transition probabilities, extending the follow-up duration would enhance the robustness of estimates for lifetime diabetes risk. The Markov model assumed that individuals transitioning to diabetes would remain diabetic. This assumption does not account for the possibility of diabetes remission or reversal through intensive interventions, although such occurrences are relatively infrequent. The absence of information on dietary habits, physical activity, and other modifiable risk factors restricts the ability to assess the impact of lifestyle interventions on diabetes risk.

The study's findings highlight critical implications for clinicians in India and other high-risk populations. Early screening for prediabetes, especially in individuals over 40 or with a BMI of ≥23 kg/m², is crucial to maximize the extended window of normoglycemia for preventive interventions. Given the rapid progression of IGT to diabetes, intensive lifestyle interventions should be prioritized for these individual. Recognizing the distinct pathophysiology of IGT and iIFG enables phenotype-specific management. Educating patients about the potential for regression to normoglycemia can enhance adherence to lifestyle changes, and integrating age, sex, and BMI into risk stratification models can help clinicians allocate resources more effectively.

Long-term follow-up studies are needed to assess lifetime progression rates and diabetes incidence. Research on the effectiveness of lifestyle interventions in reversing prediabetes in iIFG versus IGT is critical. Investigating genetic predisposition and molecular mechanisms specific to Indian populations can provide deeper understanding. Comparisons between rural and urban populations would improve the generalizability of findings, while examining the impact of comorbidities such as hypertension and dyslipidemia on glycemic progression could enhance risk prediction models.

3. Association of Baseline Factors with Glycemic Outcomes in GRADE: A Comparative Effectiveness Randomized Clinical Trial

Ref: Garvey WT, Cohen RM, Butera NM, Kazemi EJ, Younes N, Rosin SP, et al.; GRADE Research Group. Association of Baseline Factors With Glycemic Outcomes in GRADE: A Comparative Effectiveness Randomized Clinical Trial. Diabetes Care. 2024;47(4):562-70.

ABSTRACT

Objective: To characterize the separate and combined relationships between baseline variables and glycemia as well as the varying efficacy of drugs taken in addition to metformin.

Design and methods of research: The Glycemia Reduction Approaches in Diabetes: A Comparative Effectiveness Study (GRADE) participants ($n = 5,047$) with type 2 diabetes diagnosed within the last 10 years, taking metformin, and having a hemoglobin A1c (HbA1c) of 6.8–8.5% were randomized to receive either glimepiride, a sulfonylurea, liraglutide, or sitagliptin, a dipeptidyl peptidase-4 inhibitor, or basal insulin (glargine). The glycemic result, which was later verified, was HbA1c ≥ 7.0%.

The relationship between baseline characteristics and the glycemic result at years 1 and 4 was evaluated using univariate and multivariate regression as well as classification and regression tree (CART) analysis.

Outcomes: According to univariate analyses at baseline, the glycemic outcome at years 1 and/or 4 was linked to younger age (<58 years), Hispanic ethnicity, higher HbA1c, fasting glucose, and triglyceride levels, lower insulin secretion, and relatively higher insulin resistance. By the fourth year, there were no variables linked to the drugs' varying efficacy. In multivariate analyses, the glycemic result at year 4 was jointly associated with treatment group, younger age, and higher baseline HbA1c and fasting glucose.

When several baseline characteristics were taken into account, the superiority of glargine and liraglutide at year four remained. According to CART analyses, younger participants and those with a baseline HbA1c of 7.4% were more likely to fail to maintain HbA1c < 7% by year 4.

Conclusion: A number of baseline variables were linked to the glycemic result, but not to the four drugs' varying levels of efficacy. Younger age and greater baseline HbA1c were major factors in the failure to maintain HbA1c < 7%. Targeting patients for more aggressive care may be made easier by factors that predict early glucose worsening.

CRITICAL APPRAISAL

The management of type 2 diabetes mellitus (T2DM) often involves a stepwise approach to glycemic control, with metformin being the first-line therapy. However, many patients fail to maintain optimal glycemic control with metformin monotherapy, necessitating the addition of second-line agents. Previous studies have demonstrated the efficacy of different classes of glucose-lowering medications, such as basal insulin, sulfonylureas, glucagon-like peptide-1 receptor agonists (GLP-1 RAs), and dipeptidyl peptidase-4 (DPP-4) inhibitors, in achieving glycemic targets. The Glycemia Reduction Approaches in Diabetes: A Comparative Effectiveness Study (GRADE) evaluated the long-term glycemic control achieved by adding one of four glucose-lowering agents—glargine U-100 (basal insulin), glimepiride (sulfonylurea), liraglutide (GLP-1 RA), or sitagliptin (DPP-4 inhibitor)—to metformin. This randomized clinical trial assessed the ability of these medications to maintain hemoglobin A1c (HbA1c) at target levels over time, revealing substantial individual variability in glycemic responses.

To guide personalized therapy, the study investigated baseline characteristics influencing glycemic failure (HbA1c ≥ 7.0%), analyzing demographics, metabolic factors, socioeconomic status, cognitive ability, and indices of insulin sensitivity and secretion. A prior analysis identified higher baseline HbA1c as a predictor of faster glycemic failure. This comprehensive study extended these findings by examining a broader set of baseline variables and their joint associations with glycemic failure at years 1 and 4, both across and within treatment groups. These insights aim to enhance the strategic selection of second-line therapies for type 2 diabetes.

The study included 5,047 participants diagnosed with diabetes for <10 years, on metformin therapy, and with HbA1c levels between 6.8 and 8.5%. Participants were randomly assigned to one of four treatment groups: Basal insulin (glargine), sulfonylurea (glimepiride), GLP-1 RA (liraglutide), or DPP-4 inhibitor (sitagliptin). The primary outcome was failure to maintain HbA1c < 7.0%, confirmed on repeat testing, assessed at years 1 and 4.

Univariate and multivariate regression analyses were used to identify baseline factors (e.g., age, ethnicity, HbA1c, insulin secretion, and insulin resistance) associated with glycemic failure. Classification and regression tree (CART) analysis was employed to explore interactions and stratify patients based on their risk of glycemic deterioration. The study also evaluated whether baseline characteristics influenced the differential effectiveness of the four medications.

Univariate analyses identified several factors associated with poorer glycemic outcomes (HbA1c > 7%) at years 1 and/or 4: Younger age, Hispanic ethnicity, higher baseline fasting glucose and HbA1c, absence of hypertension, high triglycerides, high estimated glomerular filtration rate (eGFR), never smoking, absence of depression, lower insulin secretion, and relative insulin resistance. Notably, body mass index (BMI), waist-to-hip ratio, diabetes duration, blood pressure, neuropathy, albumin-to-creatinine ratio, socioeconomic factors, alcohol use, and cognition were not associated with glycemic outcomes.

At year 1, some baseline characteristics showed selective associations with different add-on medications. Liraglutide performed better in women and younger White participants, while sitagliptin was associated with poorer outcomes in White but not Black participants. Higher baseline HbA1c predicted glycemic failure across all treatments, but this effect was most pronounced with sitagliptin. Liraglutide was relatively more effective in insulin-resistant individuals at year 1. However, no factors predicted differential medication effectiveness at year 4.

Multivariate analyses at year 1 identified treatment group, treatment-sex interaction (glimepiride performed better in men and liraglutide better in women), and treatment-age/race interaction (specific effects in younger and older Black participants on glargine and glimepiride, respectively) as significant predictors. By year 4, only treatment group, younger age, and higher baseline HbA1c and fasting glucose remained significant. This indicates that many univariate associations were likely confounded by other predictors.

Consistent with previous GRADE findings, sitagliptin was associated with higher glycemic failure at year 1, while liraglutide and glargine were modestly more effective than sitagliptin and glimepiride at year 4, even after adjusting for baseline factors. Importantly, short-term treatment effects varied by sex, age, and race, but long-term effects were generally homogenous.

Classification and regression tree models further demonstrated how baseline factors stratify risk. Only younger age, higher HbA1c, and treatment group (at year 1 only) affected failure risk. At year 1, sitagliptin performed worse when baseline HbA1c was >7.5%. At year 4, only HbA1c and age interacted; higher HbA1c (>7.4%) and younger age (when HbA1c <7.4%) predicted poorer outcomes. By year 4, no significant associations were observed between any baseline factor and the prediction of differential responses to any of the medications.

These findings confirm the known association between higher baseline HbA1c and suboptimal treatment response. The association of Hispanic ethnicity with poorer outcomes, despite free diabetes care, suggests other contributing factors beyond access. The novel finding of poorer outcomes in younger participants is consistent with previous research showing worse glycemic control in younger-onset diabetes, possibly due to higher insulin resistance and genetic risk.

While only age and baseline HbA1c jointly predicted outcomes at year 4 in multivariate and CART analyses, the univariate associations remain relevant for identifying at-risk patients who may benefit from more aggressive initial management, such as combination therapy or weight loss interventions. This approach to risk stratification warrants further research to assess long-term outcomes.

The study's major strengths include its large and diverse cohort of 5,047 participants, enhancing generalizability, and its randomized design, which minimizes bias and ensures comparability between treatment groups. The 4-year follow-up provides robust longitudinal data on glycemic control durability, while advanced analytical techniques, such as CART analysis, allow for a comprehensive evaluation of baseline factors and outcomes. GRADE's strengths include its large, diverse cohort, long-term follow-up with minimal dropout, randomization to commonly prescribed medications, and management comparable to real-world care, making it well-designed for identifying predictors of glycemic outcomes.

However, the study has limitations, including a restricted population of patients with T2DM diagnosed for <10 years and HbA1c between 6.8 and 8.5%, limiting broader applicability. It lacks data on adverse events, which may affect long-term medication adherence, and focuses solely on HbA1c, overlooking other management aspects like weight or hypoglycemia. Self-reported data was utilized for certain baseline factors, such as depression. Validated instruments were employed to assess cognitive function, but the cohort was relatively young and cognitively intact, potentially restricting the generalizability of these findings. The unexpected univariate association between estimated glomerular filtration rate (eGFR), absence of hypertension, and never smoking and poorer glycemic outcomes was likely confounded by HbA1c and other factors, rendering it anomalous. These findings were subsequently eliminated in multivariate analysis. The study did not include thiazolidinediones, SGLT-2 inhibitors, or newer, more potent GLP-1 RAs, thereby limiting the assessment of interactions with these newer agents. The GRADE study population exhibited some underrepresentation of lower socioeconomic and educational groups compared to the general US population (as represented by NHANES), potentially diminishing the power to discern relationships with these factors.

Future research should address several gaps, including extending follow-up beyond 4 years to assess long-term glycemic control and complication prevention. Evaluating adverse event profiles is crucial for understanding medication safety and adherence Beyond HbA1c, clinically relevant outcomes such as cardiovascular events, renal function, and quality of life should be explored. Research on combination therapies could identify synergistic effects, optimizing treatment strategies.

Younger age, Hispanic ethnicity, high fasting glucose and HbA1c, triglycerides, poor insulin secretion, and insulin resistance were associated with treatment failure at in univariate analyses. However, these factors did not predict differential medication effectiveness in multivariate analysis at year 4, preventing personalized medication selection. Multivariate and CART analyses confirmed that younger age and higher baseline HbA1c predicted treatment failure at year 4, suggesting early and aggressive treatment for these patients.

4. The Difference between Cystatin C- and Creatinine-based Estimated Glomerular Filtration Rate and Risk of Diabetic Microvascular Complications Among Adults With Diabetes: A Population-based Cohort Study

Ref: He D, Gao B, Wang J, Yang C, Zhao MH, Zhang L. The Difference Between Cystatin C- and Creatinine-Based Estimated Glomerular Filtration Rate and Risk of Diabetic Microvascular Complications Among Adults With Diabetes: A Population-Based Cohort Study. Diabetes Care. 2024;47(5):873-80.

ABSTRACT

Objective: It is unknown how the discrepancy in estimated glomerular filtration rate (eGFRdiff) between creatinine- and cystatin C-based measures affects diabetic microvascular complications (DMCs). We looked into how eGFRdiff related to both general DMCs and their subtypes, such as diabetic neuropathy (DN), diabetic kidney disease (DKD), and diabetic retinopathy (DR).

Design and methods of research: 25,825 individuals with diabetes who were free of DMCs at baseline (2006–2010) were included in this prospective cohort study from the UK Biobank. Both the absolute difference (eGFRabdiff) and the ratio (eGFRrediff) between creatinine- and cystatin C-based computations were used to determine eGFRdiff. Electronic health data were used to determine the prevalence of DMCs.

The relationships between eGFRdiff and total DMCs and subtypes were assessed using Cox proportional hazards regression models.

Outcomes: DMCs developed in 5,753 participants over a median follow-up of 13.6 years, comprising 1,149 instances of DN, 3,203 cases of DKD, and 2,752 cases of DR. A 28% increased risk of total DMCs, a 14% increased risk of DR, a 56% increased risk of DKD, and a 29% increased risk of DN were linked to each SD drop in eGFRabdiff. The associated hazard ratios [95% confidence intervals (CIs)] were 1.16 (1.14, 1.18) for overall DMCs, 1.08 (1.05, 1.11) for DR, 1.29 (1.26, 1.33) for DKD, and 1.17 (1.12, 1.22) for DN for every 10% drop in eGFRrediff. None of the sensitivity analyses showed a significant change in the size of connections.

Conclusion: Risk of DMCs and its subtypes was independently linked to a large eGFRdiff. According to our research, tracking eGFRdiff in people with diabetes may help identify high-risk individuals.

CRITICAL APPRAISAL

Diabetic microvascular complications (DMCs)—including diabetic retinopathy (DR), diabetic kidney disease (DKD), and diabetic neuropathy (DN)—affect over 50% of individuals with diabetes, leading to vision loss, end-stage renal disease, pain, and reduced quality of life. The estimated glomerular filtration rate (eGFR), calculated using serum creatinine or cystatin C, is a standard marker for renal function and prognostication in diabetes care. Recent research has highlighted concerns over the intraindividual differences between cystatin C-based eGFR (eGFRcys) and creatinine-based eGFR (eGFRcr), known as discrepancy in estimated glomerular filtration rate (eGFRdiff), which has been linked to adverse outcomes such as kidney failure and mortality. However, no prior studies have explored the relationship between eGFRdiff and DMCs.

This study utilized data from the UK Biobank, a large cohort of over 0.5 million participants aged 40–69 recruited from 22 sites in the UK between 2006 and 2010. From this cohort, 31,642 participants with diabetes were identified based on self-reported or physician-diagnosed diabetes, use of glucose-lowering medication, or hemoglobin A1c (HbA1c) > 6.5%. After excluding participants with missing creatinine or cystatin C data, baseline DMCs, or eGFR < 60 mL/min/1.73 m², 25,825 participants were included in the analysis.

Baseline data included sociodemographics, medical history, anthropometrics, and biochemical measurements. Outcomes were derived from ICD-10 codes for DR, kidney disease, and neuropathy, identified through linkage with hospital and death records. Cox regression models estimated hazard ratios for DMCs associated with eGFRdiff, calculated as both absolute and relative differences between cystatin C- and creatinine-based eGFR. Models adjusted for confounders such as HbA1c, cholesterol, blood pressure, and medication use.

The study demonstrated that differences between cystatin C- and creatinine-based eGFR (eGFRdiff) are significantly associated with the risk of DMCs and their subtypes: DR, DKD, and DN. Each standard deviation decrease in absolute eGFRdiff increased the risk of overall DMCs by 28%, DR by 14%, DKD by 56%, and DN by 29%. Similarly, a 10% reduction in relative eGFRdiff was associated with a 16% higher risk of overall DMCs and varying increases for DR, DKD, and DN. These associations were consistent across subgroups and robust in sensitivity analyses, confirming eGFRdiff as an independent predictor. DKD showed the strongest correlation with eGFRdiff. These findings highlight the potential of eGFRdiff as a clinical marker to identify high-risk diabetes patients and guide prevention and management strategies for DMCs.

This study uniquely investigates the predictive value of the difference between cystatin C- and creatinine-based eGFR at baseline for incident DMCs. The large sample size, prospective nature, and robust findings (confirmed by sensitivity analyses) are notable strengths. This study has several limitations that should be noted. First, the observational design precludes definitive conclusions about causality. Second, despite adjusting for various confounding factors, others may still influence the results. Third, the predominantly White British composition of the study population limits the applicability of findings to more diverse groups. Fourth, the reliance on single baseline measurements of serum creatinine and cystatin C may result in inaccuracies or misclassification of eGFR differences. Finally, the use of ICD-10 codes for identifying DMCs may not fully capture early-stage conditions or ensure precise categorization of outcomes.

Future studies are needed to investigate the causal relationship between the difference in eGFR estimations and microvascular complications. It is necessary to explore the modifiable factors contributing to significant discrepancies in GFR estimations and to assess the effectiveness of interventions aimed at these factors.

5. The Effect of City-level Sugar-sweetened Beverage Taxes on Longitudinal HbA1c and Incident Diabetes in Adults with Prediabetes

Ref: Lee C, Sidell MA, Young DR, Hedderson MM, Cohen DA, Liu EF, et al. The Effect of City-Level Sugar-Sweetened Beverage Taxes on Longitudinal HbA1c and Incident Diabetes in Adults With Prediabetes. Diabetes Care. 2024;47(7):1220-6.

ABSTRACT

Objective: More than one-third of adults in the United States suffer from prediabetes, a disease marked by elevated blood glucose levels below the threshold for diabetes. Sugar-sweetened beverage (SSB) excise taxes are a proposed policy intervention to reduce SSB consumption in the population and provide money for health-related initiatives, which could postpone or prevent the onset of diabetes in people with prediabetes. We used Kaiser Permanente data from California to investigate how SSB taxes affected incident diabetes rates and mean hemoglobin A1c (HbA1c) levels at the person level.

Research design and methods: Using data gathered in the 6 years before and 4 years after the SSB tax was implemented, we compared two outcomes, mean HbA1c levels and incidence diabetes rates, among a matched cohort of prediabetic persons who lived and did not live in SSB excise tax cities. We examined longitudinal mean HbA1c and discrete-time survival models for incident diabetes using multivariable linear mixed effects models.

Results: The analysis comprised 68,658 adults. When compared to control persons, the longitudinal mean HbA1c in the tax cities was 0.007% [95% confidence interval (CI) 0.002, 0.011] higher in adjusted models; although the estimated difference was statistically significant, it was not clinically relevant (HbA1c < 0.5%). The likelihood of incident diabetes was not significantly different for residents of tax and control cities.

Conclusion: In the 4 years after the SSB tax was put into effect, we did not find a clinically meaningful correlation between SSB taxes and incident diabetes or longitudinal mean HbA1c among persons with prediabetes.

CRITICAL APPRAISAL

Sugar-sweetened beverages (SSBs) have been identified as a key dietary contributor to the rising rates of obesity, type 2 diabetes, and metabolic syndrome. These drinks, which include sodas, fruit juices, and sports drinks, are high in calories and sugar, contributing to weight gain and insulin resistance. As a public health intervention, excise taxes on SSBs have been proposed and implemented in various cities across the United States. These taxes aim to discourage SSB consumption by increasing their price, potentially generating revenue for health-related programs.

The study conducted a longitudinal natural experiment to evaluate the impact of SSB taxes on hemoglobin A1c (HbA1c) levels and diabetes incidence among individuals with prediabetes. Four cities with SSB taxes (intervention cities) were compared to ten matched control cities without such taxes, accounting for demographic and socioeconomic factors. Data from Kaiser Permanente (KP) electronic health records (EHRs) for 68,658 matched pairs (34,329 individuals from each group) were analyzed. Participants were adults aged 20–65 years with prediabetes, defined as HbA1c 5.7–6.4%, and had at least one HbA1c measurement pre- and post-SSB tax implementation.

To ensure balance, individuals were matched by demographics, clinical variables, and neighborhood characteristics using propensity score methods. Two outcomes were evaluated: individual-level mean HbA1c over time and incident diabetes within 4 years post-SSB tax. Difference-in-differences analyses assessed HbA1c changes, while discrete-time survival models examined diabetes incidence, with adjustments for covariates including body mass index (BMI), age, and poverty levels.

Results showed no clinically significant changes in mean HbA1c levels associated with SSB taxes. The adjusted mean HbA1c difference between tax and control cities was 0.007% [95% confidence interval (CI) 0.002–0.012], which was statistically but not clinically significant. Similarly, there was no overall association between SSB taxes and incident diabetes. Subgroup analyses by race, ethnicity, and age also revealed no significant effects, except for small increases in diabetes risk among Asian/Pacific Islander and Hispanic subgroups.

The key finding that SSB taxes did not have a clinically significant effect on HbA1c, or incident diabetes suggests that the current size of SSB excise taxes in California may not be sufficient to meaningfully impact prediabetes progression or diabetes prevention. This finding has important implications for public health policy and diabetes prevention efforts.

The study's strengths include its large sample size, matched cohort design, and detailed EHRs. The large sample size provides adequate statistical power, while the matched cohort design controls for confounding factors such as age, sex, race/ethnicity, and socioeconomic status.

However, the study also has limitations. First, the generalizability of the findings may be limited, as the study population consisted of members of KP, a large integrated healthcare system in California. The results may not be applicable to other populations or healthcare settings. Second, there is a possibility of exposure misclassification, as some individuals living in tax cities may have purchased SSBs in neighboring non-tax cities. This could underestimate the true impact of the SSB taxes. Third, the 4-year follow-up period may not be long enough to observe a significant impact on diabetes incidence, as the progression from prediabetes to diabetes can take many years. Finally, the study focused on SSB taxes alone and did not account for the potential synergistic effects of combining SSB taxes with other interventions, such as public health campaigns or improved access to healthy foods.

The lack of a strong impact of SSB taxes on diabetes-related outcomes highlights the need for comprehensive strategies beyond taxation to effectively prevent diabetes in individuals with prediabetes. Clinicians should continue to emphasize lifestyle interventions, such as healthy eating, regular physical activity, and weight management, as the cornerstone of prediabetes management.

This study highlights key areas for future research on SSB taxes. Longer-term studies are needed to assess their impact on diabetes incidence over extended periods. Research should also explore the effects of combining SSB taxes with public health measures such as education campaigns and nutrition labeling. Investigating subgroup differences by socioeconomic status, race/ethnicity, and age can clarify the heterogeneity of effects. Direct measurement of changes in SSB consumption behaviors post-tax implementation is essential to understand behavioral responses. Additionally, cost-effectiveness analyses are crucial to evaluate the economic and health benefits of SSB taxes as a strategy for diabetes prevention.

6. Association of Glucagon-like Peptide-1 Receptor Agonists with Suicidal Ideation and Self-injury in Individuals with Diabetes and Obesity: A Propensity-weighted, Population-based Cohort Study

Ref: Hurtado I, Robles C, Peiró S, García-Sempere A, Sanfélix-Gimeno G. Association of glucagon-like peptide-1 receptor agonists with suicidal ideation and self-injury in individuals with diabetes and obesity: a propensity-weighted, population-based cohort study. Diabetologia. 2024;67(11):2471-80.

ABSTRACT

Objectives and hypotheses: After the Icelandic Medicines Agency reported in July 2023 that people using liraglutide and semaglutide were experiencing suicidal ideation and self-injury (SIS), regulators around the world are examining safety data on glucagon-like peptide-1 receptor agonists (GLP-1 RA). Our goal was to evaluate the risk of SIS in new GLP-1 RA users in comparison to those on sodium-glucose cotransporter-2 inhibitors (SGLT-2i), which are used to treat type 2 diabetes in obese people.

Techniques: This cohort study, which combines many population-wide databases, covers five million people in Spain, including all obese individuals who started using SGLT-2i or GLP-1 RA for type 2 diabetes between 2015 and 2021.

We used a new user, active comparator design, and multivariable Cox regression modeling with inverse probability of treatment weighting (IPTW) based on propensity scores to determine the comparative effect of GLP-1 RA on the risk of SIS. We conducted a number of sensitivity and stratified analyses.

Findings: We included 11,627 patients starting SGLT-2i treatment and 3,040 patients starting GLP-1 RA treatment. Patients in the GLP-1 RA group were younger (55 vs. 60 years old, $p < 0.001$), more likely to have anxiety (49.4% vs. 41.5%, $p < 0.001$), sleep disorders (43.2% vs. 34.1%, $p < 0.001$), depression (24.4% vs. 19.0%, $p < 0.001$), and obesity [35.1% of people with body mass index (BMI) ≥ 40 vs. 15.1%, $p < 0.001$] than patients treated with SGLT-2i.

Standardized mean differences across groups were <0.1 for all covariates following propensity score weighting, indicating sufficient group balance at baseline following adjustment. There was no indication that GLP-1 RA enhanced the incidence of SIS in the primary per-protocol analyses [hazard ration (HR) 1.04; 95% confidence interval (CI) 0.35, 3.14]. The HR from intention-to-treat studies was 1.36 (95% CI 0.51, 3.61). The corresponding HRs in analyses that used imputation for BMI missing values and excluded people without BMI information were 0.89 (95% CI 0.26, 3.14) and 1.29 (95% CI 0.42, 3.92). There were no differences between subgroups according to stratified analysis.

Conclusion and interpretation: Although our results do not support a higher risk of SIS in people with type 2 diabetes and obesity who take GLP-1 RA, it is important to interpret them cautiously due to the rarity of SIS events and the wide uncertainty of effect size (although null, effect may be compatible with a risk as high as threefold). To rule out a causative relationship between GLP-1 RA and suicidality, more research is required, including final regulatory body assessments.

CRITICAL APPRAISAL

Glucagon-like peptide-1 receptor agonists (GLP-1 RAs) have become a cornerstone in the treatment of type 2 diabetes, particularly for patients with established cardiovascular disease, chronic kidney disease, or other related comorbidities. Beyond their glycemic effects, GLP-1 RAs have demonstrated significant benefits in weight loss, reducing cardiovascular events and improving renal outcomes, further solidifying their role in managing complex metabolic and cardiovascular conditions.

Recently, concerns have emerged regarding a potential association between GLP-1 RA use and an increased risk of suicidal ideation and self-injury (SIS). These concerns were initially triggered by reports from the Icelandic Medicines Agency, prompting regulatory agencies worldwide to initiate reviews of the available safety data. While preliminary analyses conducted by these agencies have not provided conclusive evidence of a causal link between GLP-1 RAs and SIS, the possibility of such an association warrants careful investigation and monitoring. Observational studies, which analyze real-world data from large populations, play a critical role in evaluating the potential risk of rare adverse events like SIS in the context of widespread drug use. Therefore, this study aimed to investigate the potential association between GLP-1 RA use and SIS in a large population-based cohort of individuals with diabetes and obesity.

This study employed a real-world, population-based cohort design, utilizing data from the Valencia Health System Integrated Database (VID) in Spain. The VID is a comprehensive electronic health record system that captures data on a large and diverse population, providing a valuable resource for conducting epidemiological research. The study population consisted of adult individuals ($\geq$18 years) with obesity who initiated treatment with either GLP-1 RAs or sodium-glucose cotransporter-2 inhibitors (SGLT-2i) for type 2 diabetes between 2015 and 2021. SGLT-2i medications, another class of glucose-lowering drugs with distinct mechanisms of action, served as the active comparator group.

The researchers implemented a new user, active comparator design which ensures that all participants were new users of the respective medications, reducing the potential for pre-existing conditions or prior treatment experiences to influence the outcomes. To further address potential confounding factors, the researchers employed multivariable Cox regression modeling with inverse probability of treatment weighting (IPTW). IPTW is a statistical technique that creates balanced groups by weighting each participant based on their probability of receiving each treatment, effectively mimicking a randomized controlled trial.

The study included a substantial number of participants, with 3,040 initiating treatment with GLP-1 RAs and 11,627 initiating treatment with SGLT-2i. Baseline characteristics revealed some differences between the two groups. The GLP-1 RA group was generally younger, more likely to be female, and had a higher prevalence of psychiatric comorbidities, such as anxiety, sleep disorders, and depression. They were also more likely to be obese. After applying IPTW, the baseline characteristics were well-balanced between the two groups, reducing the influence of these confounding factors on the study results.

The primary analysis, conducted according to a per-protocol approach, found no statistically significant association between GLP-1 RA use and an increased incidence of SIS [hazard ratio (HR) 1.04; 95% confidence interval (CI) 0.35, 3.14]. This result suggests that individuals treated with GLP-1 RAs did not experience a higher rate of SIS compared to those treated with SGLT-2i. To further validate these findings, the researchers performed several sensitivity analyses, including an intention-to-treat analysis and analyses excluding individuals with missing body mass index (BMI) data. These analyses consistently yielded similar results, reinforcing the lack of association between GLP-1 RA use and SIS. Additionally, stratified analyses were conducted to examine the potential influence of specific subgroups, such as those with preexisting psychiatric comorbidities, different sexes, and varying levels of obesity. These stratified analyses also did not reveal any significant differences between the GLP-1 RA and SGLT-2i groups.

This study contributes important new knowledge to the ongoing discussion about the safety of GLP-1 RAs and their potential association with SIS. This population-based cohort in Spain provides further evidence that no link exists between GLP-1 RA use and an increased risk of SIS in individuals with type 2 diabetes and obesity. This study adds valuable real-world data from a large population, strengthening the overall evidence base.

The population-based design, with its large sample size, provides substantial statistical power and increases the generalizability of the results to similar populations. The use of an active comparator (SGLT-2i) and a new user design helps to minimize bias and confounding. The application of propensity score weighting (IPTW) is a robust statistical method for addressing potential confounding by indication. The limitations of this study are listed below. Firstly, the data source (VID) comprises real-world clinical data not specifically collected for research, introducing potential biases such as differential recording, misclassification, and missing data. Secondly, despite using IPTW and adjusting for many covariates, residual confounding cannot be ruled out, as some relevant information may be missing. Indication bias, a type of confounding where a symptom influences both treatment and outcome, is also a concern. Thirdly, the rarity of suicidal outcomes means the study cannot definitively rule out a substantial increase or decrease (up to threefold) in SIS among GLP-1 RA users, necessitating cautious interpretation of association estimates. Fourthly, variability in coding practices in real-world settings is a potential bias. Fifthly, the lack of information on inpatient medication in the VID may lead to minor misestimation. Sixthly, some stratified analyses had small sample sizes, making those results exploratory. Finally, generalizability outside of Spain should be approached cautiously. However, the findings are consistent with other pharmacovigilance and pharmacoepidemiologic studies that also do not find an increased risk of SIS associated with GLP-1 RAs.

The results provide some reassurance regarding the safety of GLP-1 RAs in terms of SIS risk. Future studies are needed to confirm these findings in more diverse populations and settings, including different ethnicities, healthcare systems, and cultural contexts. Studies with longer follow-up periods are necessary to assess the long-term effects of GLP-1 RAs on mental health outcomes. Further research should explore potential risk factors for SIS among individuals using GLP-1 RAs to identify any specific subgroups that may be more vulnerable. Studies should also examine the impact of different GLP-1 RA medications and dosages on SIS risk. Finally, further investigation is needed to understand the underlying biological or psychological mechanisms that may potentially link GLP-1 RAs to mental health outcomes. It is crucial to remember that final evaluations from regulatory bodies are still pending, and continuous monitoring of the safety profile of GLP-1 RAs remains essential.

7. Associations between Diabetes and Cancer: A 10-year National Population-based Retrospective Cohort Study

Ref: Safadi H, Balogh Á, Lám J, Nagy A, Belicza É. Associations between diabetes and cancer: A 10-year national population-based retrospective cohort study. Diabetes Res Clin Pract. 2024;211:111665.

ABSTRACT

Goals: To learn more about the temporal correlation between diabetes and cancer at the national level and to examine the risk of cancer in individuals with diabetes in comparison to those without the disease.

Methods: Using data on population service use and antidiabetic prescriptions from 2010 to 2021, a retrospective cohort analysis was carried out to examine the contribution of diabetes to the development of cancer. Diabetes status, age, and sex were examined in connection to the time to cancer diagnosis using univariate and multivariate Cox regression.

Results: Based on a population analysis of 3,681,774 people, individuals with diabetes are consistently at a greater risk of being diagnosed with cancer for every cancer site examined. Diabetes adds the lowest, but still significant, risk for breast cancer (HR = 1.137, 99% CI: 1.055; 1.227) and prostate cancer (HR = 1.171, 99% CI: 1.071; 1.280). It adds the highest risk for pancreatic cancer (HR = 2.294, 99% CI: 2.099; 2.507) and liver cancer (HR = 1.830, 99% CI: 1.631; 2.054). The younger age group (40–54 years: 5.4% for diabetic patients against 4.4% for controls; 70–89 years: 12.7% for diabetic patients versus 12.4% for controls) is the main cause of the disparity in cancer rates. There are conflicting findings about whether diabetes affects men and females differently in terms of their likelihood of receiving a cancer diagnosis.

Prior to the diagnosis of diabetes, the incidence of cancer begins to rise, reaching its peak the year after. The incidence is 114/10,000 population in the control group and 195/10,000 population in the diabetic group by the year after the start of the inclusion date. The incidence then declines in the vicinity of the control group.

Conclusion: Given that the incidence of cancer is highest around the time of diabetes diagnosis, screening programs should be updated and diabetes guidelines should be supplemented with cancer prevention suggestions. Our findings for prostate cancer run counter to numerous earlier investigations; more research is advised to elucidate this.

CRITICAL APPRAISAL

Epidemiological studies have consistently demonstrated a higher incidence of certain cancers, including colorectal, liver, pancreatic, endometrial, breast, and bladder cancers, among individuals with diabetes. Several mechanisms have been proposed to explain this association, including hyperinsulinemia (elevated insulin levels), insulin resistance, chronic inflammation, hyperglycemia (high blood sugar), and alterations in growth factors and sex hormones.

Previous studies have explored these associations using various study designs, including cohort studies, case-control studies, and meta-analyses. While these studies have provided valuable insights, some limitations remain. These include variations in study populations, follow-up periods, cancer types investigated, and methods used to adjust for confounding factors. Furthermore, many studies have focused on specific cancer types or have not adequately accounted for the influence of other risk factors, such as obesity, smoking, and physical activity. Therefore, there was a need for large-scale, population-based studies with long follow-up periods to comprehensively assess the associations between diabetes and a broad range of cancers, while carefully considering potential confounding factors.

This study was a 10-year national population-based retrospective cohort study conducted in Hungary. The researchers used data from the National Health Insurance Fund Administration (NHIFA) database, which covers the entire Hungarian population. The study cohort included all individuals aged 18 years or older who were registered in the NHIFA database between 2008 and 2017.

The study population was followed from the date of cohort entry (2008) until the date of cancer diagnosis, death, or the end of the study period (2017), whichever occurred first. The researchers calculated incidence rates of various cancers in individuals with and without diabetes and used Cox proportional hazards regression models to estimate hazard ratios (HRs) for the association between diabetes and cancer risk, adjusting for age, sex, smoking status, alcohol consumption, and socioeconomic status.

In study 1 a total of 3,681,774 individuals were analyzed, with 86,537 diagnosed with diabetes (dispensing antidiabetic medications in 2014–2015) and 3,595,237 in the control group without diabetes. None had prior cancer diagnoses. The diabetes group was older (average age: 61.4 years vs. 58.0 years in the control group) and had a slightly higher male proportion. During the observation period, 10.1% of individuals with diabetes were diagnosed with cancer compared to 8.6% in the control group. The risk was notably higher in younger individuals (40–54 years: 5.4% vs. 4.4%) but less pronounced in older individuals (70–89 years: 12.7% vs. 12.4%).

The diabetes group consistently exhibited higher cancer incidence across all sites, with the greatest risks observed for pancreatic cancer (HR 2.294) and liver cancer (HR 1.830), and the lowest for breast cancer (HR 1.137) and prostate cancer (HR 1.171). Males had higher cancer rates for most cancer types, but risk patterns varied by site and sex. Diabetes, age, and male sex (where applicable) were significant risk factors. The effect of diabetes was more pronounced in younger individuals (40–54 years) for most cancer types. No significant sex differences in diabetes-related cancer risk were found for most sites, though some variability was observed for kidney and liver cancer. The influence of diabetes on cancer risk decreased with age for kidney, prostate, and colon cancer but remained consistent for pancreatic and breast cancer.

Study 2 analyzed the cancer diagnosis timing. Cancer incidence increased before the diabetes inclusion date, peaking one year after (195/10,000 for the diabetes group vs. 114/10,000 for the control group). Incidence subsequently declined but remained higher in the diabetes group. Most cancer types followed a similar temporal pattern, with pronounced peaks in pancreatic and liver cancer. Breast cancer showed no pre-inclusion increase, and prostate cancer incidence in the diabetes group aligned with controls four years post-inclusion. Diabetes is consistently associated with higher cancer risk, especially for pancreatic and liver cancer, with pronounced effects in younger individuals. The temporal relationship suggests cancer screening and prevention efforts should consider the timing of diabetes diagnosis. No significant association was found for lung cancer, prostate cancer, melanoma, or non-Hodgkin lymphoma.

The study's key strength is the use of over a decade of population-based administrative health data, enabling the creation of large cohorts, including the entire population aged 40+ with incident diabetes in 2014–2015. This extensive dataset allowed for significance evaluation at 1% and an analysis of the temporal relationship between diabetes and cancer, including annual breakdowns before and after diabetes diagnosis.

The limitations include the lack of clinical and prognostic factor data which limited the analysis to age- and sex-adjusted calculations. The inability to differentiate between type 1 and type 2 diabetes, with an assumption that most cases were type 2 needs to be noted. Potential inaccuracies in cancer diagnosis codes affected both cohorts. Limited data availability (from 2010) prevented exclusion of malignancies diagnosed before this period. Inclusion of untreated diabetes patients and those using non-reimbursed antidiabetic medications in the control group could bias results. However, this likely underestimates the diabetes-cancer association, strengthening the study's findings. Results are not generalizable to populations with pregnancy-related conditions or polycystic ovary syndrome (PCOS), as these groups were excluded.

The findings of this study reinforce the importance of cancer screening and prevention efforts in individuals with diabetes. Cancer incidence begins to rise prior to a diabetes diagnosis, reaches its highest point in the year following diagnosis, and then subsequently declines to levels comparable to those without diabetes. This pattern suggests a need for diabetes-specific adjustments to cancer screening protocols and the integration of cancer prevention strategies into existing diabetes management guidelines. Promoting healthy lifestyle choices, such as maintaining a healthy weight, engaging in regular physical activity, and avoiding smoking, is crucial for both diabetes management and cancer prevention.

Several key areas require further investigation to better understand the complex relationship between diabetes and cancer. First, research should delve into the specific biological mechanisms that connect diabetes to the development of different cancer types. Second, it's crucial to examine how factors such as the duration and severity of diabetes, as well as the specific treatments used to manage it, influence cancer risk. Third, studies are needed to evaluate the effectiveness of targeted interventions, including lifestyle modifications (like diet and exercise) and pharmacological approaches, in reducing cancer risk among individuals with diabetes. Fourth, research should assess the cost-effectiveness of various cancer screening strategies in diabetic populations to optimize resource allocation and improve patient outcomes. Finally, international collaborative studies are essential to validate these findings in more diverse populations, considering potential variations in this association across different regions and ethnicities, which could be influenced by genetic, environmental, and sociocultural factors.

8. 5-year Follow-up of the Randomised Diabetes Remission Clinical Trial (DiRECT) of Continued Support for Weight Loss Maintenance in the UK: An Extension Study

Ref: Lean ME, Leslie WS, Barnes AC, Brosnahan N, Thom G, McCombie L, et al. 5-year follow-up of the randomised Diabetes Remission Clinical Trial (DiRECT) of continued support for weight loss maintenance in the UK: an extension study. Lancet Diabetes Endocrinol. 2024;12(4):233-46.

ABSTRACT

Context: After 2 years, the weight management intervention in Diabetes Remission Clinical Trial (DiRECT), a randomized controlled efficacy trial, led to a mean weight loss of 7.2 kg, and 36% of individuals had type 2 diabetes in remission. 29 (81%) of the 36 participants in the intervention group who continued to lose >10 kg of weight after 2 years were in remission. In order to sustain weight loss and achieve clinical benefits, intervention participants were then given ongoing low-intensity dietary support for up to 5 years after baseline. The purpose of this extension study was to present observed results after 5 years.

Techniques: In the UK, primary care providers hosted the DiRECT experiment. Participants were people between the ages of 20 and 65 years who did not take insulin, had a body mass index (BMI) of >27 kg/m^2, and had type 2 diabetes for <6 years. Stepped food reintroduction (2–8 weeks), complete diet replacement (825–853 kcal/day formula diet for 12–20 weeks), stopping hypertension and antidiabetic medications, and finally structured assistance for weight-loss maintenance comprised the intervention. Following the dissemination of the 2-year results to all participants, data from the UK National Health Service was gathered every year until year 5 from the original randomly assigned groups, intervention withdrawals, and the remaining intervention participants who got low-intensity nutritional support.

Remission of type 2 diabetes was the main goal; this was expected for the extension study as it was shown in the DiRECT experiment that sustained weight loss was the main factor for remission. The International Standard Randomised Controlled Trial Number (ISRCTN) registry has the trial listed under registration number 03267836.

Results: In the initial DiRECT trial, 149 participants were randomly allocated to the intervention group and 149 to the control group between July 25, 2014, and August 5, 2016. All intervention participants who were still enrolled in the experiment after 2 years [101 (68%) of 149] were asked to continue receiving low-intensity care for an additional three years. Of the 101 participants, 95 (94%) were able to continue, gave their agreement, and were assigned to the DiRECT extension group. The nonextension group consisted of 54 participants, where intervention was withdrawn.

Participants in the DiRECT extension ($n = 85$) dropped an average of 6.1 kg at 5 years, with 11 (13%) of those in remission. Participants in DiRECT extension had more visits with hemoglobin A1c (HbA1c) <48 mmol/mol (<6.5%; 36% vs. 17%, $p = 0.0004$), without glucose-lowering medication (62% vs. 30%, $p < 0.0001$), and in remission (34% vs. 12%, $p < 0.0001$) than those in the nonextension group in comparison. Five (5%) of the 93 original control subjects ($n = 149$) were in remission, and the mean weight decrease was 4.6 kg ($n = 82$). More visits were made by original intervention participants who were in remission (27% vs. 4%, $p < 0.0001$), without antidiabetic medication (51% vs. 16%, $p < 0.0001$), had a weight more than 5% below baseline (61% vs. 29%, $p < 0.0001$), and had a HbA1c below 48 mmol/mol (29% vs. 15%, $p = 0.0002$). 26% of those in remission at year 2 were still in remission after 5 years. Compared to the control group (10.2 occurrences per 100 patient-years, $p = 0.0080$), the original intervention group experienced 4.8 serious adverse events per 100 patient-years, which was less than half.

Interpretation: Over a 5-year period, the prolonged DiRECT intervention was linked to larger absolute and aggregate weight loss and suggested improved health status.

CRITICAL APPRAISAL

Type 2 diabetes was traditionally considered a chronic, progressive disease requiring lifelong medication. However, recent evidence has challenged this view, suggesting that substantial weight loss can induce remission, especially in individuals with early-stage diabetes. The Diabetes Remission Clinical Trial (DiRECT) demonstrated that a structured weight-loss intervention could achieve remission in 36% of participants after two years, with 81% remission among those maintaining over 10 kg weight loss. These findings positioned dietary and lifestyle changes as viable alternatives to medication, with weight loss identified as a primary driver of remission.

The DiRECT study was a 2-year, open-label, cluster-randomized controlled trial conducted between July 2014 and August 2016, involving 298 participants aged 20–65 years with type 2 diabetes diagnosed within the previous 6 years. Participants, living in Scotland and northeast England, had a body mass index (BMI) of 27–45 kg/m² and were not using insulin. The trial was approved by ethical and health boards in the UK (ISRCTN 03267836).

The intervention included:
- *Withdrawal of medications*: Antidiabetic and antihypertensive drugs were discontinued.
- *Total diet replacement*: A nutritionally complete formula providing 825–853 kcal/day was prescribed for 12 weeks, extended to 5 months based on individual needs.
- *Stepped food reintroduction*: Meals were gradually reintroduced over 6–8 weeks.
- *Structured weight maintenance support*: Participants attended 30-minute appointments with National Health Service (NHS) nurses or dietitians biweekly during food reintroduction and monthly thereafter.

After the trial, 2-year results were shared with all participants, who were encouraged to focus on weight control. Routine data from GP surgeries were collected annually.

At the 2-year follow-up, 101 of 149 intervention participants were offered low-intensity dietary support for an additional 3 years, with 95 agreeing to continue. Review appointments were held quarterly, lasting 15–30 minutes, with a local nurse, dietitian, or study staff. Coronavirus disease 2019 (COVID-19) restrictions necessitated remote follow-ups via phone, text, or email. Participants self-reported weight and monitored blood pressure or glucose at their GP surgery if they regained >5 kg within 3 months.

The study extended its follow-up to 5 years, offering low-intensity dietary support to intervention participants while tracking outcomes for all groups. Primary outcomes included weight change, hemoglobin A1c (HbA1c) levels, and diabetes remission, defined as HbA1c below 48 mmol/mol without medication.

Findings

- At 5 years, the intervention group maintained an average weight loss of 6.1 kg, compared to 4.6 kg in the control group.
- 13% of intervention participants were in remission at 5 years, significantly higher than 5% in the control group.
- HbA1c levels and time spent off glucose-lowering medications were consistently better in the intervention group.
- Serious adverse events were fewer in the intervention group (4.8 per 100 patient-years) compared to the control group (10.2 per 100 patient-years).

This study provided long-term evidence of the sustainability of weight loss and its role in diabetes remission. The durability of remission is strongly linked to sustained weight loss. Participants maintaining over 10 kg of weight loss had the highest remission rates. Aggregated exposure to lower HbA1c levels and reduced medication use correlated with better health outcomes. Remission rates were higher with continued dietary support, highlighting the importance of sustained interventions. Weight regain remains a critical challenge, emphasizing the need for strategies to address relapse in weight management programs.

This study boasts strengths including a 5-year follow-up period, providing valuable data on long-term diabetes remission; implementation within routine primary care, enhancing generalizability; and comprehensive annual data collection encompassing clinical metrics, medication use, and participant-reported outcomes. However, limitations include potential self-selection bias in the extension phase due to a likely more motivated participant group; inconsistent follow-up leading to missing data and attrition, which weakens comparisons; the disruptive impact of the COVID-19 pandemic on support sessions; and the lack of investigation into underlying physiological mechanisms contributing to weight regain or variations in remission based on sex and age.

The study highlights the need for further research into the mechanisms of weight regain to improve intervention designs and explores personalized approaches considering factors such as age, sex, and ethnicity to tailor treatments effectively. Developing cost-effective, sustained support models is essential for maintaining weight loss beyond structured programs. Additionally, investigating the role of mental health and social determinants can offer holistic insights into weight management success. Exploring alternative approaches, such as pharmacological agents, could enhance and sustain diabetes remission outcomes.

9. Adiposity and Metabolic Health in Asian Populations: An Epidemiological Study Using Dual-energy X-ray Absorptiometry in Singapore

Ref: Mina T, Xie W, Low DY, Wang X, Lam BCC, Sadhu N, et al. Adiposity and metabolic health in Asian populations: an epidemiological study using dual-energy X-ray absorptiometry in Singapore. Lancet Diabetes Endocrinol. 2024;12(10):704-15.

ABSTRACT

Context: The Asia-Pacific area is seeing a sharp rise in type 2 diabetes, cardiovascular disease, and associated cardiometabolic disorders. We looked into the relationship between Asian ethnic subgroups' unfavorable cardiometabolic profiles and excess adiposity, a major risk factor for type 2 diabetes and cardiovascular disease.

Techniques: Multiethnic Asian men and women aged 30–84 years who reside in Singapore make up the population-based cohort of the Health for Life in Singapore (HELIOS) study. We conducted a cross-sectional analysis of data from people whose body composition was evaluated using metabolic characterization and dual-energy X-ray absorptiometry.

Using multivariable regression analyses, we examined the association between body mass index (BMI) and visceral fat mass index (vFMI) and cardiometabolic phenotypes (glycemic indices, lipid levels, and blood pressure), disease outcomes (type 2 diabetes, hypercholesterolemia, and hypertension), and metabolic syndrome score in a subgroup of participants who were not taking medication for these conditions.

Results: 10,004 people gave their agreement to be part of the HELIOS cohort between April 2, 2018, and January 28, 2022; 9,067 of them were included in the study [5,404 (59.6%) female, 3,663 (40.4%) male; 6,224 (68.6%) Chinese, 1,169 (12.9%) Malay, 1,674 (18.5%) Indian; mean age 52.8 years (SD 11.8)]. Type 2 diabetes was present in 8.2% of the population ($n = 744$), 27.2% of the population ($n = 2,469$), and 18.0% of the population ($n = 1,630$).

Compared to Chinese participants, Malay and Indian participants exhibited negative metabolic and adiposity profiles and had three to four times the chances of obesity and type 2 diabetes. Type 2 diabetes and other detrimental cardiometabolic health indices were linked to excess adiposity ($p < 0.0001$). Higher vFMI did not, however, account for higher glucose levels, less insulin sensitivity, or a greater risk of type 2 diabetes among Indian participants, even if it did account for the variations in blood pressure and triglycerides among the Asian ethnic groups.

Interpretation: A significant portion of type 2 diabetes patients in each of the ethnic groups under study are caused by visceral adiposity, which is also an independent risk factor for metabolic disease in Asian populations.

Adiposity, however, does not always account for the difference in insulin resistance and type 2 diabetes risk among Asian subgroups, suggesting that there are other mechanisms at play that contribute significantly to Asian populations' vulnerability to cardiometabolic disease.

CRITICAL APPRAISAL

Type 2 diabetes, cardiovascular disease (CVD), and related cardiometabolic disturbances are leading causes of morbidity and mortality globally, with a pronounced burden in the Asia-Pacific region. Over the past three decades, these diseases have increasingly shifted toward emerging economies in Asia, where urban environments and lifestyle changes have contributed to rising prevalence. Asian populations are particularly prone to type 2 diabetes and insulin resistance due to factors such as visceral adiposity, which is closely linked to metabolic dysfunction. While observational studies have established the role of adiposity in these conditions, there is limited understanding of how different fat depots, particularly visceral fat, contribute to cardiometabolic disparities among Asian ethnic groups. The Health for Life in Singapore (HELIOS) study aimed to address this gap by evaluating the relationships between adiposity and cardiometabolic health across Chinese, Malay, and Indian populations living in Singapore.

The HELIOS study is a population-based cohort involving multiethnic Asian participants aged 30–84 years residing in Singapore. Researchers performed a cross-sectional analysis of data from 9,067 participants, recruited between April 2018 and January 2022. The study included assessments of body composition using dual-energy X-ray absorptiometry (DEXA) and metabolic characterizations. Participants were categorized into three major ethnic groups—Chinese, Malay, and Indian—and their metabolic health indices, such as glycemic measures, lipid profiles, and blood pressure, were evaluated.

Participants had a mean age of 52.8 years, with 59.6% females and ethnic distributions of 68.6% Chinese, 12.9% Malay, and 18.5% Indian. Obesity prevalence was highest among Malay (49.9%) and Indian (40.6%) participants, compared to Chinese participants (14.2%). The prevalence of type 2 diabetes was similarly elevated in Malay (13.4%) and Indian (17.3%) participants, nearly four times that of Chinese participants (4.8%).

Researchers used multivariable regression analyses to examine the associations between body mass index (BMI), visceral fat mass index (vFMI), and cardiometabolic outcomes. Excess adiposity was consistently associated with adverse outcomes, including elevated fasting glucose, insulin resistance (HOMA-IR), triglycerides, and reduced high-density lipoprotein (HDL) cholesterol. A 1-SD increase in vFMI was linked to a twofold increase in the risk of type 2 diabetes and hypertension.

However, ethnic differences persisted after adjusting for adiposity. While vFMI explained disparities in triglycerides and blood pressure between groups, it did not fully account for elevated glucose levels, insulin resistance, or type 2 diabetes risk in Indian participants. This suggests that additional mechanisms beyond adiposity contribute to their heightened metabolic risk. Conversely, adiposity largely explained the metabolic differences between Malay and Chinese participants.

Sensitivity analyses confirmed the robustness of findings across various covariates, including socioeconomic status, lifestyle factors, and genetic ancestry.

The HELIOS study revealed that visceral adiposity is a major risk factor for metabolic diseases in Asian populations, contributing significantly to type 2 diabetes and hypertension. However, the findings highlight that adiposity alone does not fully explain the heightened cardiometabolic risks among Indian participants compared to Chinese and Malay groups. These results underscore the need to investigate additional pathophysiological mechanisms underlying ethnic disparities in metabolic health.

The study's strengths include its large sample size and representation of three major Asian ethnic groups living in a shared urban environment, reducing confounding factors related to geography or culture. The use of DEXA provided precise measurements of visceral fat, distinguishing it from overall body fat. Standardized methodologies ensured reliable comparisons across ethnic groups. Additionally, the study's analyses excluded participants on medications for metabolic conditions, avoiding treatment-related confounders.

As a cross-sectional study, the HELIOS study cannot establish causal relationships between adiposity and cardiometabolic outcomes. The reliance on self-reported ethnicity, though validated, may introduce bias. While visceral adiposity was robustly assessed, other potential contributors, such as hepatic fat levels, dietary habits, and physical activity, were not fully accounted for. The findings may also be influenced by recruitment biases, as healthier individuals may be more likely to participate.

The findings of the HELIOS study emphasize the critical role of visceral adiposity in driving cardiometabolic diseases among Asian populations, underscoring the need for targeted interventions. Clinicians should prioritize the early identification and management of visceral adiposity, particularly in Malay and Indian populations, who exhibit higher risks. Strategies to reduce visceral fat, such as dietary modifications and lifestyle interventions, could significantly lower the burden of type 2 diabetes and related conditions. Public health initiatives should focus on preventive measures that integrate community-specific dietary and behavioral recommendations. Lastly, the study supports the inclusion of advanced imaging techniques such as DEXA in clinical and research settings to enhance the understanding and management of adiposity-related risks.

Future research should explore additional mechanisms contributing to the heightened metabolic risks in Indian populations, including hepatic fat levels and developmental adversity. Longitudinal studies are needed to establish causal pathways between adiposity and cardiometabolic outcomes. Investigating the interplay between genetic predisposition, lifestyle factors, and adiposity could yield deeper insights into ethnic disparities. Furthermore, incorporating comprehensive dietary and physical activity assessments may clarify their independent and interactive effects on metabolic health. Addressing these gaps will inform more effective, culturally tailored interventions to reduce the burden of metabolic diseases in diverse Asian populations.

10. Association of Glycaemic Index and Glycaemic Load with Type 2 Diabetes, Cardiovascular Disease, Cancer, and All-cause Mortality: A Meta-analysis of Mega Cohorts of more than 100,000 Participants

Ref: Jenkins DJA, Willett WC, Yusuf S, Hu FB, Glenn AJ, Liu S, et al.; Clinical Nutrition & Risk Factor Modification Centre Collaborators. Association of glycaemic index and glycaemic load with type 2 diabetes, cardiovascular disease, cancer, and all-cause mortality: a meta-analysis of mega cohorts of more than 100,000 participants. Lancet Diabetes Endocrinol. 2024;12(2):107-18.

ABSTRACT

Context: The relationship between chronic disease and a food's glycaemic index is up for dispute. Our goal was to evaluate the relationships between type 2 diabetes, cardiovascular disease, diabetes-related malignancies, and all-cause mortality and glycaemic index (GI) and glycaemic load (GL).

Techniques: We conducted a meta-analysis of large cohorts from the Richard Doll Consortium (≥100,000 individuals). We looked for cohorts that prospectively investigated relationships between GI or GL and chronic illness outcomes published between the database's creation and August 4, 2023, in the Cochrane Library, MEDLINE, PubMed, Embase, Web of Science, and Scopus. Three separate reviewers reviewed the entire article and extracted the summary estimates data.

All-cause mortality, diabetes-related malignancies (bladder, breast, colorectal, endometrial, hepatic, pancreatic, and non-Hodgkin lymphoma), incident type 2 diabetes, and total cardiovascular disease (including mortality) were the main outcomes. After controlling for dietary variables and aggregating their most adjusted relative risk (RR) estimates using a fixed-effects model, we evaluated comparisons between the lowest and highest quantiles of GI and GL. We also evaluated the relationships between the four primary outcomes and diets rich in whole grains and fiber. The PROSPERO registration number for the study protocol is CRD42023394689.

Results: We found 48 studies reporting associations between GI or GL and the outcomes of interest from ten prospective large cohorts (six from the USA, one from Europe, two from Asia, and one international): 34 (71%) on various cancers, nine (19%) on cardiovascular disease, five (10%) on type 2 diabetes, and three (6%) on all-cause mortality. Type 2 diabetes {relative risk (RR) 1.27 [95% confidence interval (CI) 1.21–1.34]; $p < 0.0001$}, total cardiovascular disease [1.15 (1.11–1.19); $p < 0.0001$], diabetes-related cancer [1.05 (1.02–1.08); $p = 0.0010$], and all-cause mortality [1.08 (1.05–1.12); $p < 0.0001$] were all linked to the use of high GI foods.

Similar correlations were seen between overall cardiovascular disease [1.15 (1.10–1.20); *p* < 0.0001] and diabetes [RR 1.15 (95% CI 1.09–1.21); *p* < 0.0001]. Similar to low GI diets, there were correlations between the four major outcomes and diets rich in whole grains and fiber.

Interpretation: The impact of dietary recommendations to lower GI and GL on health outcomes may be comparable to those of recommendations to increase intake of whole grains and fiber.

CRITICAL APPRAISAL

The role of the glycemic index (GI) and glycemic load (GL) of foods in chronic disease development has been a subject of ongoing debate. GI ranks carbohydrates based on how quickly they raise blood sugar levels, while GL considers both the GI and the quantity of carbohydrates in a food. Some research suggests high GI/GL diets are linked to increased risk of type 2 diabetes, cardiovascular disease (CVD), and certain cancers, possibly due to mechanisms such as oxidative stress and inflammation triggered by blood sugar spikes. However, the 2019 WHO-sponsored report in The Lancet downplayed the relevance of GI/GL in chronic disease prevention, emphasizing fiber and whole grains instead. This sparked controversy, as other studies and meta-analyses have shown associations between high GI/GL diets and adverse health outcomes. This context highlights the need for further investigation into the independent roles of GI/GL in chronic disease, particularly in comparison to established factors such as fiber and whole grains.

This study was a meta-analysis of large cohort studies (each with at least 100,000 participants) identified from the Richard Doll Consortium. The researchers searched multiple databases (Cochrane Library, MEDLINE, PubMed, Embase, Web of Science, and Scopus) to identify studies that prospectively examined associations between GI or GL and chronic disease outcomes (type 2 diabetes, CVD, diabetes-related cancers, and all-cause mortality). Data extraction and quality assessment of included studies were performed by independent reviewers.

The primary outcome was the relative risk (RR) of the outcome in the highest quantile of GI or GL intake compared to the lowest quantile, adjusted for various dietary and lifestyle factors. The researchers used a fixed-effects model to pool RR estimates from the included studies. They also assessed associations between high-fiber and whole-grain diets and the outcomes of interest.

The study analyzed 48 GI or GL studies from ten large prospective cohorts within the Richard Doll Consortium, encompassing 104,000–567,000 participants. These cohorts included six from the USA, one from Europe, two from Asia, and one international. The studies assessed associations between GI/GL and type 2 diabetes, CVD, diabetes-related cancers, and all-cause mortality. Of these, 71% focused on cancer outcomes, 19% on CVD, 10% on type 2 diabetes, and 6% on mortality. Cohort sizes ranged from approximately 104,000–567,000 participants, with a mean follow-up of 12.6 years.

High GI consumption was associated with an increased risk of:
- *Type 2 diabetes*: RR 1.27 (95% CI 1.21–1.34)
- *Total CVD*: RR 1.15 (95% CI 1.11–1.19)
- *Diabetes-related cancers*: RR 1.05 (95% CI 1.02–1.08)
- *All-cause mortality*: RR 1.08 (95% CI 1.05–1.12)

Subgroup analysis revealed some variation in results based on cohort size, follow-up duration, and location, but these differences were minor and unlikely to affect clinical relevance. The E-values for most associations exceeded 1.2, indicating robust findings, though some cancer-related associations had E-values lower than 1.2, suggesting potential confounding factors. No publication bias was observed, and the study's data quality was high, with most cohorts scoring 7 or higher on the Newcastle–Ottawa Scale (NOS). Similar associations were observed for high GL and type

2 diabetes [RR 1.15 (95% CI 1.09–1.21)] and total CVD [RR 1.15 (95% CI 1.10–1.20)]. Importantly, diets high in fiber and whole grains showed similar protective associations for the four main outcomes as low GI diets.

This meta-analysis provides compelling evidence that high GI diets are associated with an increased risk of several major chronic diseases, including type 2 diabetes, CVD, diabetes-related cancers, and all-cause mortality. Importantly, the study demonstrates that the magnitude of these associations is comparable to the well-established benefits of high-fiber and whole-grain diets. This challenges the previous downplaying of GI/GL's importance and suggests it should be considered alongside fiber and whole grains in dietary recommendations.

Strengths of this study are the inclusion of large cohorts with high participant numbers, increasing statistical power and generalizability; direct comparison of GI/GL associations with those of fiber and whole grains in the same cohorts; and assessment of dose-response relationships and use of GRADE and NutriGrade to evaluate the certainty of evidence. It has certain limitations too. Some analyses had few assessments, and the absence of certain data or positive effects in some cases may have contributed to a lack of studies on outcomes such as cancer, myocardial infarction (MI), stroke, and CVD deaths, which are serious adverse events. This limitation could affect the estimation of heterogeneity, publication bias, and the influence of uncontrolled confounders. The robustness of the findings is limited by small differences in RRs, which could be influenced by confounders that could not be fully adjusted. While GI results for diabetes and CVD were consistent, GL associations differed for all-cause mortality and diabetes-related cancers, suggesting that the GL-cancer relationship requires further investigation.

Additionally, comparing GI with fiber and whole grain exposure for disease outcomes involved only one or two cohorts for most outcomes. Future studies should evaluate differences by sex, as some sex-based differences have been observed, although our limited data did not show a sex difference for diabetes. It would also be valuable to control for diabetes in CVD and cancer outcomes, though this might lead to over-adjustment.

Despite these limitations, low GI diets were linked to a reduced risk of diabetes, CVD, diabetes-related cancers, and all-cause mortality in large international cohorts. Comparing these effects with fiber and whole grain intake showed similar results. Therefore, despite ongoing debates, diets low in GI may offer benefits for chronic diseases, similar to those associated with higher fiber and whole grain consumption. More comprehensive studies using a harmonized federated meta-analysis approach, along with long-term randomized controlled trials, are needed. Nevertheless, current evidence supports the importance of managing postprandial glycemic excursions and suggests that GI, GL, fiber, and whole grains are crucial markers of carbohydrate quality for dietary recommendations.

11. Associations of the Glycaemic Index and the Glycaemic Load with Risk of Type 2 Diabetes in 127,594 People from 20 Countries (PURE): A Prospective Cohort Study

Ref: Miller V, Jenkins DA, Dehghan M, Srichaikul K, Rangarajan S, Mente A, et al.; Prospective Urban and Rural Epidemiology (PURE) study investigators. Associations of the glycaemic index and the glycaemic load with risk of type 2 diabetes in 127 594 people from 20 countries (PURE): a prospective cohort study. Lancet Diabetes Endocrinol. 2024;12(5):330-8.

ABSTRACT

Context: There is debate over the relationship between the incidence of type 2 diabetes and the glycemic index and glycemic load. In an international cohort with a range of glycemic load and glycemic index meals, we sought to assess this association.

Techniques: 127,594 adults between the ages of 35 and 70 from 20 high-, middle-, and low-income nations participated in the Prospective Urban and Rural Epidemiology (PURE) project, which is a prospective cohort study. Using validated food frequency questionnaires tailored to each nation, diet was evaluated at baseline. The consumption of seven types of foods that include carbohydrates was used to assess the glycemic index and the glycemic load. Participants were divided into glycemic load and glycemic index quintiles. Type 2 diabetes was the main consequence. Multiple-variable Cox hazard ratios (HRs) was calculated using frailty models with random intercepts for the study center.

Results: Over the course of a median follow-up of 11.8 years (IQR 9.0–13.0), 7,326 (5.7%) type 2 diabetes incident cases were reported. A diet with a higher glycemic index was substantially linked to an increased risk of diabetes in multivariable adjusted analyses [quintile 5 vs. quintile 1; HR 1.15 (95% CI 1.03–1.29)]. The incidence of incident type 2 diabetes was higher for individuals in the highest quartile of the glycemic load than for those in the lowest quintile (HR 1.21; 95% CI 1.06–1.37). People with a higher body mass index (BMI) [quintile 5 vs. quintile 1; HR 1.23 (95% CI 1.08–1.41)] had a stronger correlation between the glycemic index and diabetes than people with a lower BMI [quintile 5 vs. quintile 1; 1.10 (0.87–1.39); p interaction = 0.030].

Interpretation: In an international population across five continents, diets with a high glycemic load and index were linked to an increased risk of occurrence type 2 diabetes. According to our research, eating a diet low in glycemic index and low in glycemic load may help avoid type 2 diabetes.

CRITICAL APPRAISAL

Preventing diabetes is a global priority due to its significant health and economic burden. Randomized controlled trials have demonstrated that lifestyle changes, including dietary modifications, are effective in preventing and managing diabetes. Diets high in glycemic index (GI) and glycemic load (GL) have been linked to increased insulin resistance and impaired β-cell function, which may raise diabetes risk. GI ranks carbohydrate-containing foods by their postprandial glucose response, while GL accounts for both the quality and quantity of carbohydrates in a food.

Contradictory findings from various studies have highlighted the uncertainty regarding the role of GI and GL in diabetes prevention. This study sought to investigate their association with the incidence of type 2 diabetes, utilizing data from 127,594 participants from 20 countries participating in the Prospective Urban and Rural Epidemiology (PURE) study. The hypothesis posited that higher GI and GL diets would be associated with an increased incidence of diabetes due to their postprandial glycemic effects.

This study was a prospective cohort study conducted within the PURE study, which enrolled 127,594 adults aged 35–70 years from 20 high-income, middle-income, and low-income countries. Dietary intake was assessed at baseline using country-specific validated food frequency questionnaires (FFQs). The GI and GL were estimated based on the intake of seven categories of carbohydrate-containing foods: Nonlegume starchy foods, sugar-sweetened beverages, fruit, fruit juice, nonstarchy vegetables, legumes, and dairy. Participants were categorized into quintiles of GI and GL.

The primary outcome was incident type 2 diabetes, defined as a physician diagnosis, use of oral antidiabetic agents or insulin, or a documented fasting plasma glucose level of 7.0 mmol/L or more during follow-up in individuals without a history of diabetes at baseline. Multivariable Cox frailty models with random intercepts for study center were used to calculate hazard ratios (HRs) for incident diabetes, adjusting for various demographic, socioeconomic, lifestyle, and dietary factors.

In this study, data on GI and GL were available for 145,895 participants. After excluding individuals with implausible energy intake or baseline diabetes, 127,594 participants were included in the analysis. Over a median follow-up of 11.8 years, 7,326 (5.7%) new cases of type 2 diabetes occurred. The median GI was 85.9, with the highest values seen in China, Southeast Asia, and Africa. The median GL ranged from 177.1 in North America and Europe to 346.0 in South Asia.

Participants consuming high-GI diets were more likely to be less educated, live in rural areas, smoke, have lower physical activity, and have a lower body mass index (BMI), with a higher intake of starchy foods and lower intake of fruits, vegetables, dairy, and unprocessed meats. In fully adjusted models, higher GI and GL were both positively associated with an increased risk of type 2 diabetes.

In multivariable-adjusted analyses, higher GI was associated with a higher risk of diabetes:
- *Quintile 5 versus quintile 1*: HR 1.15 (95% CI 1.03–1.29)
- *HR per 10-unit GI increment*: 1.09 (95% CI 1.02–1.16)

Similarly, higher GL was associated with a higher risk of diabetes:
- *Quintile 5 versus quintile 1*: HR 1.21 (95% CI 1.06–1.37)
- *HR per 50-unit GL increment*: 1.01 (95% CI 1.00–1.03)

The association between GI and diabetes was stronger among individuals with higher BMI [HR 1.23 (95% CI 1.08–1.41) for quintile 5 vs. quintile 1] compared to those with lower BMI [HR 1.10 (95% CI 0.87–1.39) for quintile 5 vs. quintile 1; p interaction = 0.030].

This large, multinational study provides further evidence that high GI and GL diets are associated with an increased risk of type 2 diabetes. The findings are consistent with most observational studies but contrast with the 2023 WHO guideline on carbohydrate intake, which downplayed the importance of GI and GL. The study also highlights that the association between GI and diabetes risk may be stronger among individuals with higher BMI.

This analysis has several strengths, including the use of validated, country-specific FFQs, a long follow-up duration, a large sample size, and diverse participant representation from high, middle, and low-income countries. This provides broader insights into GI and GL than studies focused solely on North American or European populations. However, there are also limitations to consider. Diet was assessed at baseline, and changes over time may have occurred, especially in lower-income and middle-income countries undergoing economic transitions. Diets were self-reported, which may introduce measurement errors and lead to exposure misclassification, potentially weakening the observed associations. The GI values of foods can vary, which might also bias the findings toward the null hypothesis. Despite this, the study used internationally recognized GI tables to estimate values based on the foods most consumed across cultures.

As an observational study, it is subject to potential unmeasured or residual confounding, though extensive adjustments were made for known diabetes risk factors. The HR could vary with longer follow-up periods, and regional subgroup analyses had limited power due to smaller sample sizes, making them susceptible to sparse-data bias. Additionally, diabetes diagnosis might have been missed or misclassified in some participants, though the study found high agreement between self-reported diabetes and fasting blood glucose measures.

Healthcare professionals should advise patients to consume low GI and GL diets, especially those with higher BMI. This could involve promoting dietary changes such as choosing whole grains over refined grains, increasing consumption of fruits, vegetables, and legumes, and limiting sugary drinks and processed foods. Incorporating GI and GL into dietary guidelines could have significant public health implications for reducing the burden of type 2 diabetes globally.

Randomized controlled trials are crucial for establishing causal relationships between low GI/GL diets and reduced diabetes risk. Mechanistic studies are needed to elucidate the biological pathways through which

GI/GL influence glucose metabolism, insulin sensitivity, and other relevant factors. Further research should explore potential interactions between GI/GL and other dietary components (such as fiber, fat, and protein), as well as lifestyle factors such as physical activity and sleep. Finally, developing and evaluating culturally tailored interventions to promote the adoption and maintenance of low GI/GL dietary patterns in diverse populations is essential for translating research findings into effective public health strategies.

12. Daily Low-dose Aspirin and Incident Type 2 Diabetes in Community-dwelling Healthy Older Adults: A Post-hoc Analysis of Efficacy and Safety in the ASPREE Randomised Placebo-controlled Trial

Ref: Zoungas S, Zhou Z, Owen AJ, Curtis AJ, Espinoza SE, Ernst ME, et al. Daily low-dose aspirin and incident type 2 diabetes in community-dwelling healthy older adults: a post-hoc analysis of efficacy and safety in the ASPREE randomised placebo-controlled trial. Lancet Diabetes Endocrinol. 2024;12(2):98-106.

ABSTRACT

Context: Diabetes etiology has been linked to inflammation. This study examined the impact of low-dose aspirin as a randomized treatment on incident type 2 diabetes and fasting plasma glucose (FPG) levels in older persons.

Techniques: A double-blind, placebo-controlled study of daily oral low-dose aspirin was called Aspirin in Reducing Events in the Elderly (ASPREE). The study population consisted of community-dwelling people in the USA and Australia who were 70 years of age or older (≥65 years for US minority ethnic groups) and free of dementia, cardiovascular illness, or physical disabilities that limited their independence. Participants with diabetes at baseline or those with missing or incomplete incident diabetes data throughout follow-up were not included in the post-hoc analysis.

Oral 100 mg enteric-coated aspirin or a placebo was given to participants at random. Self-reported diabetes, the start of glucose-lowering medication, or an FPG concentration of 7.0 mmol/L or above measured at yearly follow-up visits among individuals without diabetes at baseline were all considered incident diabetes. We evaluated the impact of aspirin on incidence diabetes and FPG concentrations in the intention-to-treat population using mixed-model repeated measures and Cox proportional hazards models. Participants who had taken at least one dose of the study drug were evaluated for severe bleeding.

Results: A total of 16,209 people were included between March 10, 2010, and December 24, 2014 [8,086 (49.9%) were randomly assigned to aspirin and 8,123 (50.1%) were randomly assigned to placebo]. 995 (in 6.1% of the population) incident cases of type 2 diabetes were reported over a median follow-up of 4.7 years (IQR 3.6–5.7) (459 in the aspirin group and 536 in the placebo group). At year 5, the aspirin group's FPG concentration increased more slowly {between-group difference estimate –0.048 mmol/L [95% confidence interval (CI) –0.079 to –0.018]; $p = 0.0017$} and their risk of incident diabetes was 15% lower than that of the placebo group [hazard ratio 0.85 (95% CI 0.75–0.97); $p = 0.013$].

Of the 16,104 patients, 510 (3.2%) experienced major bleeding (major gastrointestinal bleeding, cerebral bleeding, and clinically significant bleeding at other locations); the aspirin group experienced 300 (3.7%) and the placebo group experienced 210 (2.6%). The risk of severe bleeding was 44% higher in the aspirin group than in the placebo group [hazard ratio 1.44 (95% CI 1.21–1.72); $p < 0.0001$].

Interpretation: While aspirin treatment delayed the rise in FPG concentration and decreased the prevalence of type 2 diabetes, it increased severe bleeding in older persons living in the community. The potential of anti-inflammatory drugs like aspirin to prevent type 2 diabetes or improve glucose levels is worth more research, with a thorough evaluation of all possible safety events, considering the rising incidence of type 2 diabetes in older persons.

CRITICAL APPRAISAL

Type 2 diabetes is a growing global health concern, particularly among older adults. Inflammation is increasingly recognized as a key player in the development of diabetes. Aspirin, with its anti-inflammatory properties, has been proposed as a potential preventive agent. Previous studies, like the Physicians' Health Study, have shown that aspirin might reduce diabetes risk, while others, like the Women's Health Study, showed no effect. However, these studies were conducted over 20 years ago, used different aspirin dosages and regimens, and primarily included middle-aged adults. Therefore, there is a need for more contemporary research investigating the effect of low-dose aspirin on incident diabetes, specifically in older populations.

This study is a post-hoc analysis of the Aspirin in Reducing Events in the Elderly (ASPREE) trial, a large, randomized, and placebo-controlled trial that investigated the effects of daily low-dose aspirin (100 mg enteric-coated) on various health outcomes in community-dwelling older adults. The ASPREE trial included 19,114 participants aged 70 years or older (or 65 years or older for US minority groups) without cardiovascular disease, disability, or dementia at baseline.

For this post-hoc analysis, participants with diabetes at baseline or with incomplete diabetes data during follow-up were excluded, leaving 16,209 participants (8,086 in the aspirin group and 8,123 in the placebo group). The primary outcome was incident type 2 diabetes, defined as self-reported diabetes, starting glucose-lowering medication, or having a fasting plasma glucose (FPG) concentration of 7.0 mmol/L or more at annual follow-up visits. Secondary outcomes included changes in FPG concentration over time. Major bleeding events were also assessed as a safety outcome.

The researchers used Cox proportional hazards models to analyze the effect of aspirin on incident diabetes and mixed-model repeated measures to assess changes in FPG concentrations.

Key findings included:
- *Reduced diabetes risk*: The aspirin group had a 15% lower risk of developing diabetes compared to the placebo group [hazard ratio (HR) 0.85; 95% confidence interval (CI) 0.75–0.97; $p = 0.013$].
- *Slower FPG increase*: Aspirin was associated with a slower rate of increase in FPG concentration over 5 years (between-group difference estimate −0.048 mmol/L, 95% CI −0.079 to −0.018; $p = 0.0017$).
- *Increased bleeding risk*: The aspirin group had a 44% higher risk of major bleeding events (HR 1.44; 95% CI 1.21–1.72; $p < 0.0001$), primarily gastrointestinal bleeding.

This study provides new evidence that daily low-dose aspirin can reduce the incidence of type 2 diabetes and slow the progression of elevated FPG levels in healthy older adults. However, this benefit comes with an increased risk of major bleeding events. This highlights the importance of weighing the potential benefits of aspirin against its risks when considering its use for diabetes prevention in older individuals.

This study had several strengths, including a large sample size of healthy, community-dwelling older adults without prior cardiovascular events, dementia, or major disabilities. Participants were followed for a median of 4.7 years with detailed annual data collection, yielding a substantial number of incident diabetes cases. High adherence to treatment (≥50% of study pills taken by over 70% of participants) supports the robustness of the findings.

However, limitations include the diabetes definition, which relied on self-report, initiation of glucose-lowering medication, or a single FPG measurement, without confirmatory tests or routine hemoglobin A1c (HbA1c) or oral glucose tolerance testing. Subgroup analyses [e.g., by sex, country, or body mass index (BMI)] lacked power to detect nuanced differences. Although aspirin reduced the incidence of diabetes and slowed FPG increases, it also raised the risk of major bleeding.

Despite these limitations, the study demonstrated that aspirin reduced the incidence of type 2 diabetes and slowed the rate of FPG increase, but at the cost of a significantly higher risk of major bleeding. These findings highlight the need for a careful balance between potential benefits and risks when considering aspirin as a preventive strategy for diabetes in older adults.

Given the rising global prevalence of diabetes, this study underscores the potential of anti-inflammatory agents like aspirin in preventing or delaying diabetes onset and improving glucose regulation. However, further research, including long-term follow-up and trials involving diverse populations, is necessary to fully understand the benefits and risks, particularly in high-risk groups and across varying clinical contexts.

13. Early Findings from the NHS Type 2 Diabetes Path to Remission Programme: A Prospective Evaluation of Real-world Implementation

Ref: Valabhji J, Gorton T, Barron E, Safazadeh S, Earnshaw F, Helm C, et al. Early findings from the NHS Type 2 Diabetes Path to Remission Programme: a prospective evaluation of real-world implementation. Lancet Diabetes Endocrinol. 2024;12(9):653-63.

ABSTRACT

Context: Type 2 diabetes can be remitted with total diet replacement (TDR), according to randomized controlled trials. The National Health Service (NHS) Type 2 Diabetes Path to Remission (T2DR) program, a 12-month behavioral intervention to support weight loss that involves an initial 3-month period of TDR, was developed after the NHS committed in 2019 to establishing a TDR-based interventional program delivered at scale in real-world environments. We evaluated the patients' type 2 diabetes remission.

Techniques: Those in England between the ages of 18 and 65 who had been diagnosed with type 2 diabetes within the previous 6 years were referred to the program between September 1, 2020, and December 31, 2022, as part of this nationwide prospective service evaluation of program implementation.

In order to determine hemoglobin A1c (HbA1c) readings and prescriptions for glucose-lowering drugs, program data were connected to the National Diabetes Audit. Remission of type 2 diabetes at 1 year was the main outcome, which was defined as two HbA1c readings of <48 mmol/mol taken at least 3 months apart and without the prescription of any glucose-lowering drugs for 3 months prior to the first HbA1c reading and the second HbA1c reading taken 11–15 months after the program's start date. Results were evaluated for two groups; those who began TDR on the 12-month program prior to January 2022 and for whom no data was missing, and those who began TDR on the 12-month program prior to January 2022 and had finished the program (i.e., had a valid weight recorded at month 12) by December 31, 2022, for whom there were no missing data.

Results: 7,540 persons were referred to the program between September 1, 2020, and December 31, 2022; 1,740 of those individuals began TDR prior to January 2022, giving them a full 12-month window to complete the program by the time data extraction took place at the end of December 2022. 960 (55%) of those who began TDR prior to January 2022 finished the treatment, as indicated by a weight measurement at 12 months. 8.3% [95% confidence interval (CI) 7.9–8.6] or 9.4 kg (8.9–9.8) was the mean weight loss for the 1,710 participants who began the program prior to January 2022 and had no missing data, and 9.3% (8.8–9.8) or 10.3 kg (9.7–10.9) was the mean weight loss for the 945 participants who finished the program and had no missing data.

The mean weight loss for the subgroup of 710 (42%) of 1,710 participants who began the treatment before to January 2022 and had two HbA1c measures recorded was 13.4% (12.3–14.5) or 14.8 kg (13.4–16.3). Of them, 190 (27%) experienced remission. 450 (48%) of the 945 participants who finished the program had two HbA1c measures taken; 145 (32%) of them experienced remission and lost an average of 14.4% (13.2–15.5) or 15.9 kg (14.3–17.4) of their body weight.

Interpretation: Results from the NHS T2DR program demonstrate that at-scale service delivery can result in type 2 diabetes remission outside of research settings. However, compared to randomized controlled trials, the rate of remission attained is lower and data ascertainment is more constrained when used in the real world.

CRITICAL APPRAISAL

Randomized controlled trials (RCTs) like the Diabetes Remission Clinical Trial (DiRECT) have demonstrated that total diet replacement (TDR), using low-calorie, nutritionally complete formulas, can lead to significant weight loss and remission of type 2 diabetes. These trials showed that TDR, combined with behavioral support, was more effective than usual care in achieving remission. However, RCTs are conducted in controlled settings with rigorous protocols and highly motivated participants. It remained unclear whether similar remission rates could be achieved when TDR programs are implemented at scale in real-world settings, with less intensive support and a broader range of participants. This knowledge gap led to the establishment of the National Health Service (NHS) Type 2 Diabetes Path to Remission (T2DR) program in England, aiming to deliver a TDR-based intervention within routine primary care.

This study was a prospective service evaluation of the NHS T2DR program, a 12-month behavioral intervention involving an initial 3-month period of TDR followed by food reintroduction and weight maintenance phases. The program was delivered by commercial providers across different regions in England. Participants were adults aged 18–65 years with type 2 diabetes diagnosed within the past 6 years and a body mass index (BMI) of 27 kg/m² or more (or 25 kg/m² or more for non-White ethnic groups). They were referred to the program by their general practitioners. The primary outcome was remission of type 2 diabetes at 1 year, defined as two hemoglobin A1c (HbA1c) measurements below 48 mmol/mol (6.5%) at least 3 months apart, with no glucose-lowering medications prescribed. Data were collected from the T2DR program records and linked to the National Diabetes Audit (NDA) to obtain HbA1c measurements and medication prescription data.

Between September 1, 2020 and December 31, 2022, 7,540 individuals with type 2 diabetes were referred to the NHS T2DR program. Among them, 4,340 (58%) initiated the TDR phase, and 1,740 participants began TDR before January 2022, allowing a full 12-month follow-up. Of these, 960 (55%) completed the program, defined as having a recorded weight at 12 months. The mean duration on the program was 8 months. The referred participants had a mean age of 50 years, a mean baseline weight of 109.2 kg, a BMI of 38.0 kg/m², and a mean HbA1c of 58.5 mmol/mol.

Weight loss outcomes were significant. Participants who completed the program achieved an average weight loss of 9.3% (10.3 kg). Among those with no missing data, 35% lost at least 10% of their baseline weight, and 16% lost 15% or more. Remission of type 2 diabetes, defined as two HbA1c measurements under 48 mmol/mol without glucose-lowering medication, was achieved by 27% of participants with complete data and two HbA1c readings. Higher remission rates correlated with greater weight loss (average 13.4%, or 14.8 kg). Logistic regression analysis revealed that remission was more likely for participants referred within 1 year of diagnosis and those with lower baseline HbA1c.

Variations in outcomes were observed by ethnicity, BMI, and deprivation level. White participants and those with a BMI of 30–40 kg/m² showed better weight loss outcomes. The analysis underscores the effectiveness of TDR in real-world settings, though outcomes were influenced by demographic and clinical factors.

This study demonstrates that remission of type 2 diabetes is achievable outside of research settings, through a TDR-based program delivered at scale in routine primary care. However, the remission rates observed in this real-world implementation were lower than those reported in RCTs. This highlights the challenges of translating research findings into clinical practice and the need to optimize program delivery and support to maximize effectiveness in real-world settings.

This study is notable for its size, encompassing the largest cohort referred to a diabetes remission program to date. However, limitations exist, including its observational nature, lack of a control group, and reliance on self-reported weights for some participants, which can lead to underreporting. Remission was calculated for only 42% of participants due to the availability of HbA1c measurements and prescribing data, potentially introducing selection bias.

The program's lower BMI limit was based on earlier evidence, although recent data suggest higher remission rates for those with lower BMIs. The real-world implementation often shows attenuated effect sizes and poorer data ascertainment compared to RCTs. Despite these challenges, 27% of participants with applicable HbA1c measurements achieved remission, with an average HbA1c reduction of 12.0 mmol/mol and weight loss of 13.4% (14.8 kg).

The findings provide valuable insights for clinicians and policymakers regarding the implementation of TDR programs for diabetes remission. While remission is achievable in real-world settings, it is essential to optimize program delivery and support to improve completion rates and maximize weight loss. Strategies to enhance participant engagement and adherence, such as personalized support and addressing barriers to participation, are crucial. Further research is needed to identify factors that predict success in real-world TDR programs and to tailor interventions to individual needs and preferences.

The findings demonstrate that type 2 diabetes remission is feasible through large-scale real-world delivery, although at lower rates than in controlled trials. Insights from this study have shaped a revised program now available nationwide, with future evaluations planned to track remission rates, mortality, and complications.

Future research should focus on identifying factors that influence program completion and remission rates in real-world settings. Developing and evaluating strategies to improve participant engagement and adherence. Assessing the long-term sustainability of remission achieved through real-world TDR programs and investigating the cost-effectiveness of TDR programs in different healthcare systems.

14. Food Additive Emulsifiers and the Risk of Type 2 Diabetes: Analysis of Data from the NutriNet-Santé Prospective Cohort Study

Ref: Salame C, Javaux G, Sellem L, Viennois E, de Edelenyi FS, Agaësse C, et al. Food additive emulsifiers and the risk of type 2 diabetes: analysis of data from the NutriNet-Santé prospective cohort study. Lancet Diabetes Endocrinol. 2024;12(5):339-49.

ABSTRACT

Context: Emulsifiers may have negative impacts on gut flora, inflammation, and metabolic disturbances, according to experimental research. In a sizable prospective cohort of French individuals, we sought to examine the relationships between exposures to food additive emulsifiers and the risk of type 2 diabetes.

Techniques: Data from 104,139 persons who participated in the French NutriNet-Santé prospective cohort research between May 1, 2009, and April 26, 2023, were analyzed; the mean age was 42.7 years (SD 14.5), and 82,456 (79.2%) were female. Every 6 months, three 24-hour dietary records were taken over 3 nonconsecutive days to evaluate nutritional intakes. Ad hoc laboratory tests and a variety of food composition databases were used to assess exposure to added emulsifiers.

Multivariable proportional hazards Cox models were used to characterize the relationships between cumulative time-dependent exposures to food additive emulsifiers and the risk of type 2 diabetes after controlling for known risk variables. ClinicalTrials.gov has registered the NutriNet-Santé study (NCT03335644).

Results: During follow-up, 1,056 out of 104,139 participants [mean follow-up duration 6.8 years (SD 3.7)] received a type 2 diabetes diagnosis.

The following emulsifier intakes were linked to a higher risk of type 2 diabetes: total carrageenans {hazard ratio (HR) 1.03 [95% confidence interval (CI) 1.01–1.05] per increment of 100 mg/day, $p < 0.0001$}, carrageenans gum [E407; HR 1.03 (1.01–1.05) per increment of 100 mg/day, $p < 0.0001$], tripotassium phosphate [E340; HR 1.15 (1.02–1.31) per increment of 500 mg/day, $p = 0.023$], acetyl tartaric acid esters of monoglycerides and diglycerides of fatty acids [E472e; HR 1.04 (1.00–1.08) per increment of 100 mg/day, $p = 0.042$], sodium citrate [E331; HR 1.04 (1.01–1.07) per increment of 500 mg/day, $p = 0.0080$], guar gum [E412; HR 1.11 (1.06–1.17) per increment of 500 mg/day, $p < 0.0001$], gum arabic [E414; HR 1.03 (1.01–1.05) per increment of 1,000 mg/day, $p = 0.013$], and xanthan gum [E415, HR 1.08 (1.02–1.14) per increment of 500 mg/day, $p = 0.013$].

Interpretation: In a large prospective cohort of French individuals, we discovered direct correlations between exposure to certain food additive emulsifiers commonly used in industrial meals and the incidence of type 2 diabetes. For improved consumer safety, more research is required to spur a reassessment of the laws controlling the use of added emulsifiers in the food sector.

CRITICAL APPRAISAL

Food additives, particularly emulsifiers, are widely used in processed foods to improve texture, stability, and shelf life. Recent experimental studies have raised concerns about the potential impact of emulsifiers on gut microbiota, inflammation, and metabolic health. These studies suggest that emulsifiers may disrupt the gut microbiome, leading to increased intestinal permeability, inflammation, and metabolic disturbances that could contribute to the development of type 2 diabetes. However, epidemiological evidence on the association between food additive emulsifiers and diabetes risk in humans has been limited. This gap in knowledge highlights the need for large-scale prospective studies to investigate the potential link between emulsifier consumption and diabetes risk in real-world settings.

This study was conducted within the NutriNet-Santé cohort, a large prospective cohort study in France that investigates the relationship between nutrition and health. The study included 104,139 participants who were free of diabetes at baseline. Dietary intake was assessed using repeated 24-hour dietary records, and exposure to food additive emulsifiers was evaluated by linking these records to multiple food composition databases and conducting laboratory assays.

The primary outcome was incident type 2 diabetes, ascertained through self-reported diagnoses, medical records, and linkage with the national health insurance system database. Multivariable Cox proportional hazard models were used to assess the associations between cumulative intakes of individual emulsifiers and the risk of type 2 diabetes, adjusting for various sociodemographic, lifestyle, and dietary factors.

The median follow-up duration was 6.8 years, during which 1,056 participants developed type 2 diabetes. The study found that higher intakes of several emulsifiers were associated with an increased risk of type 2 diabetes, including:

- *Total carrageenans*: Hazard ratio (HR) 1.03 [95% confidence interval (CI) 1.01–1.05] per 100 mg/day increment
- *Carrageenan gum*: HR 1.03 (95% CI 1.01–1.05) per 100 mg/day increment
- *Tripotassium phosphate*: HR 1.15 (95% CI 1.02–1.31) per 500 mg/day increment
- *Acetyl tartaric acid esters of mono- and diglycerides of fatty acids*: HR 1.04 (95% CI 1.00–1.08) per 100 mg/day increment
- *Sodium citrate*: HR 1.04 (95% CI 1.01–1.07) per 500 mg/day increment
- *Guar gum*: HR 1.11 (95% CI 1.06–1.17) per 500 mg/day increment
- *Gum arabic*: HR 1.03 (95% CI 1.01–1.05) per 1,000 mg/day increment
- *Xanthan gum*: HR 1.08 (95% CI 1.02–1.14) per 500 mg/day increment

This study provides the first large-scale epidemiological evidence linking the consumption of several commonly used food additive emulsifiers to an increased risk of type 2 diabetes in humans. These findings support the concerns raised by experimental studies and suggest that emulsifiers may contribute to the development of diabetes through their effects on gut microbiota and inflammation.

This study has notable strengths, including its prospective design, large sample size, and detailed assessment of dietary exposures. It is the first to evaluate both qualitative and quantitative exposures to food additives using repeated 24-hour dietary records, multiple food composition databases, ad hoc laboratory assays, and dynamic tracking of industrial food reformulations. Findings were robust across sensitivity analyses.

However, several limitations exist. The observational design cannot establish causality, and unmeasured or residual confounding may persist despite extensive adjustments for confounding variables. Measurement errors in emulsifier exposure are possible, particularly for products exempt from labeling or naturally occurring emulsifiers like lecithin, which lack comprehensive databases. The absence of specific biomarkers for emulsifier exposure further complicates validation efforts. Some emulsifiers had insufficient intake levels for individual analysis, and intakes reported were lower than those estimated by the European Food Safety Authority (EFSA) but aligned with US data from the CPS-3 Diet Assessment Substudy.

The generalizability of findings is limited by the demographic characteristics of the cohort, which included a higher proportion of women and health-conscious individuals. Potential biases in HR estimates, selection processes, and competing event assumptions must also be acknowledged.

The study identified associations between food additive emulsifiers and increased type 2 diabetes risk, providing the first epidemiological evidence on this topic. These findings underscore the need for additional long-term observational studies, short-term interventions, and preclinical research to strengthen the evidence. If confirmed, the results could lead to regulatory re-evaluations of emulsifier use in industrial food for improved consumer protection.

15. Meat Consumption and Incident Type 2 Diabetes: An Individual-participant Federated Meta-analysis of 1.97 Million Adults with 100,000 Incident Cases from 31 Cohorts in 20 Countries

Ref: Li C, Bishop TRP, Imamura F, Sharp SJ, Pearce M, Brage S, et al. Meat consumption and incident type 2 diabetes: an individual-participant federated meta-analysis of 1.97 million adults with 100,000 incident cases from 31 cohorts in 20 countries. Lancet Diabetes Endocrinol. 2024;12(9):619-30.

ABSTRACT

Context: Consuming meat may make type 2 diabetes more likely. The majority of the evidence, however, comes from research on populations in North America and Europe, with varying methods of study and a stronger emphasis on red meat than poultry. Using data from global cohorts and standardized analytical techniques, we sought to examine the relationships between type 2 diabetes and the consumption of unprocessed red meat, processed meat, and poultry.

Techniques: 31 cohorts that took part in the InterConnect project provided data for this individual-participant federated meta-analysis. There were 12 cohorts from the Americas, and there were also 2 from the Eastern Mediterranean, 9 from Europe, 1 from South-East Asia, and 7 from the Western Pacific.

Each cohort provided access to individual-participant data; participants were excluded if they had a diagnosis of any type of diabetes at baseline or if there were missing data, and they were eligible for inclusion if they were 18 years of age or older and had available data on dietary consumption and incident type 2 diabetes. Using a random-effects meta-analysis and meta-regression to look into possible causes of heterogeneity, cohort-specific hazard ratios (HRs) and 95% confidence intervals (CIs) were calculated for each type of meat, adjusted for potential confounders [such as body mass index (BMI)], and aggregated.

Results: Over a median follow-up of 10 (IQR 7–15) years, 107,271 incident cases of type 2 diabetes were found among the 1,966,444 people who were eligible to participate. For unprocessed red meat, the median daily consumption was 0–110 g; for processed meat, it was 0–49 g; and for poultry, it was 0–72 g. With HRs of 1.10 (95% CI 1.06–1.15) per 100 g/day of unprocessed red meat ($I^2 = 61\%$), 1.15 (1.11–1.20) per 50 g/day of processed meat ($I^2 = 59\%$), and 1.08 (1.02–1.14) per 100 g/day of poultry ($I^2 = 68\%$), higher consumption of all three types of meat was linked to an increased incidence of type 2 diabetes.

In North America, Europe, and the Western Pacific, there were positive correlations between eating meat and type 2 diabetes; in other regions, the CIs were large. There was no proof that age, sex, or BMI could account for the heterogeneity. Under different modeling assumptions, the results for poultry consumption were less compelling. A decreased incidence of type 2 diabetes was linked to substituting unprocessed red meat or fowl for processed meat.

Interpretation: Across all populations, eating meat—especially processed and unprocessed red meat—raises the risk of type 2 diabetes. These results should guide dietary recommendations and emphasize the significance of lowering meat consumption for the general public's health.

CRITICAL APPRAISAL

Previous research has suggested a link between meat consumption and an increased risk of type 2 diabetes. However, this evidence has been largely based on studies from European and North American populations, with inconsistent methodologies and a primary focus on red meat. There is limited and conflicting evidence regarding the association of poultry consumption with diabetes risk. Moreover, the generalizability of these findings to diverse populations worldwide remains unclear. This highlights the need for large-scale studies with harmonized analytical approaches to investigate the associations of different types of meat (unprocessed red meat, processed meat, and poultry) with type 2 diabetes across diverse populations.

This study was an individual-participant federated meta-analysis involving data from 31 cohorts participating in the InterConnect project. These cohorts represented diverse populations from 20 countries across the Americas, Europe, the Western Pacific, the Eastern Mediterranean, and South-East Asia. The study included 1,966,444 adults aged 18 years or older with available data on dietary consumption and incident type 2 diabetes. Participants with prevalent diabetes at baseline or missing data were excluded.

Dietary information was collected using various methods, including food frequency questionnaires, dietary history, and dietary records. The primary exposures were consumption levels of unprocessed red meat (e.g., beef, pork, and lamb), processed meat (e.g., bacon, ham, and sausage), and poultry (e.g., chicken and turkey). The primary outcome was incident type 2 diabetes, defined as a confirmed diagnosis through registry linkage, medication use, or self-report verified by additional sources.

Cohort-specific hazard ratios (HRs) and 95% confidence intervals (CIs) were estimated for each meat type, adjusted for potential confounders [including body mass index (BMI)], and pooled using a random-effects meta-analysis. Meta-regression was used to investigate potential sources of heterogeneity.

Key findings included:
- *Increased diabetes risk with all meat types*: Higher consumption of each meat type was associated with an increased incidence of type 2 diabetes. The HRs per 100 g/day increment were 1.10 (95% CI 1.06–1.15) for unprocessed red meat, 1.15 (1.11–1.20) for processed meat, and 1.08 (1.02–1.14) for poultry.
- *Regional differences*: Associations for unprocessed red and processed meat were significant in the Americas, Europe, and the Western Pacific, but not in the Eastern Mediterranean or South Asia. Poultry consumption was significantly associated with type 2 diabetes only in Europe. CIs were wider in other regions, suggesting less certainty in those associations.
- *No explanation for heterogeneity by age, sex, or BMI*: Meta-regression did not find evidence that these factors explained the heterogeneity in the associations.
- *Weaker association for poultry*: The association between poultry consumption and diabetes was weaker and more heterogeneous than that for red meat.
- *Benefit of replacing processed meat*: Replacing processed meat with unprocessed red meat or poultry was associated with a lower incidence of type 2 diabetes.

This federated meta-analysis included data from 1,966,444 individuals across 31 cohorts in the InterConnect project, 18 of which had not previously published findings on this topic. Cohorts included women-only, men-only, and mixed-gender populations, with participants' median ages ranging from under 40 to over 60 years. Meat consumption varied widely across cohorts.

Over a median follow-up of 10 years, 107,271 cases of type 2 diabetes were recorded. Higher consumption of unprocessed red meat, processed meat, and poultry was positively associated with an increased risk of type 2 diabetes.

This study provides robust evidence from a large and diverse global population that consumption of all types of meat, particularly processed meat and unprocessed red meat, is associated with an increased risk of type 2 diabetes. This reinforces the importance of reducing meat consumption, especially processed meat, for diabetes prevention. The study also highlights the need for further investigation into the association between poultry consumption and diabetes risk.

This study is the largest meta-analysis to date, examining individual-level data from diverse populations. The study's strengths include harmonizing data and analysis methods across cohorts, reducing heterogeneity, but some degree of variation persists due to study design differences, meat intake assessment, and regional differences in cooking methods. However, the findings' generalizability to regions such as Africa and the Middle East remains uncertain, where type 2 diabetes prevalence is particularly high. Further research in these regions is needed to understand the specific effects of meat consumption on diabetes risk, considering regional dietary patterns and cooking methods.

Despite attempts to harmonize variables, the study faced limitations, such as inconsistencies in dietary consumption data and diabetes outcomes across cohorts, which could have contributed to heterogeneity. Additionally, baseline-only dietary data might have led to an underestimation of the association between meat consumption and type 2 diabetes, as shown by previous studies that corrected for measurement error. The observational design also raises the possibility of residual confounding due to unaccounted factors, such as the influence of cooking methods or sociocultural factors.

There is a research gap in regions such as Africa, the Middle East, and South Asia, emphasizing the need for future studies in these areas. Overall, the findings suggest that higher meat consumption, particularly unprocessed red and processed meats, is associated with a higher incidence of type 2 diabetes globally. However, further research is needed to better understand the role of poultry consumption. The study also highlights the need to explore sustainable dietary patterns to reduce meat consumption and its impact on public health, other diseases, and environmental health.

Section 3: COMORBIDITIES

Section Editor: Pritam Biswas

1. Comparative Effectiveness of Aspirin Dosing in Cardiovascular Disease and Diabetes Mellitus: A Subgroup Analysis of the ADAPTABLE Trial

Ref: Narcisse DI, Kim H, Wruck LM, Stebbins AL, Muñoz D, Kripalani S, et al. Comparative effectiveness of aspirin dosing in cardiovascular disease and diabetes mellitus: A subgroup analysis of the ADAPTABLE trial. Diabetes Care. 2024;47(1):81-8.

ABSTRACT

Objective: To reduce the risk of further adverse cardiovascular events, patients with diabetes mellitus (DM) and associated atherosclerotic cardiovascular disease (ASCVD) need to be taking as much dose of aspirin as is recommended by their doctor.

Research design and methods: Patients with stable, chronic ASCVDs were randomized to either 81 mg or 325 mg of aspirin daily as part of the open-label, pragmatic ADAPTABLE trial. The primary effectiveness outcome, a composite of all-cause death, hospitalization for myocardial infarction or stroke, and the primary safety outcome of hospitalization for serious bleeding were evaluated in order to determine the impact of aspirin dosage. For the primary effectiveness and safety outcome, we compared aspirin dosage in patients with and without DM using Cox proportional hazards models in this predetermined analysis.

Results: Out of 15,076 patients, 5,676 (39%) had DM; 2,820 (49.7%) of these patients were prescribed 81 mg of aspirin, and 2,856 (50.3%) were prescribed 325 mg. The composite cardiovascular outcome (9.6% vs. 5.9%; $p < 0.001$) and bleeding events (0.78% vs. 0.50%; $p < 0.001$) were more common in patients with DM than in those without. There was no change in the primary effectiveness result [9.3% vs. 10.0%; hazard ratio (HR) 0.98 (95% CI 0.83–1.16); $p = 0.265$] or safety outcome [0.87% vs. 0.69%; subdistribution HR 1.25 (95% CI 0.72–2.16); $p = 0.772$] between individuals with DM who took 81 mg and 325 mg of aspirin.

Conclusion: This study demonstrates that people with DM are at a higher risk regardless of their aspirin dosage. According to our research, even in a more susceptible group, a higher aspirin dosage has no additional therapeutic benefits.

CRITICAL APPRAISALS

Based on evidence from prior clinical evidences, the efficacy of aspirin is proven beneficial for secondary prevention in patients with established atherosclerotic cardiovascular disease (ASCVD). However, it is not clear what the optimal long-term aspirin dose is for secondary prevention. Recent European guidelines gave recommendation for daily low-dose (81 mg) aspirin, whereas, the American College of Cardiology/American Heart Association (ACC/AHA) guidelines have not taken a definitive stance on dosing strategies (81 vs. 325 mg), they suggested lowest possible daily aspirin dose in patients with diabetes mellitus (DM) and ASCVD to minimize adverse effects, particularly gastrointestinal (GI) bleeding. This subgroup analysis of ADAPTABLE trial adds after adjustment for baseline characteristics, patients with DM and established ASCVD would have clear benefits of giving aspirin irrespective of its dosage with comparable safety outcomes. ADAPTABLE participants with DM had higher rates of adverse cardiovascular outcomes regardless of aspirin dosing compared with patients without DM which corroborates to previous reports.

Major limitations were, this trial primarily included patients with stable patients, which may limit the applicability of the results to other populations, such as those with acute conditions or different comorbidities. The primary focus was on cardiovascular events and bleeding complications, which may not capture all relevant outcomes, such as quality of life or other health impacts. While adaptive designs can improve efficiency, they also introduce complexities in trial management and analysis, which can lead to potential biases if not properly controlled.

Major strength of this study was, it included a significant number of participants, which enhances the statistical power and reliability of the findings; being a randomized controlled trial (RCT), it reduces bias and allows for more reliable comparisons between the different aspirin dosing regimens. However, the intensity of antithrombotic therapy in terms of number of drugs, doses, frequency, and duration remains unclear. Data regarding adjustment for DM medications (particularly insulin), variability in control, or in duration of the disease were not analyzed as the part of study, which would have provide further understanding of therapeutic efficacy and safety limits.

---

2. A Methodological Framework for Meta-analysis and Clinical Interpretation of Subgroup Data: The Case of Major Adverse Cardiovascular Events With GLP-1 Receptor Agonists and SGLT-2 Inhibitors in Type 2 Diabetes

Ref: Karagiannis T, Tsapas A, Bekiari E, Toulis KA, Nauck MA. A Methodological framework for meta-analysis and clinical interpretation of subgroup data: The case of major adverse cardiovascular events with GLP-1 receptor agonists and SGLT2 inhibitors in type 2 diabetes. Diabetes Care. 2024;47(2):184-92.

ABSTRACT

We offer a methodological framework for doing and analyzing meta-analyses of subgroups. Evaluation of clinical heterogeneity in relation to subpopulation definition, subgroup meta-analysis credibility assessment, and conversion of relative into absolute treatment effects were among the methodological procedures. We used subgroup data for patients with established cardiovascular disease (CVD) and those at high cardiovascular risk without obvious CVD from type 2 diabetes cardiovascular outcomes trials (CVOTs) using sodium-glucose cotransporter-2 (SGLT-2) inhibitors and glucagon-like peptide 1 (GLP-1) receptor agonists.

Using the incidence of major adverse cardiovascular events (MACEs) in the placebo arm as a stand-in for baseline cardiovascular risk, we first assessed the variation in subpopulation definitions across CVOTs. We performed subgroup meta-analyses of hazard ratios (HRs) for MACE and evaluated the validity of a potential effect modification because baseline risk did not vary significantly between CVOTs. The findings indicated that the two subgroups should be treated with the same overall relative effect (HR 0.85; 95% CI 0.80–0.90, for GLP-1 receptor agonists, and HR 0.91; 95% CI 0.85–0.97, for SGLT-2 inhibitors). Lastly, we determined the 5-year absolute treatment effects, or the number of patients who experienced an event per 1,000.

In the subgroup of individuals with known cardiovascular illness, GLP-1 receptor agonist treatment led to 30 fewer events, while in patients without obvious CVD, the number of events decreased by 14. 18 and 8 fewer patients experienced an incident per 1,000 patients, respectively, as a result of SGLT-2 inhibitors. Subgroup meta-analyses can use this approach independent of the modification variables or results.

CRITICAL APPRAISALS

Glucagon-like peptide 1 receptor agonists and sodium–glucose cotransporter-2 (SGLT-2) inhibitors are recommended for patients with type 2 diabetes at increased risk for cardiovascular complications. These recommendations are based on the findings of placebo-controlled cardiovascular outcomes trials (CVOTs). Some of these studies exclusively recruited patients with established cardiovascular disease (CVD), while most CVOTs also included participants at high cardiovascular risk (with CV risk factors only or subclinical CVD). Study parameters among different CVOT trials had minor variations, seen in ELIXA, LEADER, SUSTAIN-6, and PIONEER-6 trials, like age cut-off, primary composite outcomes, hypertension, albuminuria, dyslipidemia, and current tobacco use. High cardiovascular risk definition also shown to be varied across the eight CVOT trials. Here, they present a practical 4-stepped framework for performing and interpreting subgroup meta-analyses of relative effects (HR), credibility assessment (ICEMAN analysis), and 5-year absolute effects compared to placebo, in the context of CVOTs with GLP-1 receptor agonists and SGLT-2 inhibitors. Main implication in this analysis is absolute benefits for major adverse cardiovascular events (MACEs) were approximately twofold higher in patients with established CVD compared with those with indicators of high cardiovascular risk only. Strength of this analysis, they evaluated the definition and baseline risk separately for each subpopulation of interest and used outcome data from post hoc reports of trials that used more consistent definitions for cardiovascular risk; emphasized the importance of reporting both relative and absolute treatment effects. Limitations were also addressed here, as there was a constant annual risk over the duration of 5-year frame, which was considered acceptable, and may not accurately reflect the dynamic nature of CVD and its risk factors, which is expected to change over time in a real-world setting. It is also important to emphasize that ICEMAN was designed for evaluation of claims of potential subgroup effects and not for making claims of the absence of a subgroup effect. In fact, the developers of ICEMAN specifically report that its use is not warranted when the $P_{interaction}$ value is ≥ 0.1, especially seen this effect in case of SGLT-2i. They aptly said that "absence of evidence is not evidence of absence", and in the context of subgroup analyses it means that a nonsignificant $P_{interaction}$ (≥ 0.1) should not be interpreted as conclusive evidence of absence of a subgroup effect. Therefore, in the subgroup meta-analysis for SGLT-2i should be interpreted as currently available data from CVOTs do not provide sufficient evidence to support the presence of an effect modification between the two subpopulations rather than suggesting that there is evidence of the absence of a subgroup effect. Meta-analysis for GLP-1 receptor agonists resulted in a significant $P_{interaction}$, which facilitates to conduct further credibility assessment using ICEMAN, which suggested that there is likely no effect-modification. It is essential to recognize that the interpretation remains ambiguous even after the use of ICEMAN. This uncertainty is intrinsic to all subgroup studies, as they are fundamentally observational, even when performed within a meta-analysis of randomized controlled trials. Subgroup meta-analyses, like to subgroup analyses of individual randomized controlled trials, function as hypothesis-generating instruments rather than hypothesis-testing mechanisms, providing insights into the existence of a possible subgroup effect rather than confirming causality between a modifying variable and a treatment effect.

3. Effect of Semaglutide on Regression and Progression of Glycemia in People with Overweight or Obesity but without Diabetes in the SELECT Trial

Ref: Kahn SE, Deanfield JE, Jeppesen OK, Emerson SS, Boesgaard TW, Colhoun HM, et al. Effect of Semaglutide on Regression and Progression of Glycemia in People With Overweight or Obesity but Without Diabetes in the SELECT Trial. Diabetes Care. 2024;47(8):1350-9.

ABSTRACT

Objective: To find out if semaglutide decreases the rise of blood sugar in individuals with cardiovascular disease who are overweight or obese but do not have diabetes.

Research design and methods: Participants in a multicenter, double-blind study who were 45 years of age, had a body mass index (BMI) of 27 kg/m^2, had cardiovascular disease but no diabetes [glycated hemoglobin (HbA1c) <6.5%], and were randomly assigned to receive subcutaneous semaglutide (2.4 mg weekly) or a placebo. HbA1c and the percentages reaching biochemical normoglycemia (HbA1c < 5.7%) and developing biochemical diabetes (HbA1c ≥ 6.5%) were the main glycemic outcomes.

Results: 8,803 of the 17,604 participants received semaglutide, whereas 8,801 received a placebo. The follow-up period was 176 ± 40 weeks, and the mean ± SD exposure to the intervention was 152 ± 56 weeks. Participants' mean nadir HbA1c was 20 weeks for both treatment arms. Following this, HbA1c rose in both arms in a comparable manner, with a mean difference of 20.32 percentage points [95% CI 20.33–20.30; 23.49 mmol/mol (23.66–23.32)], preferring semaglutide for the course of the research ($p < 0.0001$). Semaglutide caused an 8.9% decrease in body weight, which plateaued after 65 weeks. By week 156, a smaller percentage developed biochemical diabetes (1.5% vs. 6.9%; $p < 0.0001$) and a larger percentage were normoglycemic (69.5% vs. 35.8%; $p < 0.0001$).

In order to avoid developing diabetes, 18.5 was the figure that needed to be treated. Glycemia at baseline influenced both regression and progression, with the extent of weight loss playing a significant role in mediating 27.1% of regression and 24.5% of progression.

Conclusion: Long-term semaglutide enhances regression to biochemical normoglycemia and decreases advancement in individuals with preexisting cardiovascular disease who are overweight or obese but do not have diabetes.

CRITICAL APPRAISALS

Development of diabetes risk has been studied using approaches that included lifestyle, medications, and bariatric procedures. The glucose-lowering agents, such as insulin sensitizers: thiazolidinediones and metformin; insulin secretagogues; endogenous insulin replacement therapy; and weight loss medication orlistat and angiotensin receptor blocker: valsartan, were being evaluated. These "prevention studies," outcome, has ranged in reductions of progression of diabetes onset and/or progression from 72% with thiazolidinediones to 58% with intensive lifestyle intervention, 37% with orlistat, 31% with metformin, 20% with insulin glargine, and 14% with valsartan. Nateglinide was associated with a slightly increased risk of progression to diabetes. Weight loss therapy significantly improves insulin sensitivity and represents an attractive approach for "beta-cell rest". Such an effect could be beneficial if maintained long-term. Furthermore, with weight loss in combination with an approach to enhance only the required amount of prandial insulin release, it should be possible to slow the progression of dysglycemia. Such a benefit has been suggested for glucagon-like peptide 1 receptor agonists (GLP-1 RA) agents, in some of their post-study analyses, of liraglutide for weight reduction in pre-diabetes patients and of semaglutide in its weight reduction studies. It has also been implied from a nonrandomized study of bariatric surgery. Here in the SELECT trial, 3P-MACE was reduced by 20%. In this study, the research questions were expanded on the previously reported secondary end points of glycemic status at 52 and 104 weeks by evaluating glycemia through 156 weeks to ask the patterns of glycemia; effects on glucose metabolism to normalize glycemia in people with prediabetes, and progression of prediabetes to diabetes, and how does this relate to body size at baseline as well as in the follow-up. Body weight reduction became plateaued at 65 weeks and was 8.9% lower with semaglutide arm compared to placebo. At week 156, a greater proportion (69.5%) were remained normoglycemic, in semaglutide arm, only 1.5% had biochemical diabetes. The number needed to treat was 18.5, that was quite high. Adverse effects were the major limitations of long-term semaglutide administration. Large number of samples, follow-up for a longer duration, controlled trial, lesser drop-outs were the strength of this study. Despite variability in responses to semaglutide regarding both regression and progression, its advantageous effects were associated with baseline glycemia and the extent of weight reduction. This indicates that while the influence of semaglutide on islet function is crucial, its perceived impact on insulin sensitivity, mediated by weight loss, is also significant.

4. Semaglutide and Cardiovascular Outcomes by Baseline HbA1c and Change in HbA1c in People with Overweight or Obesity but without Diabetes in SELECT

Ref: Lingvay I, Deanfield J, Kahn SE, Weeke PE, Toplak H, Scirica BM, et al; SELECT Trial Investigators. Semaglutide and Cardiovascular Outcomes by Baseline HbA1c and Change in HbA1c in People With Overweight or Obesity but Without Diabetes in SELECT. Diabetes Care. 2024;47(8):1360-9.

ABSTRACT

Objective: In a predetermined analysis of Semaglutide Effects on Cardiovascular Outcomes in People with Overweight or Obesity (SELECT), the cardiovascular effects of semaglutide are assessed by baseline glycated hemoglobin (HbA1c) and changes in HbA1c.

Design and methods of research: Individuals with atherosclerotic cardiovascular disease without diabetes who were overweight or obese were randomly assigned to receive semaglutide 2.4 mg or a placebo once a week in the SELECT study. Semaglutide was 20% less likely than a placebo to cause cardiovascular mortality, nonfatal myocardial infarction, or stroke, the main endpoint of first major adverse cardiovascular events (MACE).

All-cause mortality by baseline HbA1c subgroup and categories of HbA1c change (<20.3, 20.3–0.3, and >0.3 percentage points) from baseline to 20 weeks using the intention-to-treat principle with Cox proportional hazards were included in the analysis of outcomes, along with first MACE, its individual components, expanded MACE (cardiovascular mortality, nonfatal myocardial infarction or stroke; coronary revascularization; or hospitalization for unstable angina), and a heart failure composite (heart failure hospitalization or urgent medical visit or cardiovascular mortality).

Results: The baseline HbA1c was < 5.7% for 33.5%, 5.7% to <6.0% for 34.6%, and 6.0% to <6.5% for 31.9% of 17,604 participants (mean age 61.6 years, 72.3% male). For all end goals, with the exception of all-cause mortality, the cardiovascular risk reduction with semaglutide compared to placebo was consistent with the whole study and did not differ across baseline HbA1c groups. Additionally, cardiovascular outcomes were consistent among HbA1c change subgroups.

Conclusion: Regardless of baseline or altered HbA1c, semaglutide decreased cardiovascular events in individuals with overweight or obesity and established atherosclerotic cardiovascular disease but not diabetes. People with pre-existing atherosclerotic cardiovascular disease who are normoglycemic at baseline and/or who do not have improvements in their HbA1c are therefore anticipated to benefit cardiovascularly from semaglutide.

CRITICAL APPRAISALS

Elevated glucose levels independently facilitate the onset of coronary artery disease, peripheral arterial disease, stroke, and heart failure. Interventions that mitigate the progression to diabetes (such as lifestyle modifications, metformin, thiazolidinediones, and various glucose-lowering and nonglucose-lowering medications) have demonstrated improvements in cardiovascular risk factors; however, none of these studies indicated a reduction in cardiovascular events among individuals with prediabetes. The cardiovascular advantages of these medicines arise from pleiotropic actions. The SELECT study demonstrated that, among persons with overweight or obesity and pre-existing cardiovascular illness, but without a diabetes history and irrespective of baseline glycated hemoglobin (HbA1c) levels, semaglutide [a glucagon-like peptide 1 receptor agonist (GLP-1 RA)] decreased the risk of a major adverse cardiovascular event (MACE) by 20%. There was two-thirds of the population had prediabetes with the other one-third being normoglycemic. An expanded MACE version which includes cardiovascular mortality, nonfatal myocardial infarction, or stroke; coronary revascularization; or hospitalization for unstable angina, along with a heart failure composite (heart failure hospitalization or urgent medical visit or cardiovascular mortality), coronary revascularization, and all-cause mortality were assessed compositely. Here, the cardiovascular benefits of semaglutide were consistent across baseline HbA1c subgroups and across change in HbA1c subgroups. Those who were normoglycemic, its effect is not impacted by changes in HbA1c, strongly suggests that semaglutide's nonglucose-lowering effects mediate these kind of benefits. In addition, they also analyzed well-recognized benefits of semaglutide as GLP-1 RA class effects for traditional cardiovascular risk factors including body fat distribution, blood pressure, low-density lipoprotein (LDL) and high-density lipoprotein (HDL) cholesterol, and triglycerides along with a near 40% reduction in C-reactive protein. Renal function, hepatic steatosis, microvascular and coronary flow, and plaque stability, had not been measured, was one of the limitations. Another limitation of the study was these findings apply only to individuals with established cardiovascular disease and overweight or obesity who did not have a history of diabetes, and cannot be extrapolated to those with overweight or obesity but who do not have established cardiovascular disease. These studies have limited study power and necessitate cautious interpretation. Individuals with more significant metabolic abnormalities at baseline and those with normoglycemia at baseline may have been sourced from distinct clinics. Considering the substantial sample size of the study, the extensive variety of participating sites, the significant number of locations, and the site-level randomization, it is improbable that any selection bias would have influenced the results.

5. Metabolomic Fingerprints of Medical Therapy versus Bariatric Surgery in Patients with Obesity and Type 2 Diabetes: The STAMPEDE Trial

Ref: Axelrod CL, Hari A, Dantas WS, Kashyap SR, Schauer PR, Kirwan JP. Metabolomic Fingerprints of Medical Therapy Versus Bariatric Surgery in Patients With Obesity and Type 2 Diabetes: The STAMPEDE Trial. Diabetes Care. 2024;47(11):2024-32.

ABSTRACT

Objective: Sleeve gastrectomy (SG) and Roux-en-Y gastric bypass (RYGB) are successful treatments for type 2 diabetes (T2D). The underlying metabolic changes that mediate improvements in glucose homeostasis are still mostly unknown, though. Finding metabolic markers linked to the biochemical resolution of T2D following medical treatment (MT) or bariatric surgery was the aim of this investigation.

Research design and methods: Ultra performance liquid chromatography with tandem mass spectrometry was used to retrospectively perform untargeted metabolomic analysis on plasma samples from 90 patients (age 49.9 ± 7.6 years; 57.7% female) who were randomly assigned to MT ($n = 30$), RYGB ($n = 30$), or SG ($n = 30$) at baseline and 24 months of treatment. Supervised machine learning was used to determine phenotypic significance. A linear mixed effects model was used to evaluate correlations between changes in glucose homeostasis and circulating metabolites.

Results: Following SG and RYGB, the circulating metabolome underwent a significant transformation, and following MT, the signatures mainly overlapped. As a result of reduced medication use, SG and RYGB significantly increased the levels of metabolites linked to lipid and amino acid signaling while reducing xenobiotic metabolites. According to random forest analysis, 2-hydroxydecanoate is the most distinctive characteristic between MT, SG, and RYGB and has a selective importance for RYGB. Accordingly, after RYGB but not SG or MT, changes in 2-hydroxydecanoate were associated with decreases in fasting glucose.

Conclusion: The longer-term responses to MT, RYGB, and SG were characterized by a new metabolomic fingerprint. Significantly, the metabolomic profiles of the SG and RYGB procedures differed, suggesting that different effects on metabolism could result in comparable weight loss.

CRITICAL APPRAISAL

Metabolic surgery is now broadly recognized as the gold standard for treating moderate to severe obesity and type 2 diabetes (T2D). Nonetheless, significant contention persists on whether the metabolic and glycemic advantages are chiefly attributable to the surgical procedure or the resultant weight loss, essentially questioning whether they stem solely from "weight-dependent" alterations or if there are supplementary effects involved. Extensive clinical trials with prospective randomization have demonstrated that the metabolic advantages conferred by bariatric surgery are both synergistic with and potentially independent of weight reduction. However, if surgical processes differ from lifestyle and/or medicinal therapies, there exists significant potential to employ combinatorial techniques to improve long-term patient outcomes. Thorough analysis of metabolites, referred to as metabolomics. Bariatric surgery has been recognized as a safe and effective intervention for obesity and associated conditions, including T2D. Nonetheless, the response to surgical treatments aimed at treating T2D is inconsistent, historically ascribed to changes in caloric consumption, physical activity, and/

or modifications in gut hormone responses. Roux-en-Y gastric bypass (RYGB) and sleeve gastrectomy (SG) profoundly altered the circulating metabolome and specifically identified 2-hydroxydecanoate as having selective importance related to improvements in glucose homeostasis after RYGB. All three interventions increased 1,5-anhydroglucitol (AG). Plasma 1,5-AG reflects short-term glucose status, unlike HbA1c, which is a marker of longer-term glycemic control. Increased 1,5-AG with lower glucose also indicates improved insulin sensitivity, because 1,5-AG competes with glucose for reabsorption in the kidney. In the context of this study, the greatest changes were observed with RYGB and SG (6.5-fold), reflective of the vastly greater improvements in fasting glucose and glycated hemoglobin (HbA1c). There were variable changes also noticed among plasma branched-chain amino acids, leucine, isoleucine, and valine after SG and RYGB compared to MT, which signifies differences in insulin sensitivity. Strength of the study was, the samples were taken for this comparative study, collected in randomized pattern, which eliminates some bias along with it had a longer follow-up period and high compliance. Furthermore, this study is one of the first to report the long-term adaptations of the metabolome in a procedure-dependent manner including RYGB and SG. Potential limitations include the lack of an interim metabolomic data set and the differential use of medications that may affect whole-body metabolism. They did not observe associations between 2-hydroxydecanoate and changes in HbA1c indicating that the relationship may be limited to fasting conditions. Future research would be enhanced by integrating short-term metabolomic data with extended phenotypic observations to facilitate the prediction of remission and/or recurrence of T2D.

6. Cardiovascular and Mortality Outcomes with GLP-1 Receptor Agonists versus Other Glucose-lowering Drugs in Individuals with NAFLD and Type 2 Diabetes: A Large Population-based Matched Cohort Study

Ref: Krishnan A, Schneider CV, Hadi Y, Mukherjee D, AlShehri B, Alqahtani SA. Cardiovascular and mortality outcomes with GLP-1 receptor agonists vs other glucose-lowering drugs in individuals with NAFLD and type 2 diabetes: a large population-based matched cohort study. Diabetologia (2024) 67:483-93.

ABSTRACT

Objectives and hypotheses: In contrast to other glucose-lowering medications, we sought to ascertain whether the use of glucagon-like peptide 1 receptor agonists (GLP-1 RA) in people with nonalcoholic fatty liver disease (NAFLD) and type 2 diabetes mellitus lowers the risk of new-onset adverse cardiovascular events (CVEs) and the mortality rate in a real-world population setting.

Techniques: We used TriNetX to do a population-based propensity-matched retrospective cohort analysis. Patients over 20 who received new glucose-lowering medication treatment between January 1, 2013, and December 31, 2021, and were monitored until September 30, 2022, made up the cohort.

1:1 propensity matching with other glucose-lowering medications was used to match new GLP-1 RA users according to their age, demographics, comorbidities, and medication use. The composite incidence of major adverse cardiovascular events (MACE; defined as unstable angina, myocardial infarction, or coronary artery procedures or surgeries) and composite cerebrovascular events (defined as the first occurrence of stroke, transient ischemic attack, cerebral infarction, carotid intervention, or surgery) combined with the new onset of adverse CVEs, such as heart failure, were the primary outcome.

All-cause mortality was the secondary outcome. To estimate hazard ratios (HRs), Cox proportional hazards models were employed.

Results: 2,835,398 participants with type 2 diabetes and NAFLD participated in the study. There was no discernible difference between the GLP-1 RAs group and the sodium-glucose cotransporter-2 (SGLT-2) inhibitors group in terms of cerebrovascular events (HR 0.99; 95% CI 0.94, 1.03), MACE (HR 0.95; 95% CI 0.90, 1.01), or new-onset heart failure (HR 0.97; 95% CI 0.93, 1.01). Additionally, there was no indication of a difference in the death rate between the two groups (HR 1.06; 95% CI 0.97, 1.15). The outcomes of the various sensitivity studies were comparable. The GLP-1-RAs showed a lower rate of adverse CVEs, such as heart failure (HR 0.88; 95% CI 0.85, 0.92), MACE (HR 0.89; 95% CI 0.85, 0.94), cerebrovascular events (HR 0.93; 95% CI 0.89, 0.96), and all-cause mortality rate (HR 0.70; 95% CI 0.66, 0.75), when compared to other second- or third-line glucose-lowering drugs.

Conclusion and interpretation: When compared to metformin or other second- and third-line glucose-lowering drugs, GLP-1 RAs are linked to decreased rates of adverse CVEs and all-cause mortality in people with NAFLD and type 2 diabetes. However, when compared to those using SGLT-2 inhibitors, there was no discernible difference in all-cause mortality or unfavorable CVEs.

CRITICAL APPRAISALS

Research indicates a bidirectional link between nonalcoholic fatty liver disease (NAFLD) and type 2 diabetes, suggesting that NAFLD may precede and/or facilitate the onset of type 2 diabetes. NAFLD is mostly managed by weight reduction and enhancement of insulin sensitivity by lifestyle modifications. The application of glucagon-like peptide 1 receptor agonists (GLP-1 RAs), a category of medications sanctioned for the management of type 2 diabetes, has been investigated in individuals with NAFLD, with pioglitazone. GLP-1 RAs have been shown to have pleiotropic cardiovascular and renal protective benefits in adults with type 2 diabetes, making them a compelling therapeutic alternative for patients with NAFLD. Nonetheless, there are no direct comparisons between GLP-1 RAs and other noninsulin glucose-lowering agents for individuals with NAFLD and type 2 diabetes. The objective is to ascertain whether GLP-1 RAs, in comparison to sodium-glucose cotransporter-2 (SGLT-2) inhibitors, metformin, or other second- or third-line glucose-lowering agents, are linked to a reduced incidence of new-onset adverse cardiovascular events (CVEs) in patients with NAFLD and type 2 diabetes. Research on SGLT-2 inhibitors revealed no indication of a disparity in cardiovascular outcomes and death rates among individuals with type 2 diabetes mellitus and NAFLD. GLP-1 RAs demonstrated a markedly greater decrease in cardiovascular outcomes compared to metformin. The mortality rate was much lower in the GLP-1 RAs group compared to the metformin group. Moreover, GLP-1 RAs demonstrated a much greater decrease in cardiovascular outcomes compared to other second- or third-line glucose-lowering agents. The mortality rate was much lower in the GLP-1 RAs group compared to those receiving second- or third-line medicines. This study included several strengths, including a large population-based sample and multicenter data gathered nationwide from healthcare organizations. Baseline characteristics and possible confounders were adjusted to establish a strong control group. A novel user cohort research design was employed as a comparison, mitigating the risk of unmeasured confounding. They also excluded alcohol-related disorders, alcohol misuse, alcohol dependence, and alcohol-related liver illnesses. This is perhaps the most extensive published study comparing adverse cardiovascular events in individuals with NAFLD and type 2 diabetes, both with and without GLP-1 RA medication. The study has limitations due to its retrospective approach and dependence on an external database. Comorbid conditions were not assessed at baseline, potentially introducing selection bias in the cohorts. Imaging techniques to validate the NAFLD diagnosis were also excluded. Future research should ideally associate NASH and type 2 diabetes independently with the frequency of unfavorable cardiovascular events and death rates.

7. Circulating Metabolomic Markers Linking Diabetic Kidney Disease and Incident Cardiovascular Disease in Type 2 Diabetes: Analyses from the Hong Kong Diabetes Biobank

Ref: Jin Q, Lau ESH, Luk AO, Tam CHT, Ozaki R, Lim CKP, et al; Hong Kong Diabetes Biobank Study Group. Circulating metabolomic markers linking diabetic kidney disease and incident cardiovascular disease in type 2 diabetes: Analyses from the Hong Kong Diabetes Biobank. Diabetologia. 2024;67:837-49.

ABSTRACT

Aim/Hypothesis: This study sought to find predictive biomarkers and characterize the metabolome in diabetic kidney disease (DKD) and its relationship to incident cardiovascular disease (CVD) in type 2 diabetes.

Techniques: Using NMR spectroscopy, baseline sera ($n = 1,991$) from a prospective cohort of people with type 2 diabetes were measured for 170 metabolites with a median follow-up of 5.2 years. After controlling for multiplicity and confounders, linear regression was used to look for associations between each metabolite with either chronic kidney disease [CKD, estimated glomerular filtration rate (eGFR) < 60 mL/min/1.73 m^2] or significantly elevated albuminuria. Cox regressions were used to look at relationships between incident CVD and metabolites associated with DKD (CKD or substantially elevated albuminuria). Two separate cohorts were used to replicate the identification and evaluation of metabolomic biomarkers for CVD prediction.

Results/Findings: False detection rate (FDR) < 0.05 linked 156 metabolites, including apolipoprotein B-containing lipoproteins, high-density lipoprotein (HDL), fatty acids, phenylalanine, tyrosine, albumin, and glycoprotein acetyls, to DKD (151 for CKD and 128 for substantially elevated albuminuria). 75 metabolites were linked to incident CVD at FDR < 0.05 throughout 5.2 years of follow-up. A model with age, sex, and three metabolites (albumin, triglycerides in large HDL, and phospholipids in small LDL) performed similarly to traditional risk factors (C statistic 0.765 vs. 0.762, $p = 0.893$). Including the three metabolites also enhanced discrimination and reclassification and improved the prediction of CVD (C statistic from 0.762 to 0.797, $p = 0.014$). The three-metabolite score was verified in separate Dutch and Chinese cohorts.

Conclusion and Interpretation: Modified metabolomic profiles in DKD increase the risk of CVD and are linked to event CVD.

CRITICAL APPRAISALS

Chronic kidney disease (CKD) occurs in around 40% of individuals with type 2 diabetes and is linked to a two- to fourfold elevated risk of cardiovascular disease (CVD) and death. In CKD, triglyceride-rich lipoproteins (TRLs) are elevated due to diminished lipoprotein lipase activity, reduced Apo-CII levels, and increased Apo-CIII activity. Lipoprotein fluxes traverse the endothelium and get sequestered in the subendothelial region of the artery wall, accompanied by activated macrophages, hence beginning and exacerbating atherosclerosis. CKD alters the structure and content of high-density lipoprotein. The metabolomic signature of diabetic kidney disease (DKD) was studied in relation to its correlation with incident CVD in individuals with type 2 diabetes. Metabolomic biomarkers were identified from metabolites. The results underwent external validation. Significant disparities in triglyceride-rich lipoproteins (TRLs), along with reduced estimated glomerular filtration rate (eGFR), were seen in individuals with diabetes compared to those without, indicating a possible association of TRLs with residual CVD risk in individuals with DKD. Among the analyzed TRLs, very-low-density lipoprotein (VLDL) exhibited the most significant connection with the incidence of CVD. Insulin resistance enhances hepatic VLDL synthesis and secretion. Unlike low-density lipoprotein (LDL), which often necessitates oxidative alteration prior to phagocytosis, bigger TRLs can be more readily captured and promptly phagocytized by macrophages, resulting in the formation of foam cells. Furthermore, the breakdown of triglycerides in triglyceride-rich lipoproteins by lipoprotein lipase might release nonesterified fatty acids, hence inciting inflammation and facilitating atherosclerosis. In our prospective research, high-density lipoprotein (LDL) exhibited an adverse relationship with CVD, with the link being confined to medium and small HDL particles. Sphingomyelins were linked to DKD, although none were correlated with the onset of CVD. The study's strength lies in its extensive cross-sectional analysis of metabolites associated with DKD, identifying many metabolites connected to DKD. A robust metabolomics infrastructure was in place, with rigorous quality control and reliable outcomes across sensitivity analyses. The group had a modest predominance of men over women. The effects of ongoing lipid-lowering treatment were not taken into account. The finding analysis exclusively comprised Chinese individuals. The urinary albumin-to-creatinine ratio (uACR) was derived from a singular measurement to address intraindividual variability. Fasting samples were analyzed, along with dietary consumption and physical activity that may influence the metabolome. Metabolomic biomarkers had equivalent predictive value to conventional risk variables and enhanced CVD risk categorization beyond previous prediction models. Additional research on the pathophysiology and predictive capabilities of metabolites is necessary.

8. Effect of Sodium-glucose Cotransporter-2 Inhibitors on Myocardial Infarction Incidence: A Systematic Review and Meta-analysis of Randomized Controlled Trials and Cohort Studies

Ref: Huang X, Dannya E, Liu X, Yu Y, Tian P, Li Z. Effect of sodium-glucose cotransporter-2 inhibitors on myocardial infarction incidence: A systematic review and meta-analysis of randomized controlled trials and cohort studies. Diabetes Obes Metab. 2024;26(3):1040-9.

ABSTRACT

Goal: To determine if people with or without type 2 diabetes experience fewer myocardial infarctions (MI) when taking sodium-glucose cotransporter-2 (SGLT-2) inhibitors.

Methods: Up until May 7, 2022, searches were conducted using PubMed, Embase, Web of Science, the Cochrane Library, and https://ClinicalTrials.gov. Included were cohort studies and randomized controlled trials (RCTs) that examined how SGLT-2 inhibitor therapy affected the incidence of MI. For the incidence of MI, relative risks (RRs) were extracted and aggregated with a 95% CI. To investigate the heterogeneity, meta-regression and subgroup analysis were used.

Results: Data from six SGLT-2 inhibitors and 3,394,423 people were included in this meta-analysis, which also comprised 54 RCTs and 32 cohort studies. Overall, SGLT-2 inhibitors significantly decreased the incidence of MI in cohort studies (RR 0.89; 95% CI 0.83–0.94) and RCTs (RR 0.9; 95% CI 0.84–0.96). Subgroup analysis results in RCTs showed no significant differences in outcomes according to sources of outcome extraction, cardiovascular disease (CVD) status, control drug types, and different types of SGLT-2 inhibitors ($P_{interaction} > 0.05$). In cohort trials, SGLT-2 inhibitors had comparable benefits on lowering the risk of MI in the presence or absence of CVD ($P_{interaction} = 0.179$).

However, in cohort studies, differences in outcomes were noted according to the kind of control group ($P_{interaction} = 0.036$). The results of meta-regression showed no correlation between the incidence of MI, follow-up duration, or baseline cardiovascular risk variables.

Conclusion: SGLT-2 inhibitors decreased the incidence of MI in both RCTs and cohort studies. Patients with and without a history of CVD were found to benefit from SGLT-2 inhibitors' cardioprotective effects.

CRITICAL APPRAISALS

The most critical and life-threatening form of ischemic heart disease is myocardial infarction (MI). Sodium-glucose cotransporter-2 (SGLT-2) inhibitors, a category of innovative antihyperglycemic agents often employed in the management of type 2 diabetes mellitus (T2DM), have garnered significant attention in several cardiovascular outcomes trials (CVOTs) in recent years. These trials have demonstrated that SGLT-2 inhibitors can enhance cardiorenal outcomes in patients with atherosclerotic cardiovascular disease (CVD), heart failure, and chronic kidney disease, irrespective of T2DM status. Given that MI is the predominant cause of heart failure, the capacity of SGLT-2 inhibitors to enhance outcomes in MI is plausible. The EMBODY and EMMY studies shown advantages in acute MI. This systematic review and meta-analysis aim to thoroughly examine the association between SGLT-2 inhibitors and the incidence of MI. The research employed a stringent search approach, precise criteria, and an evaluation of methodological quality, synthesizing data from both randomized controlled trials (RCTs) and cohort studies. Reduction in MI incidence by 10% in RCTs and 11% in cohort studies, respectively. The outcome indicates that the kind of SGLT-2 inhibitors did not alter the impact. The results differed according on the type of control group included in cohort studies. Empirical investigations have also demonstrated no significant disparity in the incidence of MI among T2DM patients treated with glucagon-like peptide 1 (GLP-1) receptor agonists compared to SGLT-2 inhibitors. The impact of SGLT-2 inhibitors on MI incidence was independent of the patient's CVD state. The strength of the study lies in its knowledge of the impact of SGLT-2 inhibitors on the incidence of MI. The inclusion of both RCTs and cohort studies in the study enabled a thorough evaluation of the treatment impact in controlled and cohort environments, while also employing subgroup analysis and the function of $p_{interaction}$. The study's limitations include significant variability in patient numbers between studies, coupled with disparities in patient selection, sample size, and follow-up time, which contribute to the heterogeneity of the results. Consequently, The cardioprotective benefits were seen in individuals regardless of their CVD history.

9. Prediction of New-onset Heart Failure in Patients with Type 2 Diabetes Derived from ALTITUDE and CANVAS

Ref: Said F, Arnott C, Voors AA, Heerspink HJL, Ter Maaten JM. Prediction of new-onset heart failure in patients with type 2 diabetes derived from ALTITUDE and CANVAS. Diabetes Obes Metab. 2024;26(7):2741-51.

ABSTRACT

Objective: The objective is to develop and evaluate a prediction model that will identify individuals with type 2 diabetes (T2D), including those receiving treatment with sodium-glucose cotransporter-2 (SGLT-2) inhibitors, who are at high risk of developing new-onset heart failure (HF).

Methods: The Aliskiren Trial in Type 2 Diabetes Using Cardiorenal Endpoints (ALTITUDE), which involved T2D patients with cardiovascular disease or albuminuria, was used to create a prediction model. 5,081 patients without a history of HF who had baseline measurements of N-terminal prohormone of brain natriuretic peptide (NT-proBNP) were included. The model was created using Cox regression and externally validated in patients receiving canagliflozin treatment as well as in the placebo arm of the Canagliflozin Cardiovascular Assessment Study (CANVAS), which comprised 996 participants with T2D who had established cardiovascular disease or high cardiovascular risk.

Findings: The median serum NT-proBNP level for ALTITUDE participants (mean age 64 ± 9.8 years) was 157 (25th–75th percentile 70–359) pg/mL. In both cohorts, higher body mass index (BMI), troponin T (TnT) level, and NT-proBNP level were found to be significant and independent predictors of new-onset HF. Glycated hemoglobin, age, hematocrit, urine albumin-to-creatinine ratio, and calcium channel blocker use were also included in the model. The C-statistic for a prediction model that included these variables was 0.800 (95% CI 0.720–0.880) in CANVAS and 0.828 (95% CI 0.801–0.855) in ALTITUDE. Following a year of canagliflozin treatment, the C-statistic for this model rose to 0.847 (95% CI 0.792–0.902) in patients.

Conclusion: Higher NT-proBNP, TnT, and BMI levels in T2D patients—including those using SGLT-2 inhibitors—are independent, externally verified predictors of new-onset HF. This recently created model could help detect and potentially prevent new-onset HF by identifying people who are at high risk.

CRITICAL APPRAISALS

Individuals with type 2 diabetes (T2D) had a 1.66 to almost fourfold elevated risk of developing heart failure (HF) relative to those without T2D, with a population-attributable risk of 7% in older demographics and 14% in younger demographics. Prompt identification and potential mitigation through lifestyle modifications or pharmacological intervention at the preclinical phase may alleviate this burden, alongside the timely administration of specific approved medications, such as sodium–glucose cotransporter 2 (SGLT-2) inhibitors and the nonsteroidal mineralocorticoid receptor antagonist finerenone, in patients with chronic kidney disease to avert HF. Numerous prediction models for new-onset HF have been created, although their use as a screening tool for the general population remains unestablished. This study identifies markers predictive of new-onset HF in a high-risk cardiovascular population, including individuals treated with an SGLT-2 inhibitor, to develop an accurate and clinically applicable prediction model for new-onset HF using routinely measured variables, and offers a web-based risk prediction engine to enhance clinical application of the model. The WATCH-DM model for HF has been adjusted in the ALTITUDE and CANVAS parameters, resulting in improved C-statistics following the incorporation of NT-proBNP and cTnT levels. This model score is relevant for a substantial and clearly defined group at elevated risk of cardiovascular disease with T2D. It was verified both internally and externally in a well-phenotyped, independent sample of individuals with T2D at elevated risk for cardiovascular disease. Alternative scores (TRS-HF, DM-CURE score) that emphasize these biomarkers exhibit either inferior C-statistics or are complex to calculate. The study's strengths lie in its description of a model utilizing factors that are readily accessible in clinical practice. The methodology is comprehensive, without variable preselection, incorporates both internal and external evaluation, and demonstrates exceptional discriminative accuracy. Moreover, the data utilized for model construction is of exceptional quality, as all endpoints were rigorously adjudicated. Furthermore, only hospitalization for HF was utilized as an outcome, excluding the diagnosis of HF in an outpatient clinic setting. It also generates predictive capability following 1 year of canagliflozin, an SGLT-2 inhibitor, usage. The HF guidelines now endorse the utilization of this medication class for high-risk patients. These markers may be inaccessible in certain primary care environments and might be expensive. Regrettably, data on the classification of HF[HF with decreased ejection fraction (HFrEF) versus HF with maintained ejection fraction (HFpEF)] were absent. Nonetheless, elevated BMI correlates more significantly with the development of HFpEF than with HFrEF. It may restrict its application in the younger demographic. A biomarker-guided prospective research involving HF-naïve patients with diabetes and renal failure is essential to evaluate the model's accuracy and facilitate early treatment management.

10. Impact of Glycaemic Status on the Cardiac Effects of Empagliflozin when Initiated Immediately after Myocardial Infarction: A Post-hoc Analysis of the EMMY Trial

Ref: Sourij C, Oulhaj A, Aziz F, Tripolt NJ, Aberer F, Pferschy PN, et al. Impact of glycaemic status on the cardiac effects of empagliflozin when initiated immediately after myocardial infarction: A post-hoc analysis of the EMMY trial. Diabetes Obes Metab. 2024;26(5):1971-5.

ABSTRACT

The EMPA-REG outcome trial demonstrated that empagliflozin, a sodium-glucose cotransporter-2 inhibitor (SGLT-2i), not only substantially decreased major adverse cardiovascular events but also lowered the risk of 3P-major adverse cardiovascular events (MACE) compared to placebo in individuals with type 2 diabetes (T2D). Similar cardiovascular benefits were observed in the EMPEROR trials for patients with chronic heart failure, regardless of their ejection fraction or glycemic status. Additionally, the empagliflozin in acute myocardial infarction (EMMY) trial revealed positive effects of empagliflozin on N-terminal prohormone of brain natriuretic peptide (NT-proBNP) levels and cardiac function and structure when administered immediately following an acute myocardial infarction (AMI).

CRITICAL APPRAISALS

Cardiovascular outcome studies and heart failure outcome trials utilizing Empagliflozin therapies (EMPA-REG, EMPEROR) demonstrated substantial enhancements in both primary and secondary composite outcomes. This posthoc study of the EMMY trial seeks to determine if the reported advantageous cardiac effects are contingent upon the individuals' initial glycemic condition. In the EMMY study, 48.5% of patients hospitalized after acute myocardial infarction (AMI) have decreased glucose metabolism. Glycated hemoglobin (HbA1c) values were 5.4% (IQR 5.3–5.5%) in the normoglycemic group, 5.9% (IQR 5.7–.0%) in the prediabetic group, and 6.8% (6.4–8.3%) in the type 2 diabetes group; NT-proBNP levels and left ventricular ejection fraction showed no significant differences among the three groups. The effect of empagliflozin on the alterations in NT-proBNP levels from baseline to week 26 was not influenced by baseline glycemic state ($P_{interaction} > 0.05$). The left ventricular ejection fraction had a significant interaction effect ($P_{interaction} = 0.032$) when contrasting prediabetes with normoglycemia, indicating a diminished impact in those with prediabetes. No such relationship is detected in individuals with T2D compared to those with normoglycemia. The study's strengths include its multicenter design, randomized (1:1 ratio), double-blind, and placebo-controlled methodology, focusing on heart failure biomarkers and cardiac function metrics, with medication administration commencing promptly (within 72 hours) post-AMI. The EMMY study was not a cardiovascular outcome trial and utilized the heart failure surrogate marker NT-proBNP as the primary end measure. It limits the applicability among younger generations. The cardiovascular outcome study of empagliflozin in individuals with AMI is now under progress (NCT04509674). A further drawback of the research is the absence of oral glucose tolerance testing; thus, the incidence of individuals with prediabetes or diabetes, as shown by postchallenge hyperglycemia, may be considerably greater than reported.

11. Impact of Empagliflozin on Insulin Needs in Patients with Heart Failure and Diabetes: An EMPEROR-Pooled Analysis

Ref: Talha KM, Green J, Filippatos G, Pocock S, Zannad F, Brueckmann M, et al. Impact of empagliflozin on insulin needs in patients with heart failure and diabetes: An EMPEROR-Pooled analysis. Diabetes Obes Metab. 2024;26(7):2578-87.

ABSTRACT

Objective: To evaluate the impact of empagliflozin on patients with diabetes and concomitant heart failure (HF), whether or not they have baseline insulin, and to investigate how empagliflozin affects insulin needs over time.

Materials and procedures: Pooled patient-level data from two cardiovascular outcomes trials of empagliflozin in HF (EMPEROR-Reduced and EMPEROR-Preserved trials) were subjected to a post-hoc analysis. We conducted a subgroup analysis that included all diabetic individuals and were stratified by baseline insulin use. The major composite endpoint of initial hospitalization for HF or cardiovascular death, the rate at which the estimated glomerular filtration rate declined, the composite renal outcome, and the rates of sustained insulin start were among the outcomes that were examined.

Findings: 1,333 (658 in empagliflozin and 675 in placebo) of the 4,794 diabetic individuals were using insulin at baseline. Both the treatment effect of empagliflozin on the rate of decline of the estimated glomerular filtration rate ($P_{interaction} = 0.75$) and the hazard ratio on the primary endpoint were consistent regardless of insulin use [no insulin, hazard ratio 0.74, 95% CI 0.63–0.86; using insulin, hazard ratio 0.81, 95% CI 0.66–1.00, $P_{interaction} = 0.49$]. Empagliflozin had no influence on the composite renal outcome for individuals who were on insulin or not ($P_{interaction} = 0.30$). Empagliflozin-randomized patients who did not use insulin at baseline started taking it less frequently during the follow-up period than placebo-treated patients (2.6% vs. 3.8%, odds ratio 0.66, 95% CI 0.50–0.88).

Conclusion: Regardless of baseline insulin use, empagliflozin consistently improves cardiovascular outcomes and the decrease of renal function. It also lessens the requirement for prolonged insulin introduction in patients with diabetes and HF.

CRITICAL APPRAISALS

The prevalence of type 2 diabetes (T2D) in patients with heart failure (HF) ranges from 30 to 50%, and it is associated with a mortality increase of up to 50% compared to individuals without diabetes. Individuals with T2D have a two- to fourfold increased prevalence of HF, and around 30% of patients with HF and diabetes are treated with insulin. The EMPEROR-Reduced and EMPEROR-Preserved trials demonstrated that empagliflozin, a sodium-glucose cotransporter-2 inhibitor (SGLT-2i), significantly diminished the risk of a composite primary outcome of cardiovascular death or hospitalization for HF, regardless of diabetes status or baseline glycated hemoglobin levels. The EMPA-REG Outcome study shown that empagliflozin medication significantly postponed the commencement of insulin therapy and decreased daily insulin requirements in individuals with diabetes at elevated cardiovascular risk. Both the DAPA-HF and DELIVER trials demonstrated a reduction in the commencement of new insulin therapy and avoided increases in existing insulin dosages; however, the studies did not assess the influence of baseline usage on the therapeutic efficacy of dapagliflozin. In the TOPCAT study, diabetic patients with HF with preserved ejection fraction (HFpEF) receiving aldosterone plus insulin had an elevated risk of congestive symptoms, increased natriuretic peptide levels, reduced quality of life, and a twofold risk of hospitalizations for HF and cardiovascular mortality. This study analyzes pooled individual patient-level data from the EMPEROR-Reduced and EMPEROR-Preserved trials to assess the effect of baseline insulin usage on outcomes in diabetic patients with HF and to evaluate its influence on the treatment efficacy of empagliflozin. The administration of empagliflozin in HF resulted in a notable 34% relative risk decrease in the initial sustained introduction of insulin for diabetes treatment, in comparison to placebo, among patients with prediabetes or diabetes who were not on insulin at baseline. Empagliflozin did not have a meaningful impact on the composite renal endpoint overall, and there was no notable difference in treatment effect between individuals taking insulin and those not using insulin ($P_{interaction}$ = 0.31). The present research indicated that empagliflozin markedly lowered the rate of eGFR decline overall, with effects comparable in individuals utilizing insulin and those not utilizing insulin. No significant difference in adverse events (genital infection, ketoacidosis) was seen between the empagliflozin and placebo groups, regardless of baseline insulin usage. The study's limitations stem from its exploratory patient-level analysis of the EMPEROR Preserved and EMPEROR-Reduced trials; hence, the findings are regarded as hypothesis-generating. Furthermore, the diabetic patients participating in this experiment may not accurately reflect the broader diabetic community, as the study exclusively involved individuals with diabetes and HF. These data substantiate the metabolic, cardiovascular, and renal advantages of empagliflozin in patients with HF and impaired glucose metabolism.

12. Diabetes and Risk of Heart Failure in People with and without Cardiovascular Disease: Systematic Review and Meta-analysis

Ref: Panchal K, Lawson C, Chandramouli C, Lam C, Khunti K, Zaccardi F. Diabetes and risk of heart failure in people with and without cardiovascular disease: systematic review and meta-analysis. Diabetes Res Clin Pract. 2024;207:111054.

ABSTRACT

Background: Compared to people without diabetes, people with diabetes are more likely to develop heart failure (HF). But no thorough systematic review or meta-analysis has looked into how these associations might vary depending on the prevalence of cardiovascular disease (CVD).

Goals: To calculate the risk of incident HF in those with and without diabetes in relation to those without diabetes.

Methods: Web of Science, PubMed, and Scopus were searched for observational cohort studies starting on March 22, 2023. Using a random-effects model, the pooled relative risk (RR) was determined.

Findings: Out of 11,609 publications, 31 and 6 research, respectively, reported data on individuals with type 2 diabetes (T2D) and type 1 diabetes (T1D). Regardless of the prevalence of CVD, those with T2D had a higher risk of HF 1.61 (95% CI 1.35–1.92) in people with CVD, 1.78 (1.60–1.99) in people without CVD, and 2.02 (1.75–2.33) in people with an unknown CVD prevalence. When comparing HF risk in T2D persons with and without CVD, meta-regression failed to find a significant difference ($p = 0.232$).

Conclusion: Regardless of the frequency of CVD, those with T2D had a similar elevated risk of HF as people without diabetes. Both people with and without CVD should emphasize strategies that have been shown to reduce the risk of heart attacks in those with T2D.

CRITICAL APPRAISALS

Individuals with diabetes have an elevated risk of heart failure (HF), characterized by a robust bidirectional association, which therefore heightens their likelihood of hospitalizations and fatality. A prior meta-analysis from 2018 indicated that those with diabetes possess a heightened risk of HF compared to those without diabetes; however, the study aggregated data from varied study designs, resulting in significant bias. A 2020 meta-analysis, utilizing just data from observational cohort studies, indicated that those with diabetes possess a heightened risk of new-onset HF compared to those without diabetes; however, it failed to account for at least age and sex, potentially resulting in biased outcomes. The extent to which the link between diabetes and incident HF varies between groups with and without widespread cardiovascular disease remains unclear. The results demonstrate that, regardless of cardiovascular disease (CVD) incidence, those with type 2 diabetes (T2D) had a heightened risk of developing incident HF compared to those without diabetes. This underscores the necessity of implementing efficient HF prevention and treatment measures for individuals with T2D, irrespective of any prior cardiovascular incident. Subsequent research ought to corroborate these findings utilizing individual-level data from both trials and extensive observational cohorts to get more precise estimates. The study's strength lies in its substantial sample size, encompassing numerous studies and participants, HF events, and a follow-up duration spanning from 6 months to 22.5 years. It excluded studies where "diabetes" was not the primary exposure of interest to mitigate risk and included studies with at least minimal adjustments for age and sex. They also conduct a meta-analysis of research encompassing both 2D and type 1 diabetes (T1D), albeit with a smaller sample size for T1D. Limitations encompass the significant heterogeneity among studies and the potential for publication bias; the meta-regression findings must be interpreted with caution regarding the risk of ecological fallacy; furthermore, the subgroup analysis based on CVD prevalence was constrained by inadequate reporting of baseline characteristics and/or stratification of HF, including distinctions such as hospital versus community settings, duration of diabetes, fasting glucose levels, and HF phenotype (with and without ejection fraction), which were inconsistently reported. Proven measures to reduce HF risk should be used in individuals with T2D, regardless of their cardiovascular disease history, to optimally mitigate HF risk.

13. Semaglutide in Patients with Obesity-related Heart Failure and Type 2 Diabetes

Ref: Kosiborod MN, Petrie MC, Borlaug BA, Butler J, Davies MJ, Hovingh GK, et al. Semaglutide in Patients with Obesity-Related Heart Failure and Type 2 Diabetes. N Engl J Med. 2024;390(15):1394-407.

ABSTRACT

Background: Patients with heart failure with intact ejection fraction are more likely to be obese and have type 2 diabetes, which is associated with a high burden of symptoms. In people with type 2 diabetes, there are currently no licensed treatments that particularly address obesity-related heart failure with intact ejection fraction.

Methods: Patients with heart failure with maintained ejection fraction, a body mass index of 30 or more (weight in kilograms divided by the square of height in meters), and type 2 diabetes were randomized to receive either 2.4 mg of semaglutide once a week or a placebo for 52 weeks.

The change in body weight and the clinical summary score (KCCQ-CSS) of the Kansas City Cardiomyopathy Questionnaire (which has a score range of 0–100, with higher scores indicating less symptoms and physical limitations) were the main end goals. The change in six-minute walk distance, a hierarchical composite end goal that comprised mortality, heart failure events, and variations in the change in the KCCQ-CSS and six-minute walk distance, as well as the change in the C-reactive protein (CRP) level, were all examples of confirmatory secondary endpoints.

Results: 616 participants in all were randomly assigned. The average change in body weight was −9.8% with semaglutide and −3.4% with placebo (estimated difference, −6.4 percentage points; 95% CI −7.6 to −5.2; $p < 0.001$), and the average change in the KCCQ-CSS was 13.7 points with semaglutide and 6.4 points with placebo (estimated difference, 7.3 points; 95% CI 4.1–10.4; $p < 0.001$). Semaglutide was found to be superior to placebo in the confirmatory secondary endpoints [estimated between-group difference in change in six-minute walk distance, 14.3 m (95% CI 3.7–24.9; $p = 0.008$); win ratio for hierarchical composite endpoint, 1.58 (95% CI 1.29–1.94; $p < 0.001$); and estimated treatment ratio for change in CRP level, 0.67 (95% CI 0.55–0.80; $p < 0.001$)]. 55 participants (17.7%) in the semaglutide group and 88 participants (28.8%) in the placebo group experienced serious side events.

Conclusion: Semaglutide resulted in more weight loss than a placebo at 1 year and larger improvements in heart failure-related symptoms and physical limitations among individuals with obesity-related heart failure who had maintained ejection fraction and type 2 diabetes. Novo Nordisk provided funding for this study; the STEP-HFpEF DM ClinicalTrials.gov identifier is NCT04916470.

CRITICAL APPRAISALS

Excess adiposity significantly contributes to the onset and advancement of heart failure with intact ejection fraction and type 2 diabetes, which is also linked to worse functional capacity compared to individuals without type 2 diabetes. Semaglutide, a glucagon-like peptide 1 (GLP-1) receptor agonist, is administered weekly at a dosage of 2.4 mg and has demonstrated considerable weight loss in individuals with overweight or obesity, along with beneficial impacts on cardiometabolic risk factors and a marked decrease in the probability of major adverse cardiovascular events in high-risk patients. In patients with heart failure with preserved ejection fraction and obesity, but without type 2 diabetes, treatment with semaglutide resulted in more significant reductions in heart failure-related symptoms and physical limitations, enhanced weight loss, and superior improvements in exercise function compared to placebo. In type 2 diabetes, outcomes may vary for several reasons—the extent of weight loss in antiobesity pharmacotherapy trials is consistently less in patients with type 2 diabetes; these patients are more frequently prescribed sodium-glucose cotransporter-2 (SGLT-2) inhibitors, which have become the standard treatment for heart failure with preserved ejection fraction; and they typically present with a more advanced phenotype. All these factors may influence the efficacy of therapy with semaglutide. The efficacy and safety of a once-weekly dosage of 2.4 mg semaglutide in this patient population is being evaluated. The semaglutide group had more significant decreases in heart failure-related symptoms and physical limits, as well as higher weight loss, compared to the placebo group after 52 weeks. Semaglutide also enhanced the six-minute walk distance, yielded more successes in the assessment of the hierarchical composite endpoint, and decreased CRP levels more significantly than placebo. The results of the STEP-HFpEF DM trial augment the previously reported findings of the STEP-HFpEF trial in multiple aspects, notably by extending the comprehensive clinical advantages and safety profiles of semaglutide to individuals with heart failure with preserved ejection fraction and type 2 diabetes. Heart failure manifested despite a weight reduction with semaglutide that was approximately 40% less than that observed in non-diabetic patients in the STEP-HFpEF trial, indicating that the mechanisms underlying the benefits of semaglutide may transcend mere weight loss. This trial demonstrates the reliability of semaglutide's impact on heart failure-related outcomes in patients administered SGLT-2 inhibitors. No increase in diabetic retinopathy incidents was observed with semaglutide, addressing a potential issue associated with GLP-1 receptor agonists in type 2 diabetes. Limitations of the study, they did not assess ethnic variations which limits generalizability, were not designed to evaluate events such as hospitalizations and urgent visits for heart failure, the duration of follow-up was limited to 1 year. Despite good outcomes and a signal for a potential reduction in clinical events, which requires further confirmation in heart failure outcome trials in future.

14. Effects of Empagliflozin on Progression of Chronic Kidney Disease: A Prespecified Secondary Analysis from the EMPA-KIDNEY Trial

Ref: The EMPA-KIDNEY Collaborative Group. Effects of empagliflozin on progression of chronic kidney disease: a prespecified secondary analysis from the EMPA-KIDNEY trial. Lancet Diabetes Endocrinol. 2024;12:39-50.

ABSTRACT

Context: In a variety of patients, sodium-glucose cotransporter-2 (SGLT-2) inhibitors lower the risk of cardiovascular morbidity and death as well as the progression of chronic renal disease. However, because few clinical kidney outcomes occurred among these patients in the completed trials, it is unknown how they affect the course of kidney disease in some patients with chronic kidney disease. Specifically, several guidelines stratify their recommendations for the appropriate use of SGLT-2 inhibitors according to albuminuria and diabetes status. Our goal was to evaluate the impact of empagliflozin on the course of chronic kidney disease in general and among particular participant types in the EMPA-KIDNEY study.

Techniques: Individuals aged 18 years or older with an estimated glomerular filtration rate (eGFR) of 20 to <45 mL/min/1.73 m^2, or with an eGFR of 45 to <90 mL/min/1.73 m^2 and a urinary albumin-to-creatinine ratio (uACR) of 200 mg/g or higher, were included in the randomized, controlled, phase 3 trial known as EMPA-KIDNEY, which was carried out at 241 centers across eight countries (Canada, China, Germany, Italy, Japan, Malaysia, the UK, and the USA). We investigated how 10 mg of oral empagliflozin taken once day compared to a placebo affected the primary outcome of the annualized rate of change in eGFR slope.

We looked at the acute slope (from randomization to 2 months) and chronic slope (beyond 2 months) independently. We estimated the latter using shared parameter models. Intention-to-treat analyses were performed on all randomly allocated subjects. The registration number for EMPA-KIDNEY is NCT03594110 on ClinicalTrials.gov.

Results: 6,609 participants were randomly allocated and followed up for a median of 2.0 years (IQR 1.5–2.4) between May 15, 2019, and April 16, 2021. 2,282 (34.5%) with an eGFR of <30 mL/min/1.73 m^2, 2,928 (44.3%) with an eGFR of 30 to <45 mL/min/1.73 m^2, and 1,399 (21.2%) with an eGFR of 45 mL/min per 1.73 m^2 or more were among the predefined subgroups of eGFR. 1,328 (20.1%) had an uACR of <30 mg/g, 1,864 (28.2%) had an uACR of 30–300 mg/g, and 3,417 (51.7%) had an uACR of >300 mg/g. These were the predetermined groupings of uACR. Overall, eGFR decreased by 2.12 mL/min/1.73 m^2 (95% CI 1.83–2.41) when allocated to empagliflozin, which is equivalent to a 6% (5–6) decrease in the first 2 months.

The chronic slope was then cut in half, from −2.75 to −1.37 mL/min/1.73 m^2 year (half difference, 95% CI 42–58). Diabetes status and baseline values of eGFR and uACR had a substantial impact on the absolute and relative advantages of empagliflozin on the amplitude of the chronic slope. Specifically, patients with lower baseline uACR had a smaller absolute difference in chronic slopes; however, because they progressed more slowly than those with higher uACR, this resulted in a larger relative difference in chronic slopes [86% (36–136) reduction in the chronic slope among those with baseline uACR < 30 mg/g compared with a 29% (19–38) reduction for those with baseline uACR ≥ 2,000 mg/g; P$_{trend}$ < 0.0001].

Interpretation: In the EMPA-KIDNEY experiment, empagliflozin reduced the rate of chronic kidney disease development in all participant types, including those with low albuminuria. It is not appropriate to use albuminuria alone to decide whether to use an SGLT-2 inhibitor.

CRITICAL APPRAISALS

Clinical trials in chronic kidney disease populations have conventionally employed dichotomous composite outcomes that merge kidney failure (a rare event) with a proportional decline in kidney function [assessed by changes in estimated glomerular filtration rate (eGFR)] from baseline, exceeding a specified threshold, typically 40–57%. Analyses derived from these outcomes exhibit diminished statistical sensitivity in assessing treatment effects among patient cohorts with a reduced risk of kidney failure, particularly those with relatively preserved renal function; however, they ultimately represent the predominant segment of the general population afflicted by kidney failure. Consequently, there is a keen interest in analyzing the annualized rate of deterioration of renal function (eGFR slope). The EMPA-KIDNEY study analyzed the effects of empagliflozin compared to placebo on eGFR slope, involving a diverse cohort of patients with chronic kidney disease at risk of advancement, including those with minor albuminuria, low eGFR, and both diabetic and nondiabetic patients.

The decrease in albuminuria may be the principal measurable factor contributing to the improvements noted in EMPA-KIDNEY, accounting for one-fifth of the impact on chronic slopes and two-fifths of the effect on the key composite outcome of kidney disease progression. Empagliflozin induced a little immediate reduction in eGFR, followed by a significant deceleration in the long-term advancement of chronic kidney disease. The long-term benefits differed according on diabetes status, eGFR, and most notably urinary albumin-to-creatinine ratio (uACR), along with associated features including the projected probability of renal failure. The trial was terminated prematurely due to evident advantages observed in high-risk patients; however, the analyses indicate that lower-risk patients, particularly those with reduced albuminuria levels—many of whom would likely experience kidney failure in their lifetime—could also gain from the preservation of kidney function, alongside established cardiovascular and mortality benefits. The widespread use of sodium-glucose cotransporter-2 (SGLT-2) inhibitors might significantly influence the public health consequences of chronic renal disease. The study's limitations encompass a limited number of participants with type 1 diabetes, exclusion of individuals with autosomal dominant polycystic kidney disease or kidney transplants, and the intentional omission of patients at low risk for chronic kidney disease progression (specifically, those with an eGFR of ≥45 mL/min/1.73 m² and uACR <200 mg/g). However, it illustrated that the relative benefit on the chronic slope was inversely related to the predicted risk of kidney failure. An further 2 years of off-treatment follow-up is in progress to evaluate the long-term effects of an average of 2 years of therapy.

15. Efficacy and Safety of Once-weekly Semaglutide 2.4 mg versus Placebo in People with Obesity and Prediabetes (STEP 10): A Randomised, Double-blind, Placebo-controlled, Multicentre Phase 3 Trial

Ref: McGowan BM, Bruun JM, Capehorn M, Pedersen SD, Pietiläinen KH, Muniraju HAK, et al; STEP 10 Study Group. Efficacy and safety of once-weekly semaglutide 2.4 mg versus placebo in people with obesity and prediabetes (STEP 10): A randomised, double-blind, placebo-controlled, multicentre phase 3 trial. Lancet Diabetes Endocrinol. 2024;12(9):631-42.

ABSTRACT

Context: The effects of semaglutide 2.4 mg in clinical studies on people with obesity and prediabetes are currently poorly understood. Our goal was to evaluate the safety and effectiveness of semaglutide 2.4 mg for glycemic control and weight management in individuals with prediabetes and obesity.

Techniques: In STEP 10, participants aged 18 years or older with a body mass index (BMI) of 30 kg/m² or higher and prediabetes according to UK National Institute for Health and Care Excellence criteria [defined as having at least one of the following at screening: HbA1c of 6.0–6.4% (42–47 mmol/mol) or fasting plasma glucose (FPG) of 5.5–6.9 mmol/L] were randomized, double-blind, parallel-group, phase 3 trials conducted across 30 trial sites in Canada, Denmark, Finland, Spain, and the UK.

After 52 weeks of diet and exercise counseling, participants were randomized (2:1) to receive subcutaneous semaglutide 2.4 mg once a week or a placebo. There was a 28-week break from treatment after that. Bodyweight change as a percentage and the percentage of patients who returned to normoglycemia [glycated hemoglobin (HbA1c) < 6.0% (<42 mmol/mol) and FPG < 5.5 mmol/L] at week 52 were the main outcomes. All randomly assigned participants were evaluated by intention to treat. For participants who received at least one dose of the study medication, specific safety information was gathered.

Results: 138 participants were randomly assigned to receive 2.4 mg of semaglutide and 69 to receive a placebo between September 16 and December 29, 2021. 183 (88%) were White, 60 (29%) were male, and 147 (71%) were female. Every participant who was assigned at random received at least one dosage of the research medication. HbA1c was 5.9% [0.3; 41.3 mmol/mol (3.0)], FPG was 5.9 mmol/L (0.6), waist circumference was 120.1 cm (14.7), bodyweight was 111.6 kg (22.2), and the baseline mean age was 53 years (SD 11). At week 52, semaglutide 2.4 mg resulted in a substantially higher reduction in bodyweight than placebo [−13.9% (SD 0.7) vs. −2.7% (0.6); estimated treatment difference −11.2% (95% CI −13.0 to −9.4); $p < 0.0001$]. At week 52, semaglutide 2.4 mg caused a higher percentage of patients to revert to normoglycemia than placebo [103 (81%) of 127 vs. 9 [14%] of 64; odds ratio 19.8 (95% CI 8.7–45.2); $p < 0.0001$]. Twelve (9%) participants who received semaglutide 2.4 mg experienced serious adverse events, compared to six (9%) who received a placebo. Compared to one participant in the placebo group, eight (6%) in the semaglutide 2.4 mg group experienced adverse events that resulted in treatment termination. There were no reports of any new safety signals.

Interpretation: In individuals with obesity and prediabetes, semaglutide 2.4 mg produced a greater reduction in body weight and a return to normoglycemia than a placebo. The safety and tolerability profile aligned with the GLP-1 receptor agonist class and other research. According to these results, semaglutide 2.4 mg may be used to help people with obesity and prediabetes return to normal blood sugar levels.

CRITICAL APPRAISALS

Prediabetes (nondiabetic hyperglycemia) is a worldwide health issue, affecting around 6–9% of individuals and linked to a heightened risk of acquiring type 2 diabetes. Prediabetes is linked to obesity-related problems that elevate mortality risk, including significant cardiovascular adverse events; hence, patients with prediabetes gain from weight loss. Participants with obesity in the STEP 1 and STEP 4 studies exhibited comparable outcomes regarding obesity. The STEP 2 study demonstrated that semaglutide 2.4 mg effectively reduces body weight and enhances glycemic management and cardiometabolic risk factors in individuals with type 2 diabetes and obesity. Nonetheless, a degree of weight return and a decline in cardiometabolic and glycemic advantages were noted following the discontinuation of semaglutide 2.4 mg therapy in the STEP 1 extension and STEP 4 trials. The STEP 10 trial investigated the effects of semaglutide 2.4 mg on body weight, glycemic parameters, and cardiovascular risk factors in individuals with prediabetes, as well as the persistence or regression of benefits after discontinuation. Semaglutide 2.4 mg demonstrated a significantly greater reduction in body weight and a return to normoglycemia compared to placebo in participants with obesity and prediabetes. Nonetheless, sustaining weight reduction might be challenging due to metabolic changes that counteract this process. A higher percentage of subjects achieved normoglycemia with semaglutide 2.4 mg compared to placebo. While other STEP studies did not exclusively include people with prediabetes, they did assess some outcomes within subpopulations of individuals with this disease. A reduced percentage of individuals developed type 2 diabetes at week 52 with semaglutide 2.4 mg compared to placebo. This data indicates that semaglutide 2.4 mg may prevent or postpone the development of prediabetes to type 2 diabetes in obese people; however, the trial lacked sufficient power to assess this outcome. The outcomes of the SELECT experiment substantiate this idea. Participants administered semaglutide 2.4 mg exhibited enhancements in cardiometabolic risk variables, such as waist circumference, glycated hemoglobin (HbA1c), fasting plasma glucose, systolic blood pressure, and lipid profiles, in contrast to the placebo group. The study's limitations were a predominance of female participants, a limited sample size, and a majority of white individuals, necessitating the inclusion of a more heterogeneous group. A further drawback is the inability to determine the extent to which the decrease in HbA1c resulted from weight loss versus the previously proven direct glucose-lowering action of semaglutide. The strength of STEP 10 encompasses the off-treatment interval and the elevated rates of treatment compliance and trial completion along with it was randomized, double-blind, placebo-controlled, multicenter. Ultimately, the safety and tolerability profile aligned with other trials, and these results endorse the prospective application of semaglutide 2.4 mg as a therapeutic option for persons with obesity and prediabetes to attain reversion to normoglycemia.

16. Impact of Primary Kidney Disease on the Effects of Empagliflozin in Patients with Chronic Kidney Disease: Secondary Analyses of the EMPA-KIDNEY Trial

Ref: The EMPA-KIDNEY Collaborative Group. Impact of primary kidney disease on the effects of empagliflozin in patients with chronic kidney disease: secondary analyses of the EMPA-KIDNEY trial. Lancet Diabetes Endocrinol. 2024;12:51-60.

ABSTRACT

Context: According to the EMPA-KIDNEY trial, empagliflozin primarily slowed the advancement of kidney disease, hence lowering the risk of the key composite outcome of cardiovascular death or kidney disease progression in individuals with chronic kidney disease. Our goal was to evaluate the potential differences in empagliflozin's effects by primary renal disease in its large population.

Techniques: 241 centers across eight countries (Canada, China, Germany, Italy, Japan, Malaysia, the UK, and the USA) participated in the randomized, controlled, phase 3 experiment known as EMPA-KIDNEY. Individuals who had a urinary albumin-to-creatinine ratio (uACR) of 200 mg/g or above at screening and an estimated glomerular filtration rate (eGFR) of 20 to < 45 mL/min/1.73 m² or 45 to < 90 mL/min/1.73 m² were eligible.

They were given either a matching placebo or 10 mg of oral empagliflozin once daily at random (1:1). eGFR slope studies were performed using shared parameter models, and effects on renal disease progression (defined as a sustained ≥40% eGFR drop from randomization, end-stage kidney disease, a sustained eGFR ≤ 10 mL/min/1.73 m², or death from kidney failure) were evaluated using prespecified Cox models. By adding pertinent interaction terms to the models, subgroup comparisons were carried out. EMPA-KIDNEY's ClinicalTrials.gov registration number is NCT03594110.

Results: 6,609 participants were randomly allocated and followed up for a median of 2.0 years (IQR 1.5–2.4) between May 15, 2019, and April 16, 2021. 2,057 (31.1%) participants had diabetic kidney disease, 1,669 (25.3%) had glomerular disease, 1,445 (21.9%) had hypertension or renovascular disease, and 1,438 (21.8%) had other or unknown reasons. These were predetermined subgroups by primary kidney disease. There was no indication that the relative effect size differed significantly by primary kidney disease ($P_{heterogeneity}$ = 0.62), and kidney disease progression happened in 384 (11.6%) of 3,304 patients in the empagliflozin group and 504 (15.2%) of 3,305 patients in the placebo group [hazard ratio 0.71 (95% CI 0.62–0.81)].

A 50% (42–58) decrease in the rate of chronic eGFR decline was shown by the between-group difference in chronic eGFR slopes (i.e., from 2 months to final follow-up) of 1.37 mL/min/1.73 m^2 per year (95% CI 1.16–1.59). In analyses by several primary kidney illnesses, including by type of glomerular disease and diabetes, the relative effect of empagliflozin on the chronic eGFR slope was comparable (p values for heterogeneity all > 0.1).

Interpretation: Empagliflozin decreased the risk of renal disease advancement in a wide spectrum of patients with chronic kidney disease at risk of progression, including those with a variety of nondiabetic sources of the disease. Sodium-glucose cotransporter-2 (SGLT-2) inhibitors should be a part of the standard of therapy to reduce the risk of renal failure in chronic kidney disease, according to the very similar effect sizes, regardless of the source of primary kidney disease.

CRITICAL APPRAISALS

In chronic kidney disease, many extensive placebo-controlled outcome studies have demonstrated that empagliflozin, dapagliflozin, and canagliflozin diminish the risk of main composite cardiorenal outcomes related to kidney disease progression or cardiovascular mortality. A meta-analysis of these and other extensive sodium-glucose cotransporter-2 (SGLT-2) inhibitor trials demonstrated a 37% reduction in the risk of at least a 50% sustained decline in estimated glomerular filtration rate (eGFR) from randomization, end-stage kidney disease (i.e., initiation of maintenance dialysis or receipt of a kidney transplant), a sustained low eGFR (<15 or <10 mL/min/1.73 m^2), or mortality due to kidney failure. Two studies included in this meta-analysis involved people with nondiabetic primary renal disorders (EMPA-KIDNEY and DAPA-CKD). In these supplementary analyses of the EMPA-KIDNEY trial, which encompassed a substantial cohort of patients with nondiabetic etiologies of chronic kidney disease at risk of advancement, empagliflozin diminished the likelihood of kidney disease progression, exhibiting comparably sized effects across patients with various primary kidney disorders. Analyses of the yearly rate of change of eGFR on a relative scale facilitated a more nuanced investigation into the variability of treatment effects. Such studies indicated that empagliflozin mitigated the reduction in eGFR regardless of these diagnosis. Empagliflozin was predominantly safe and well tolerated among the study cohort. Elevated intraglomerular pressure and subsequent glomerular hyperfiltration are postulated to be prevalent in several types of chronic kidney disease, particularly in cases with reduced nephron count. The data may possibly suggest other common pathways influenced by pathology in the renal tubules. SGLT-2 inhibitors reduce tubular strain and oxygen consumption by diminishing the reabsorption of glucose and salt, hence enhancing oxygen delivery capacity to the renal tubules. This may elucidate the more pronounced impact of SGLT-2 inhibitors on the course of renal disease compared to the relatively mild effects on albuminuria. This method may elucidate the beneficial benefits on acute renal damage noted in meta-analyses. The study's strengths include the design of EMPA-KIDNEY, which ensures broad generalizability of findings, the provision of the largest body of randomized data on SGLT-2 inhibition for patients with chronic kidney disease at risk of progression, and the use of various statistically sensitive methodologies (e.g., eGFR slope analyses) to evaluate treatment effects on a relative scale. This method facilitated more dependable subgroup comparisons. Limitations, the generalizability of the obtained findings is constrained by the exclusion of patients with polycystic kidney disease or those who have had kidney transplantation. While there was a significant cohort of people with immunoglobulin A

(IgA) nephropathy, the numbers for other specific etiologies of glomerular disease were comparatively less, with just 68 participants diagnosed with type 1 diabetes. This restricted capacity to evaluate treatment impacts on the spectrum of outcomes directly in these less well researched patient populations. Altogether, in a diverse cohort of individuals with chronic kidney disease at risk of progression, empagliflozin effectively decreased the risk of renal disease advancement and loss in eGFR, with comparably substantial relative effects across several categories of primary kidney disease.

Section 4: COMPLICATIONS

Section Editor: Abhranil Dhar

1. Mortality in the Glycemia Reduction Approaches in Diabetes: A Comparative Effectiveness Study (GRADE)

Ref: Banerji MA, Buse JB, Younes N, Krause-Steinrauf H, Ghazi A, Lee M, et al.; GRADE Research Group. Mortality in the Glycemia Reduction Approaches in Diabetes: A Comparative Effectiveness Study (GRADE). Diabetes Care. 2024;47(4):589-93.

ABSTRACT

Goal: In the Glycemia Reduction Approaches in Diabetes: A Comparative Effectiveness Study (GRADE), we present mortality results for individuals with type 2 diabetes who were diagnosed within the last 10 years and had no recent history of cancer or cardiovascular events.

Design and methods of research: Major causes of death and overall mortality rates were evaluated throughout a follow-up period of 5 years on average. A central committee tasked with assigning therapy determined the cause of death. We looked for correlations using the 10-year Framingham Risk Score and baseline variables.

A low mortality rate of 0.59 per 100 participant-years was the outcome. Individuals with substantial albuminuria, a history of smoking, hypertension, advanced age, and male gender were more likely to have died during follow-up. Cancer (26.8%) and "cardiovascular cause" (a composite of underlying causes) (38.6%) were the two most prevalent underlying causes of death. By treatment group, there were no differences.

Conclusion: Causes of death varied among individuals with diabetes of very short duration. It is necessary to pay attention to health dangers other than cardiovascular illnesses.

CRITICAL APPRAISAL

What was Known Prior to this Study?

Mortality rate in people with type 2 diabetes is higher compared to general population. All-cause mortality rates among people with type 2 diabetes in US and UK epidemiological studies are 1.52 and 2.8–2.9 deaths per 100 participant-years (PY). It has been shown in previous studies that intensive glucose control reduces the incidence and progression of micro- and macrovascular complications in both type 1 and type 2 diabetes, thereby reducing morbidity and mortality. With the initiation of newer glucose-lowering agents with additional cardiovascular and renal benefits, this risk is further decreasing. But most of these study populations have longer duration of diabetes and with established cardiovascular disease (CVD) or with kidney disease.

What this Study Adds?

- This study assessed the determinants of mortality in people with brief duration of diabetes (<10 years), without recent-onset cardiovascular event in past 1 year and without chronic kidney disease, which is different from previous cardiovascular and kidney outcome trials.
- Effect of glucose-lowering drugs was largely unknown in type 2 diabetes with lower cardiorenal risk.
- It also compared the effectiveness of four groups of glucose-lowering agents: Insulin glargine U-100, sulfonylurea—glimepiride, glucagon-like peptide 1 receptor agonist—liraglutide, and dipeptidyl peptidase-4 inhibitor—sitagliptin, in reducing mortality rates when they are added to metformin.

This comparative effectiveness of different glucose-lowering agents has also not been assessed in previous studies.

This study showed that there were no differences in mortality among all four glucose-lowering agents, although mortality rate was numerically lowest in the liraglutide group.
- This study has found out that 10-year Framingham Risk Score for CVD was the best predictor of cancer and "cardiovascular-cause" mortality.
- The relationship of hemoglobin A1c (HbA1c) with mortality and cardiovascular events is nonlinear and not associated with increased risk of mortality in this GRADE study (Glycemia Reduction Approaches in Diabetes: A Comparative Effectiveness Study).
- Infection, liver disease, respiratory failure, pneumonia, accidents, and suicides are among the other common causes of death apart from cardiovascular and renal cause.

Major Strengths
- GRADE study offers an opportunity to assess the determinants of mortality in a cohort of type 2 diabetes with brief duration.
- No previous study with comparative effectiveness of four glucose-lowering agents

Limitations
- High proportion of unknown cause of death
- Use of personal device technology could have identified more numbers of hypoglycemia and arrhythmia.
- This study was neither designed nor statistically powered for mortality testing, as the expected number of deaths was small.

- HbA1c at baseline (6.8–8.5%) was too narrow to demonstrate a mortality effect of baseline or on-treatment glycemic control.
- Numerically lower all-cause mortality in the liraglutide treatment group was not statistically significant.
- Very few conclusive findings to guide individualization of therapy
- The study population was limited to the US population.

Clinical Implications
- Cause of death was varied among people with relatively shorter duration of diabetes and attention to health risks beyond cardiovascular diseases is necessary, like cancer screening, smoking reduction, infection control, suicide prevention, etc.
- No difference between different glucose-lowering medications in terms of reduction of mortality
- 10-year Framingham Risk Score can be used for prediction of cardiovascular-cause mortality.

Knowledge Gaps and Scope for Future Research

Sodium-glucose cotransporter-2 inhibitors (SGLT-2i) and thiazolidinediones (TZDs) were not included in the study since, at its inception, the first SGLT-2i had not yet been licensed by the FDA. This study was not adequately powered as well to conclude on the lower number of mortality rates of liraglutide. Therefore, a long-term adequately powered study is much needed with the addition of SGLT-2i.

2. Risk of Diabetic Retinopathy and Diabetic Macular Oedema with Sodium-glucose Cotransporter-2 Inhibitors and Glucagon-like Peptide 1 Receptor Agonists in Type 2 Diabetes: A Real-world Data Study from a Global Federated Database

Ref: Eleftheriadou A, Riley D, Zhao SS, Austin P, Hernández G, Lip GYH, et al. Risk of diabetic retinopathy and diabetic macular oedema with sodium–glucose cotransporter 2 inhibitors and glucagon-like peptide 1 receptor agonists in type 2 diabetes: a real-world data study from a global federated database. Diabetologia. 2024;67:1271-82.

ABSTRACT

Objectives and hypotheses: According to some recent research, glucagon-like peptide 1 receptor agonists (GLP-1 RA) and sodium-glucose cotransporter-2 inhibitors (SGLT-2i) may have preventive effects beyond glycemic management in the development of diabetic retinopathy and diabetic macular edema. Our goal was to examine the clinical effects of GLP-1 RA and SGLT-2i treatment on the risk of diabetic macular edema and diabetic retinopathy in people with type 2 diabetes who are on insulin.

Techniques: This study uses a global federated health research network (TriNetX, Cambridge, USA) to retrospectively analyze a cohort of almost two million individuals with type 2 diabetes who are receiving insulin across 97 healthcare organizations. A control cohort (insulin without SGLT-2i/GLP-1 RA, $n = 1,922,312$) was contrasted with two intervention cohorts (SGLT-2i + insulin, $n = 176,409$; GLP-1 RA + insulin, $n = 207,034$). For every outcome, estimated hazard ratios (HRs) were presented using a Kaplan–Meier survival analysis. Age, sex, hypertension, microvascular complications, chronic renal disease, hemoglobin A1c (HbA1c), body mass index (BMI), and the use of pioglitazone, lipid-modifying drugs, antilipemic medicines, angiotensin-converting enzyme (ACE) inhibitors, angiotensin II inhibitors, and metformin were all matched 1:1 using the propensity score. Additionally, a subanalysis was conducted to compare the two intervention cohorts.

Findings: While GLP-1 RA with insulin showed no signal with no statistical relevance to the HR (1.013; 0.960, 1.069), SGLT-2i with insulin was linked to a lower HR [95% confidence interval (CI)] for diabetic macular edema when compared to the control cohort (0.835; 0.780, 0.893). While GLP-1 RA with insulin raised the risk of diabetic retinopathy (1.308; 1.261, 1.357), SGLT-2i with insulin did not increase the chance of developing diabetic retinopathy in a clinically relevant way (1.076; 1.027, 1.127). GLP-1 RA with insulin was linked to an increased risk of diabetic macular edema (1.130; 1.056, 1.208) and diabetic retinopathy (1.205; 1.153, 1.259) in comparison to SGLT-2i with insulin.

Conclusion and interpretations: According to our research, taking insulin and SGLT-2i together may reduce the incidence of diabetic macular edema. However, in people with type 2 diabetes who also take insulin, using GLP-1 RA was linked to an increased incidence of diabetic retinopathy. According to a comparative investigation, SGLT-2i and insulin had positive effects on the development of diabetic retinopathy and diabetic macular edema. To ascertain the causal link with these medicines, randomized controlled trials (RCTs) utilizing specialized retinal imaging are necessary.

CRITICAL APPRAISAL

What was Known Prior to this Study?

Diabetic retinopathy (DR) with macular edema is a well-known microvascular complication of type 2 diabetes, which can lead to blindness. Laser photocoagulation and vascular endothelial growth factor (anti-VEGF) ocular injection are the available treatment options for advanced DR and macular edema, respectively. There is limited data regarding effects of different glucose-lowering agents on development and progression of diabetic retinopathy. Previous studies have shown some benefits with sodium-glucose cotransporter-2 inhibitors (SGLT-2i) and glucagon-like peptide 1 receptor agonists (GLP-1 RA). Possible mechanisms behind this may be the reduction of retinal endothelial cell apoptosis and mitigation of gradual central retinal thinning with SGLT-2i. SGLT-2i also have been demonstrated to reduce the total circulating volume, improve sodium balance, and increase hematocrit, which may improve oxygen delivery to tissues. GLP-1 RA have shown a neuroprotective role in retinal ganglion cells, as well as a reduction in the oxidative stress and vascular remodeling. Previously, one meta-analysis suggested that canagliflozin increased diabetic retinopathy, although this effect was not present for two other SGLT-2i (empagliflozin and dapagliflozin). Post hoc analysis of the EMPA-REG OUTCOME trial showed no increased risk of retinopathy with empagliflozin versus placebo. Lin et al. demonstrated the rate of developing diabetic retinopathy was comparable between SGLT-2i and GLP-1 RA, although individuals receiving SGLT-2i had a lower risk of proliferative diabetic retinopathy. Effects of GLP-1 RA in previous studies were heterogeneous. The SUSTAIN-6 trial demonstrated that the rates of retinopathy complications, including vitreous hemorrhage, blindness were higher with semaglutide. The LEADER trial with liraglutide found a nonsignificant increased incidence of retinopathy compared to placebo. The AngioSafe Type 2 Diabetes Study demonstrated no association between GLP-1 RA and severe diabetic retinopathy.

What this Study Adds?

- This study has shown that SGLT-2i can reduce risk of development of diabetic macular edema, but clinically insignificant increased risk of diabetic retinopathy has also been demonstrated.
- GLP-1 RA have shown no significant effect on macular edema, but there is increased risk of diabetic retinopathy.

Major Strength

This is a real-world study from a global federated database, including around 2 million people with type 2 diabetes receiving insulin treatment.

Limitations

- This is a retrospective study and thus randomization and controlling of the confounding variables was not possible.
- Despite propensity score matching, unmeasured confounding variables may bias our findings.
- In propensity score matching for hemoglobin A1c (HbA1c), body mass index (BMI), and estimated glomerular filtration rate (eGFR), categorical instead of continuous values were opted, resulting in residual confounding.
- Due to lack of individual data, multivariant analysis is not possible. Also, data completeness cannot be assured.
- The sequence of initiating insulin relative to GLP-1 RA or SGLT-2i is not known. Also, the length of treatment with SGLT-2i, GLP-1 RA and/or insulin or adherence to treatment as well as the time of exposure to those medications are not known.
- Probably, the patients were having more advanced type 2 diabetes as they are already on insulin. Therefore, results may not be generalizable to other patient populations.
- Mostly the study population were US-based, limiting its generalizability.

Clinical Implications

This study supported the fact that SGLT-2i can reduce risk of development of diabetic macular edema without any risk of progression of diabetic retinopathy. Also, we need to be cautious regarding the use of GLP-1 RA in advanced retinopathy with or without macular edema.

Knowledge Gaps and Scope of Future Research

There is a clear need to evaluate the impact of SGLT-2i and GLP-1 RA on diabetic eye disease in dedicated prospective studies. Mechanisms for predisposition of GLP-1 RA toward development of diabetic retinopathy is yet to be proven. Possible hypothesis demonstrates it may be due to rapid reduction in HbA1c, which can lead to alterations in VEGF and insulin-like growth factor 1 (IGF-1) resulting in the development or early worsening of diabetic retinopathy. A Phase III clinical trial with semaglutide on diabetic ocular disease is underway. It is also not known whether the association of GLP-1 RA and diabetic retinopathy may be mitigated over time with long term glycemic control.

Randomized controlled trials (RCTs) using dedicated retinal imaging are required to determine the causal relationship with these therapies.

3. Effect of Preceding Drug Therapy on the Renal and Cardiovascular Outcomes of Combined Sodium-glucose Cotransporter-2 Inhibitor and Glucagon-like Peptide-1 Receptor Agonist Treatment in Patients with Type 2 Diabetes and Chronic Kidney Disease

Ref: RECAP study group; Tsukamoto S, Kobayashi K, Toyoda M, Tone A, Kawanami D, Suzuki D, et al. Effect of preceding drug therapy on the renal and cardiovascular outcomes of combined sodium-glucose cotransporter-2 inhibitor and glucagon-like peptide-1 receptor agonist treatment in patients with type 2 diabetes and chronic kidney disease. Diabetes Obes Metab. 2024;26(8):3248-60.

ABSTRACT

Aim: The purpose of this post-hoc subgroup analysis is to determine whether the composite renal outcome was different for patients with type 2 diabetes (T2D) from the RECAP study who were treated with sodium-glucose cotransporter-2 inhibitor (SGLT-2i) and glucagon-like peptide 1 receptor agonist (GLP-1 RA) combination therapy. This analysis will only look at patients with chronic kidney disease (CKD).

Methods: Out of the 643 T2D patients in the RECAP research, we included 438 patients with CKD (GLP-1 RA-first group, $n = 223$; SGLT-2i-first group, $n = 215$). A propensity score (PS)-matched model was used to analyze the incidence of the composite renal outcome, which is defined as a decline in estimated glomerular filtration rate (eGFR) of at least 50% and/or progression to macroalbuminuria. The win ratio was also computed for these composite renal outcomes, which were weighted as follows: (1) A decline in eGFR of ≥50% and progression to macroalbuminuria; (2) a decline in eGFR of ≥50% only; and (3) progression to macroalbuminuria only.

Results: 132 patients from each group were paired using the PS-matched model. The two groups did not vary in the incidence of renal composite outcomes [10% for the GLP-1 RA-first group and 17% for the SGLT-2i-first group; odds ratio 1.80; 95% confidence interval (CI) 0.85–4.26; $p = 0.12$]. Compared to the SGLT-2i-first group, the GLP-1 RA-first group's win ratio was 1.83 (95% CI 1.71–1.95; $p < 0.001$).

Conclusion: The win ratio of the GLP-1 RA-first group compared to the SGLT-2i-first group was considerable, despite the fact that the renal composite result was the same for both groups. These findings imply that adding an SGLT-2i to baseline GLP-1 RA treatment may result in better renal outcomes in GLP-1 RA and SGLT-2i combination therapy.

CRITICAL APPRAISAL

What was Known Prior to this Study?

Sodium-glucose cotransporter-2 inhibitors are well known to have additional renal benefit in type 2 diabetes (T2D) patients. In CREDENCE trial, canagliflozin reduced the risk of a kidney-specific composite events by 34% in T2D with albuminuric chronic kidney disease (CKD). In DAPA-CKD and EMPA-KIDNEY trial also, there is significant reduction of kidney-specific composite events in patients with or without diabetes compared to placebo.

Glucagon-like peptide 1 receptor agonists (GLP-1 RAs) have also been shown to reduce albuminuria as a secondary or exploratory outcomes in CVOT trials. In REWIND study with dulaglutide, renal composite outcome was 15% lower compared to placebo. Recently published FLOW trial is a primary kidney outcome trial, where composite of onset of kidney failure, estimated glomerular filtration rate (eGFR) decline of <50% from baseline, and kidney death were reduced significantly in injectable semaglutide group. In comparison to monotherapy, combination therapy results in greater reductions in hemoglobin A1c (HbA1c), body weight, and systolic blood pressure. Also, it is more effective in reducing cardiovascular and renal events. But, in clinical practice usually these two groups of drugs are not added simultaneously. As per ADA-KDIGO (American Diabetes Association-Kidney Disease: Improving Global Outcomes) consensus, SGLT-2i have to initiated first in addition to metformin irrespective of glycemic status. Thereafter GLP-1 RA can be added if glycemic target is not achieved or, to promote weight loss. It is not known whether premedication with SGLT-2i is preferable or not for patients who require combination therapy.

What this Study Adds?

- This post hoc subgroup study demonstrated the impact of differing preceding therapies on eGFR and albuminuria in T2D patients with CKD treated with combination of SGLT-2i and GLP-1 RAs.
- This study showed that using GLP-1 RA therapy first may provide more renal protection than using a SGLT-2i first.

Major Strength

- It is the first study to examine the renal impact of differences in treatment sequence in patients receiving SGLT-2 inhibitor and GLP-1 RA combination therapy.
- Actual clinical data were available for known background factors, which allows to evaluate treatment effects more practically.

Limitations

- It is a retrospective observational study with post hoc analysis, therefore biases, especially data dredging bias, may not have been fully removed.
- Lipid profile and electrolytes have not been assessed.
- Types and dosages of SGLT-2i and GLP-1 RA were changed during the treatment periods on many patients, which were not adjusted in this study.
- In Japan, only smaller dosages of GLP-1 RAs were approved until May 2019. Therefore, many patients received insufficient dosages of GLP-1 RA, which may have shown benefit with addition of SGLT-2i. Also, addition of insufficient dosage of GLP-1 RA may have resulted in less benefit in the SGLT-2i initiation group.
- Incidence of renal composite outcomes did not differ between the two groups as the study is underpowered.

Clinical Implications

In future, this study will guide us regarding use of combination therapy with SGLT-2i and GLP-1 RA in T2D with CKD as standard of care. In that case, there may be some benefit in using GLP-1 RAs prior to SGLT-2 inhibitors during combination treatment for patients with T2D complicated by CKD.

Knowledge Gaps and Scopes for Future Research

Mechanisms for the positive advantage trend observed in the GLP-1 RA-first have not been well understood. Possibly improving the renal microvascular environment with prior GLP-1 RA administration by its anti-atherosclerotic and anti-inflammatory effects, enhances the effects of SGLT-2i. The statement "GLP-1 RA pretreatment was better" must be applied with caution, as it is equal to the statement "SGLT-2 inhibitors as additional treatment was better". For conclusion, a larger prospective study is needed to examine which contributed more to the final outcome.

---

4. Comparing Clinical Outcomes in Patients with Type 2 Diabetes Mellitus after Ischaemic Stroke: Sodium-glucose Cotransporter-2 Inhibitors Users versus Non-users. A Propensity Score Matching National Cohort Study

Ref: Chen TY, Lee HF, Chan YH, Chuang C, Li PR, Yeh YH, et al. Comparing clinical outcomes in patients with type 2 diabetes mellitus after ischaemic stroke: Sodium–glucose cotransporter 2 inhibitors users versus non-users. A propensity score matching National Cohort Study. Diabetes Obes Metab. 2024 Oct;26(10):4501-4509.

ABSTRACT

Aim: In order to compare clinical outcomes between patients treated with sodium-glucose cotransporter-2 inhibitors (SGLT-2i) and those not receiving SGLT-2i, this nationwide cohort study assessed the effect of SGLT-2i on patients with type 2 diabetes mellitus (T2DM) following ischemic stroke (IS).

Materials and procedures: From May 1, 2016 to December 31, 2019, we used Taiwan's National Health Insurance Research Database to find 707 T2DM patients who received SGLT-2i treatment and 27,514 patients who did not receive SGLT-2i treatment following an IS. Baseline attributes were balanced using propensity score matching. The follow-up period ran from the index date (3 months after the index acute IS) until the study outcomes independently occurred, 6 months after the index medicine was stopped, or the study period expired (December 31, 2020), whichever came first.

In comparison to the non-SGLT-2i group ($n = 2,813$), the SGLT-2i group ($n = 707$) showed a significant decrease in all-cause mortality [5.396% per year vs. 7.489% per year; hazard ratio 0.58; 95% confidence interval (CI) 0.39–0.85; $p = 0.0058$] and recurrent IS rates (3.605% per year vs. 5.897% per year; hazard ratio 0.55; 95% CI 0.34–0.88; $p = 0.0131$) following propensity score matching. The incidence of lower limb amputation, heart failure hospitalization, cardiovascular (CV) death, and acute myocardial infarction (AMI) did not differ significantly.

Conclusion: Among T2DM patients undergoing SGLT-2i therapy, our results show markedly reduced rates of recurrent IS and all-cause mortality. To confirm these findings and look into the underlying mechanisms causing the impacts that have been noticed, more research is needed.

CRITICAL APPRAISAL

What was Known Prior to this Study?

One review study involving population from South, East, and Southeast Asia identified diabetes as the second most significant risk factor for stroke, following hypertension. Diabetes also triples the rate of stroke occurrence as per this study. As ischemic stroke (IS) also has been identified to increase other cardiovascular

(CV) risk factors, glucose-lowering agents like sodium-glucose cotransporter-2 inhibitors (SGLT-2i) with additional CV benefit should have some protective role in this group of patients. But, until before this study no antidiabetic agent has been conclusively proven to reduce the incidence or recurrence of IS. The CV benefits of SGLT-2i have been documented in different multiple large-scale clinical trials like EMPAREG, CANVAS, and DECLARE TIMI, showing a significant positive impact in reducing CV deaths and nonfatal CV complications.

In the EMPA-REG OUTCOME trial, an increased rate of nonfatal stroke events was observed. Although CANVAS trial reported that SGLT-2i use was associated with protective effects against hemorrhagic stroke. In DECLARE TIMI trial, dapagliflozin use had neutral outcome on IS. SGLT-2i are lipid-soluble, enabling them to cross the blood–brain barrier and via SGLT-1 and SGLT-2 coreceptors, they maintain glucose homeostasis in brain offering neuroprotective effects.

Anti-inflammatory effects of SGLT-2i may have some additional effects on neuroprotection. But diuretic effects of SGLT-2i may increase incidence of IS by reducing perfusion.

What this Study Adds?

- The study showed lower risks of IS and all-cause mortality in the SGLT-2i group.
- SGLT-2i may confer protective benefits beyond glucose control in this high-risk population.
- The study also showed the lack of significant differences between SGLT-2i group and placebo in the rates of acute myocardial infarction (AMI), CV death, and heart failure hospitalization in this population of type 2 diabetes with IS.

Major Strength

- Previously, no antidiabetic agent has been conclusively proven to reduce the incidence or recurrence of IS.

- There are limited data available regarding the use of SGLT-2i among patients with type 2 diabetes mellitus (T2DM) following IS.
- The two study groups (SGLT-2i and non-SGLT-2i) were well balanced in all characteristics in this study after propensity score matching.

Limitations

- Despite using propensity score matching, residual confounding may still exist because of unmeasured variables, such as lifestyle factors, dietary habits, and precise glycemic control levels.
- Analysis does not distinguish between different types of SGLT-2i (dapagliflozin, empagliflozin, canagliflozin) and its effects on study outcomes.
- Study assumes adherence to SGLT-2i treatment based on prescription records without directly measuring medication compliance, which may affect the results.
- Severity of IS was not specifically accounted for, which could affect patient outcomes. Patients with more severe conditions may respond differently to SGLT-2i treatment compared with those with milder forms.

Clinical Implications

This study guides us regarding use of SGLT-2i in type 2 diabetes patients with IS to prevent recurrence and to reduce all-cause mortality beyond glucose control.

Knowledge Gaps and Scope for Future Research

Future prospective or randomized studies are needed to further investigate the neuroprotective effects of SGLT-2i. Further studies are required to validate the underlying hypothesis behind this observed effect. Also, there is a need to compare outcomes between different types of SGLT-2i.

5. Uric Acid-lowering Effects of Sodium-glucose Cotransporter 2 Inhibitors for Preventing Cardiovascular Events and Mortality: A Systematic Review and Meta-analysis

Ref: Diallo A, Diallo MF, Carlos-Bolumbu M, Galtier F. Uric acid-lowering effects of sodium-glucose cotransporter 2 inhibitors for preventing cardiovascular events and mortality: A systematic review and meta-analysis. Diabetes Obes Metab. 2024;26(5): 1980-5.

ABSTRACT

Background: To assess how cardiovascular (CV) events and mortality are affected in patients receiving sodium-glucose cotransporter-2 inhibitors (SGLT-2i) when uric acid (UA) is reduced by 1 mg/dL.

Methods and design of the research: To find extensive SGLT-2i trials, we conducted a systematic evaluation of the MEDLINE and EMBASE databases that were searched until June 30, 2023 (PROSPERO, CRD42022355479). To pool the estimates, random-effects meta-analyses were employed.

Findings: A total of five SGLT-2i studies were examined, involving 31,535 patients, of whom 54% had heart failure. The mean decrease in UA over a median follow-up of 2.2 years was −0.79 mg/dL [95% confidence interval (CI) −1.03 to −0.54]. With a comparable risk of mortality, each 1 mg/dL decrease in UA was linked to a significantly decreased risk of a composite of CV death and heart failure hospitalization [hazard ratio 0.64 (95% CI 0.46–0.88)] and heart failure hospitalization (0.68; 95% CI 0.62–0.74)].

Conclusion: SGLT-2i decreased CV events and UA levels without affecting the presence of heart failure.

CRITICAL APPRAISAL

What was Known Prior to this Study?

There is a U-shaped association of uric acid (UA) to cardiovascular (CV) events and all-cause mortality. Urate-lowering effect of sodium-glucose cotransporter-2 (SGLT-2) may be mediated by urate transporter 1 and/or glucose transporter member 9 in the proximal tubule. Meta-analyses has shown that SGLT-2 inhibitors (SGLT-2i) reduce serum UA levels in patients with type 2 diabetes by an average of 0.60–0.96 mg/dL, but none of the previous studies have studied effect of this reduction on CV events and mortality.

What this Study Adds?

- SGLT-2i in this study showed a mean reduction of uric acid by 0.79 mg/dL.
- UA reduction has been associated with reduced risk of a composite of heart failure hospitalization and CV death.
- SGLT-2i significantly reduce plasma UA level as well as CV morbidity and mortality even in patients without heart failure.

Major Strength

This meta-analysis included five major SGLT-2i trials (DAPA-HF, CANVAS, EMPEROR-PRESERVED, EMPEROR-REDUCED, EMPA-REG) involving a large sample of patients. Most of the patients with type 2 diabetes had heart failure or chronic kidney disease.

Limitations

- Moderate-to-high heterogeneity was observed in the definition of CV death, all-cause mortality, and a composite of heart failure and CV death.
- Differences in participant characteristics, or in study design, may account for this heterogeneity.
- Lack of patient-level data limits the ability to explore possible sources of heterogeneity.

Clinical Implications

The study findings support the use of SGLT-2 drugs as an adjunct to UA-lowering therapy in addition to their cardiorenal protection.

Knowledge Gaps and Future Scope for Research

Beneficial effect of SGLT-2i as shown in this study is multifactorial, because of their pleiotropic effect on the regulation of glucose, sodium, and UA homeostasis. Future trials should explore the benefits of using SGLT-2i, alone or in combination, in the prevention or treatment of hyperuricemia.

---

6. A Meta-analysis of Randomized Controlled Studies Examining the Effects of Sodium-glucose Cotransporter-2 Inhibitors on Peripheral Artery Disease and Risk of Amputations

Ref: Geng L, Sun B, Chen Y. A meta-analysis of randomized controlled studies examining the effects of sodium-glucose co-transporter-2 inhibitors on peripheral artery disease and risk of amputations. Diabetes Obes Metab. 2024;26(11):5376-89.

ABSTRACT

The purpose of sodium-glucose cotransporter-2 inhibitors (SGLT-2i) is to help diabetics maintain glycemic control while also having positive benefits on their kidneys and heart. However, using some SGLT-2i has been linked to an increased risk of peripheral artery disease (PAD) and amputation. Using information from randomized controlled trials (RCTs), a meta-analysis was carried out to determine how SGLT-2i affected amputation and PAD events.

Materials and methods: Using the Medline and Central databases for RCTs including the administration of SGLT-2i against placebo/active comparators to diabetic patients, a systematic literature review was carried out. PAD and amputation events were the main results. Subgroup analyses were conducted and the pooled odds ratio was computed using a random-effects model.

Results: The meta-analysis contained data from 97,589 patients from 51 RCTs. According to a meta-analysis of the data, using SGLT-2i increased the risk of PAD significantly ($p = 0.04$) but did not significantly raise the risk of amputation when compared to placebo/active comparators ($p = 0.43$). Subgroup analyses showed no discernible difference in the incidence of PAD or amputation by SGLT-2i type, treatment duration, or patient risk factors. However, in the SGLT-2i treatment groups, a significant rise in the chances of both PAD and amputation was linked to the duration of drug treatment (>100 weeks).

Conclusion: When SGLT-2i was used for shorter treatment durations, the meta-analysis's findings revealed no discernible correlation between its use and the risks of PAD and amputation in diabetic patients.

CRITICAL APPRAISAL

What was Known Prior to this Study?

Despite the glycemic and extraglycemic benefits of sodium-glucose cotransporter-2 inhibitors (SGLT-2i), some trials, like in CANVAS trial, showed an increased risk of amputation in patients taking canagliflozin [hazard ratio (HR) 1.97; 95% confidence interval (CI) 1.41–2.75]. This leads to cautious use of canagliflozin in high-risk patients. Volume depletion and dehydration caused by the diuretic effect of SGLT-2i may lead to tissue hypoperfusion and increased amputation risk. Empagliflozin and dapagliflozin have not been shown to increase amputation rates relative to placebo. Increased degree of blood pressure reduction in canagliflozin may be responsible for greater hypoperfusion and more amputation risk. So, there is an unmet need to weigh the risk versus benefit of SGLT-2i in this population.

What this Study Adds?

- Peripheral artery disease (PAD) risks were statistically significant only for the canagliflozin group, but not for any of the other SGLT-2i drugs.
- The study also assessed type of drug, patient characteristics, and duration of drug treatment on risk profile.
- This can help guide clinical decision-making regarding the optimal length of treatment as long duration of treatment >100 weeks is associated with both PAD as well increased risk of amputation.

Major Strength

- This meta-analysis provides current and updated information regarding side effects associated with SGLT-2i in patients with type 2 diabetes, thereby shedding light on the usefulness of these agents compared to other agents.
- 51 randomized controlled trials (RCTs) involving 97,589 participants were included in this meta-analysis.
- It included male and female participants with both type 1 and type 2 diabetes, different hemoglobin A1c (HbA1c) levels, cardiovascular or renal risk factors, and patients with concomitant medication or insulin treatment.

Limitations

- RCTs included in this meta-analysis may not be of sufficient duration to capture all adverse events such as amputations and PAD.
- RCTs included in this meta-analysis may not also be adequately powered for these events.
- The high heterogeneity between studies, attributed to varying baseline characteristics of patients such as glycemic status, comorbidities, and concomitant medications.
- In most studies, the anatomic location of amputation was not specified. The differential effect that the amputation site has on patient outcome is important.
- The exact definition of PAD differed between studies, making it difficult to come to a consensus.

Clinical Implications

These data are expected to help in clinical decisions making regarding SGLT-2i over other antidiabetic agents after weighing risk versus benefits. This study also guides the safe use of SGLT-2i in high-risk population with increased risk of PAD and amputation.

Knowledge Gaps and Scope for Future Research

To provide a more comprehensive assessment regarding safety of SGLT-2i, it is important to identify patient characteristics that influence the occurrence of adverse effects. It will help to select patient groups accordingly where the drug must be avoided. Further trials should be done directed toward patient-level meta-analysis that will help overcome patient heterogeneity and which also focus on specific patient subgroups.

7. Efficacy of Aspirin for Primary Prevention among Adults with High-risk Type 2 Diabetes in the ACCORD Trial

Ref: Kazibwe R, Singleton M, Bancks MP, Namutebi J, Hammoud A, Shapiro M, et al. Efficacy of Aspirin for primary prevention among adults with high-risk type 2 diabetes in the ACCORD trial. Diabetes Obes Metab. 2024;26(9):4011-8.

ABSTRACT

With regard to incident atherosclerotic cardiovascular disease (CVD) and mortality in high-risk type 2 diabetes, the purpose of this study is to evaluate the effectiveness of aspirin therapy for primary prevention of CVD.

Techniques: We included ACCORD trial participants who did not have CVD at baseline in this post hoc analysis. After controlling for demographics, cardiovascular (CV) risk factors, and comorbidities, Cox proportional hazard analysis was used to assess the relationship between aspirin use and the primary outcome (a composite of nonfatal myocardial infarction, nonfatal stroke, or CV death) and all-cause mortality.

Findings: 3,026 (47.8%) of the eligible individuals ($n = 6,330$) used aspirin, 43.8% of the participants were female, and the participants' baseline ages were 62.8 ± 5.9 years. The number (%) of primary outcome and all-cause mortality events in aspirin users (compared to nonusers) was 196 (6.5) versus 229 (6.9) and 146 (4.8) versus 147 (4.5) over a median (interquartile range) follow-up of 4.9 (4.1–5.7) years. For the primary outcome and all-cause mortality, the adjusted hazard ratios [95% confidence interval (CI)] linked to aspirin use were 0.94 (0.77–1.14) and 1.08 (0.85–1.36), respectively.

Conclusion: Aspirin use for primary prevention did not appear to be linked to a lower incidence of incident CVD or all-cause mortality in high-risk adults with type 2 diabetes.

CRITICAL APPRAISAL

What was Known Prior to this Study?

As per the American Diabetes Association (ADA) guidelines, aspirin is considered as a primary prevention strategy for individuals with diabetes at an increased cardiovascular (CV) risk, after taking into account the potential benefit versus risk of bleeding. Recommendations are based largely on the basis of ASCEND trial, which showed absolute benefits of aspirin for primary prevention of cardiovascular disease (CVD) were largely counterbalanced by the bleeding hazard. In ASCEND trial, 15,480 participants underwent randomization and over a period of 7.4 years' follow-up, serious vascular events occurred in a significantly lower percentage of participants in the aspirin group than in the placebo group [658 participants (8.5%) vs. 743 (9.6%); rate ratio 0.88; 95% confidence interval (CI) 0.79–0.97; $p = 0.01$]. But, major bleeding events occurred in 314 participants (4.1%) in the aspirin group, as compared with 245 (3.2%) in the placebo group (rate ratio 1.29; 95% CI 1.09–1.52; $p = 0.003$). Similar recommendation have been given as per American College of Cardiology/American Heart Association and from the 2021 European Society of Cardiology guidelines. The Prevention of Progression of Arterial Disease and Diabetes (POPADAD) trial did not support the use of aspirin for primary prevention in those with diabetes. A meta-analysis in 2018, from 13 trials showed that in a subgroup of patients with diabetes, aspirin did not prevent CV events or mortality and was associated with a high bleeding risk.

Therefore, this study has been designed to identify high-risk individuals who could potentially benefit from aspirin for primary prevention and to address this unresolved conflict in the existing evidence and current guidelines.

What this Study Adds?

This post hoc analysis of ACCORD trial showed aspirin was not associated with a decreased risk of future CVD outcomes or all-cause mortality in high risk type 2 diabetes without CVD at baseline. So this study concludes that even in those with high-risk diabetes, aspirin has an uncertain role for primary prevention.

Major Strength

- A total of 6,330 patients from ACCORD trial were randomized.
- Previously very few studies have focused on individuals with a high risk of CVD. Study population from ACCORD trial had anatomical evidence of significant atherosclerosis, albuminuria, left ventricular hypertrophy, or at least two additional risk factors for CVD (dyslipidemia, hypertension, current status as a smoker, or obesity).
- This study focused on two main outcomes: (1) The primary ACCORD trial endpoint (a composite of nonfatal myocardial infarction, nonfatal stroke, or CV death) and (2) all-cause mortality.

Limitations

- As it is a post hoc analysis of a clinical trial, this study was not primarily designed with a focus on aspirin for primary prevention.
- The potential for residual confounding persists. Possibility of confounding by indication of aspirin use and possibility of misclassification of baseline CVD status is present.
- This study did not assess the association of aspirin with bleeding, as information regarding bleeding was not available in ACCORD data.
- Most studies demonstrated that low doses (75–100 mg/day) are effective for primary prevention. But, this study did not analysis aspirin dosage.
- There is limitation regarding generalizability of the results to broader populations as study population excluded type 1 diabetes and people with low CV risk.

Clinical Implications

This study highlighted the persistent uncertainties about aspirin's role in primary CVD prevention in individuals with diabetes. The study concluded that role of aspirin for primary prevention even in high-risk patients of type 2 diabetes is uncertain.

Knowledge Gaps and Scope for Future Research

Bleeding risk was not assessed in this analysis. Also, any difference between low-dose and high-dose aspirin was not evaluated. Indeed, there is utmost need for a large prospective trial with different dosages of aspirin and need to weigh the risks versus benefit, so that a conclusion can be reached, which will be reflected in the guidelines.

---

8. Glycaemic Control and Macrovascular and Microvascular Outcomes: A Systematic Review and Meta-analysis of Trials Investigating Intensive Glucose-lowering Strategies in People with Type 2 Diabetes

Ref: Kunutsor SK, Balasubramanian VG, Zaccardi F, Gillies CL, Aroda VR, Seidu S, et al. Glycaemic control and macrovascular and microvascular outcomes: A systematic review and meta-analysis of trials investigating intensive glucose-lowering strategies in people with type 2 diabetes. Diabetes Obes Metab. 2024;26(6):2069-81.

ABSTRACT

Our goal was to compare the macrovascular and microvascular effects of intensive and routine glucose-lowering techniques in people with type 2 diabetes (T2D) and look into how these effects relate to the reduction of glycated hemoglobin (HbA1c) in the experimental arm.

Materials and procedures: We found pertinent trials for this systematic review and meta-analysis by searching MEDLINE, Embase, the Cochrane Library, and bibliographies up until August, 2023. Safety results as well as macrovascular and microvascular results were assessed. We computed study-specific pooled hazard ratios (HRs) with 95% confidence intervals (CIs) and used meta-regression to examine the associations between outcomes and lowering HbA1c.

Findings: Of the 51,469 T2D patients (intensive therapy, n = 26,691; routine therapy, n = 24,778), we included 11 distinct randomized controlled trials (RCTs). While there was no difference in the risk of severe adverse cardiovascular events (HR 0.97; 95% CI 0.92–1.03) or other adverse cardiovascular outcomes, intensive therapy decreased the risk of nonfatal myocardial infarction (MI) (HR 0.84; 95% CI 0.75–0.94). The risk of retinopathy (HR 0.85; 0.78–0.93), nephropathy (HR 0.71; 0.58–0.87), and composite microvascular outcomes (HR 0.88; 0.77–1.00) was decreased by intensive therapy as opposed to routine care. Although they were not statistically significant, meta-regression studies revealed little evidence of inverse linear correlations between HbA1c reduction and the outcomes of major adverse cardiovascular events (MACE), nonfatal MI, stroke, and retinopathy.

Intense glucose management was linked to a lower incidence of nonfatal MI and a number of microvascular consequences, especially retinopathy and nephropathy, in individuals with type 2 diabetes. A more thorough approach to treating cardiovascular risk factors in addition to glycemic control is necessary because rigorous glucose-lowering has little effect on the majority of macrovascular outcomes.

CRITICAL APPRAISAL

What was Known Prior to this Study?

Glucose control is the mainstay of type 2 diabetes (T2D) management. Uncontrolled glycated hemoglobin (HbA1c) is associated with increased cardiovascular adverse events. According to the guidelines, it is recommended to keep the HbA1c below 7%. As T2D is a multifactorial disease, macrovascular complications are not always linked to glycemic control but also related to blood pressure, dyslipidemia, and weight gain. Previous studies had variable results regarding effect of intensive glucose control on microvascular and macrovascular complications. ADVANCE and UKPDS provided strong evidence supporting the importance of tight glycemic control in reducing the risk of diabetic retinopathy, nephropathy, and neuropathy. In contrast, ACCORD trial reported an increased risk of cardiovascular events among patients assigned to intensive glycemic control targeting a HbA1c level of below 6%.

Control group of meta-analysis, which included ACCORD, ADVANCE, UKPDS, and VADT showed that intensive glucose control reduced the risk of microvascular outcomes, i.e., kidney and eye events. Steno-2 study also reported 55% reduction in composite outcome of major adverse cardiovascular events (MACE) plus amputation. This positive association of glycemic control with microvascular complications is linked to the concept of "metabolic memory". Although results on microvascular outcomes are more or less consistent, the impact on macrovascular complications has been contradictory.

What this Study Adds?

- Intensive glucose control was associated with a 16% reduced risk of nonfatal

myocardial infarction (MI) compared to standard glucose control.
- Intensive glucose control also reduced incidence of retinopathy, nephropathy, composite microvascular outcomes, macroalbuminuria, and microalbuminuria.
- No strong evidence of reduction of MACE, cardiovascular death, heart failure (HF), stroke, peripheral vascular disease, amputations, overall MI, fatal MI, or all-cause mortality, compared with standard therapy

Major Strength
- This meta-analysis included 11 unique randomized controlled trials (RCTs) published between 1998 and 2021 involving 51,469 patients with T2D.
- Study provided valuable insights into the relationship between glycemic control and macrovascular and microvascular outcomes in patients with T2D.
- Subgroup analyses were conducted based on relevant clinical characteristics, enabling exploration of potential variations in treatment effects across different patient populations.

Limitations
- Some of the trials included in this study were conducted before the introduction of newer glucose-lowering agents, such as glucagon-like peptide 1 receptor agonists (GLP-1 RAs) and sodium-glucose cotransporter-2 inhibitors (SGLT-2is).
- Some outcomes were based on data from a single or few studies, which may limit the generalizability of these particular findings.
- Some outcomes had low event rates, leading to inadequate statistical power for a comprehensive evaluation.
- Apart from all-cause mortality, the number of trials available for the other evaluated outcomes was limited.

Clinical Implications
Study confirmed the established microvascular benefits of intensive versus standard therapy in patients with T2D. In addition, they also shed some light on the lack of significant benefits for several macrovascular outcomes.

These results suggest that achieving intensive glycemic control alone might not be sufficient to drive substantial improvements in macrovascular outcomes.

Knowledge Gaps and Scope for Future Research
Data on the impact of intensive glycemic control on macrovascular outcomes remain inconclusive. Lack of an effect of intensive glucose-lowering on most macrovascular outcomes calls for a more comprehensive approach to manage cardiovascular risk factors alongside glycemic control. These factors need to be addressed in larger prospective trials.

---

9. Incidence and Progression of Diabetic Retinopathy in Patients Treated with Glucagon-like Peptide-1 Receptor Agonists versus Sodium-glucose Cotransporter 2 Inhibitors: A Population-based Cohort Study

Ref: Lin DS, Lo HY, Huang KC, Lin TT, Lee JK, Lin LY. Incidence and progression of diabetic retinopathy in patients treated with glucagon-like peptide-1 receptor agonists versus sodium-glucose cotransporter 2 inhibitors: A population-based cohort study. Diabetes Obes Metab. 2024;26(10):4386-96.

ABSTRACT

Goal: Although sodium-glucose cotransporter-2 inhibitors (SGLT-2i) and glucagon-like peptide 1 receptor agonists (GLP-1 RA) are advised for diabetic patients, nothing is known about how they affect the onset or course of diabetic retinopathy (DR).

Methods: Information for this retrospective cohort analysis came from a national database. We identified diabetic patients who started taking a GLP-1 RA or SGLT-2i between May 1, 2016 and December 31, 2017. Before being grouped into the GLP-1 RA and SGLT-2i groups based on drug use, patients were separated into those who had or had not previously been diagnosed with DR. The composite of vitreous hemorrhage, tractional retinal detachment (RD), and new-onset proliferative DR was the main result of interest in the DR group.

The composite of newly diagnosed DR of any severity, vitreous hemorrhage, and RD was the main outcome in the non-DR group.

Findings: A total of 97,413 patients were found. Following matching, 3,034 patients in the DR cohort received SGLT-2i treatment and 1,517 patients received GLP-1 RA treatment. 19,098 and 9,549, respectively, started an SGLT-2i and a GLP-1 RA in the non-DR cohort. Due to mainly the elevated risk of tractional RD, the incidence of any DR progression event was substantially higher in the GLP-1 RA group than in the SGLT-2i group in patients with preexisting DR [subdistribution hazard ratio 1.50; 95% confidence interval (CI) 1.01–2.23]. The GLP-1 RA and SGLT-2i groups had comparable risks for all ocular outcomes in patients who did not have DR at baseline.

Conclusion: Compared to SGLT-2i usage, GLP-1 RA medication was linked to higher risks of DR advancement in people with diabetes mellitus and established DR.

CRITICAL APPRAISAL

What was Known Prior to this Study?

Sodium-glucose cotransporter-2 inhibitors (SGLT-2i) and glucagon-like peptide 1 receptor agonists (GLP-1 RAs) are two important glucose-lowering agents in recent times, largely known for their additional cardiovascular and renal benefits. But their effects on development and progression of diabetic retinopathy (DR) has been less studied. In SUSTAIN-6 trial with injectable semaglutide, rates of retinopathy complications were higher. In LEADER trial, liraglutide was associated with a numerically greater but statistically nonsignificant ocular events. One meta-analysis with GLP-1 RAs, concluded that GLP-1 RA treatment per se was not associated with DR events, but the magnitude of hemoglobin A1c (HbA1c) reduction was positively correlated with the risks of retinopathy.

Regarding SGLT-2i, usually they have neutral effects on DR. In the EMPA-REG OUTCOME trial, composite retinopathy outcomes were numerically lower in the empagliflozin group, although statistically neutral. Overall glycemic control may have some benefits in reducing DR progression as evident in previous studies. In ACCORD study, intensive glycemic control is associated with reduction of retinopathy progression. In UKPDS, there was 25% risk reduction in microvascular endpoints, including the need for retinal photocoagulation. One review of randomized controlled trials (RCTs) suggested that retinal benefits by intensive glycemic control were lost in patients with severe DR at baseline. The present study aimed at showing the real-world outcomes of patients with diabetes mellitus (DM) receiving GLP-1 RA compared with those treated with SGLT-2i in terms of ocular events.

What this Study Adds?

- The study concluded that GLP-1 RA use was associated with an elevated risk of DR progression compared with SGLT-2i, specially with pre-existing DR.

- The risks of DR occurrence were not different between GLP-1 RA and SGLT-2i therapy in those without pre-existing DR.

Major Strength
- No previous study with GLP-1 RA came with conclusive evidence regarding DR progression.
- Differential effects of SGLT-2i and GLP-1 RA on the basis of pre-existing DR has additional advantage in guiding clinical practice.
- Subgroup analyses were also done to examine whether the effects on the progression of DR in the DR group and any DR event in the non-DR group were consistent across different prespecified subgroup variables, which included age, gender, presence of dyslipidemia, hypertension (HTN), ischemic heart disease, chronic kidney disease (CKD), peripheral artery disease (PAD), history of ischemic stroke, duration of DM, and presence of DM neuropathy and DM nephropathy.

Limitations
- Low incidence of events in non-DR group may lead to lack of difference between treatment arms.
- As there is relatively short follow-up, possible "early worsening" of DR may have been present in this cohort and the conclusions from this study cannot be extrapolated to longer-term use of these drugs.
- This study cohort was enrolled through the National Health Insurance Research Database (NHIRD) with International Classification of Diseases (ICD) codes. The NHIRD lacks details on the severity of metabolic disease and other patient characteristics, like severity of DR, HbA1c, baseline renal function, body mass indices, and lifestyle factors (exercise, smoking, etc.). These data may be associated with prognosis, and the inability to adjust for these factors may result in confounding.
- It is a retrospective study using national database of Taiwan. Reimbursement for GLP-1 RA in Taiwan is restricted to patients with poor glycemic control or higher atherosclerotic risk, possibly leading to higher risk profiles for those using GLP-1 RA in this cohort. Patients who pay GLP-1 RA out-of-pocket will not be identified in the NHIRD and may be erroneously categorized into the SGLT-2i group.
- Unmeasured confounders related to patient or physician behavior are difficult to avoid in retrospective database studies.

Clinical Implications
The study guides us regarding avoidance of GLP-1 RA in type 2 diabetes with pre-existing DR and higher baseline risk, as it may further worsen the retinopathy status, although effect of long-term GLP-1 RA use has not been established.

Knowledge Gaps and Scope for Future Research
Whether this effect of "early worsening" of DR by GLP-1 RA is related to more rapid glycemic control or with GLP-1 RA use, that remains to be elucidated. The conclusions of this study cannot be extrapolated to longer-term use of these drugs. Further investigations with longer study periods are needed for that. Additional studies that document changes in HbA1c levels are also essential for understanding the effects of these drugs on retinopathy outcomes.

10. Normoalbuminuria—Is It Normal? The Association of Urinary Albumin within the 'Normoalbuminuric' Range with Adverse Cardiovascular and Mortality Outcomes: A Systematic Review and Meta-analysis

Ref: Sehtman-Shachar DR, Yanuv I, Schechter M, Fishkin A, Aharon-Hananel G, Leibowitz G, et al. Normoalbuminuria—is it normal? The association of urinary albumin within the 'normoalbuminuric' range with adverse cardiovascular and mortality outcomes: A systematic review and meta-analysis. Diabetes Obes Metab. 2024;26(10):4225-40.

ABSTRACT

Goal: To evaluate the relationship between mortality and unfavorable cardiovascular (CV) events and urine albumin-to-creatinine ratio (UACR) categories that fall within the normal range.

Materials and procedures: A comprehensive search for real-world evidence (RWE) studies was conducted using PubMed and Embase. Studies were assessed by hand based on predetermined eligibility standards. Cohort studies, including prospective and retrospective, that examined the relationship between CV events or mortality and UACR categories below 30 mg/g were considered. We manually gathered published data on study design, participants, UACR classification, statistical techniques, and outcomes. A two-category (UACR < 10 mg/g vs. 10–30 mg/g) and a three-category division (UACR < 5 mg/g vs. 5–10 and 10–30 mg/g) UACR categorization methods were established. Studies which qualified for the meta-analysis were subjected to a random effects meta-analysis.

Findings: 15 of the 22 publications that were selected for the systematic review qualified for the meta-analysis. The findings point to a correlation between increased UACR in the normal to slightly elevated range and increased risks of CV death, coronary heart disease, and all-cause mortality, especially in the 10–30 mg/g range. The hazard ratio [HR; 95% confidence interval (CI)] for UACR between 10 and 30 mg/g was 1.41 (1.15, 1.74) for all-cause mortality and 1.56 (1.23, 1.98) for coronary heart disease when compared to UACR < 10 mg/g. The risk of CV death for UACR between 10 and 30 mg/g was more than double that of UACR < 5 mg/g [HR (95% CI): 2.12 (1.61, 2.80)].

Additionally, a greater risk of all-cause death was linked to intermediate UACR (5–10 mg/g) [HR (95% CI): 1.14 (1.05, 1.24)]. and death from heart disease [HR (95% CI): 1.50 (1.14, 1.99)].

Conclusion: As a predictor of CV morbidity and death, we suggest taking into account a higher UACR within the normoalbuminuric range. The clinical importance of even slight elevations in albuminuria is highlighted by our findings.

CRITICAL APPRAISAL

What was Known Prior to this Study?

Abnormal urinary albumin [urine albumin-to-creatinine ratio (UACR) > 30 mg/g] has been shown to be associated with adverse kidney outcomes as well as cardiovascular (CV) outcomes and mortality. This is a well-established fact. Some studies have demonstrated that elevation of urine ACR within the range of so-called normoalbuminuria can be associated with increased risk of CV and all-cause mortality. But, so far no urine ACR threshold has been established for predicting the CV risk. Another meta-analysis with 114 studies showed that compared with UACR of <10 mg/g, higher categories (including a 10–30 mg/g category) were associated with higher rates of various CV and kidney outcomes. Previous meta-analysis has also demonstrated that this risk persists both in population with high CV risk as well as in normal population.

What this Study Adds?
- This study suggested that albuminuria within the normal range is associated with an increased risk of CV morbidity and mortality.
- Urine ACR 10–30 mg/g compared with urine ACR < 10 mg/g is specifically associated with increased CV risk.
- Albuminuria should be addressed as a continuous variable, while assessing CV risk.
- The study also underscores the lack of standardization existing in category definitions within the normoalbuminuric range.

Major Strength
- More than 186,000 subjects have been included in this meta-analysis, which enhances the broader applicability and generalizability of the results.
- The study solely focused on population with normoalbuminuria.
- In contrast to previous studies, this meta-analysis compared two different categorizations of UACR within the normal to mildly increased range.
- This meta-analysis includes only real-world evidence (RWE) studies, which provide important insights on the real-life effects and also enable generalizability of study findings.

Limitations
- There may be differences in laboratory methods in determination of urine ACR in different studies.
- A multivariable meta-regression analysis could not be performed, as individual data were missing.
- Contribution of factors that might interact with albuminuria in predicting an increased risk of adverse CV outcomes and mortality, such as estimated glomerular filtration rate (eGFR) and body mass index (BMI) are not tested as subgroup analysis could not be performed.
- There is incomplete data on patients' ethnicities across the studies and different ethnicities may interact with CV and mortality outcomes.
- Use of results calculated by different models in each study may involve differences in the adjustments.
- Use of spot urine ACR does not address the fluctuation in albumin excretion level.
- Some of the studies included in the analyses which showed high heterogeneity and the causes of this heterogeneity are not explored using a meta-regression model or subgroup analysis due to limited data availability.

Clinical Implications
In future, urine ACR can be used to predict CV and mortality risk in type 2 diabetes patients even if it is in normoalbuminuric range. Also, it will help to initiate novel treatments early which can mitigate the risk of chronic kidney disease (CKD) progression.

Knowledge Gaps and Scope for Future Research
Data is scarce regarding the use of novel treatments, which can reduce albuminuria and CKD progression at this early urine ACR threshold. Additional research is required to establish the effect of the aforementioned treatments on CVD and mortality in subjects with baseline normal to mildly increased albuminuria.

11. Comparison of Estimated Glomerular Filtration Rate Change with Sodium-glucose Cotransporter-2 Inhibitors versus Glucagon-like Peptide-1 Receptor Agonists among People with Diabetes: A Propensity-score Matching Study

Ref: Suzuki Y, Kaneko H, Nagasawa H, Okada A, Fujiu K, Jo T, et al. Comparison of estimated glomerular filtration rate change with sodium-glucose cotransporter-2 inhibitors versus glucagon-like peptide-1 receptor agonists among people with diabetes: A propensity-score matching study. Diabetes Obes Metab. 2024;26(6):2422-30.

ABSTRACT

Goal: To assess the risk of kidney outcomes in diabetics using sodium-glucose cotransporter-2 inhibitors (SGLT-2i) versus glucagon-like peptide-1 receptor agonists (GLP-1 RAs).

Materials and techniques: Using information from the JMDC claims database, we examined 12,338 diabetics who had just started taking SGLT-2i or GLP-1 RAs in this retrospective observational analysis. Changes in the estimated glomerular filtration rate (eGFR), which was calculated using a linear mixed-effects model, were the main result. The eGFR changes in GLP-1 RA and SGLT-2i users were compared using a 1:4 propensity-score-matching technique.

Results: 2,549 people [median (range) age 52 (46–58) years, 80.6% men] were analyzed using propensity-score matching (510 GLP-1 RA new users and 2,039 SGLT-2i new users). When compared to GLP-1 RA use, SGLT-2i use was linked to a smaller reduction in eGFR {−1.41 [95% confidence interval (CI) −1.63 to −1.19] mL/min/1.73 m^2 vs. −2.62 (95% CI −3.15 to −2.10) mL/min/1.73 m^2}.

Conclusion: Based on our data, SGLT-2i may be better for renal outcomes in diabetics than GLP-1 RAs.

CRITICAL APPRAISAL

What was Known Prior to this Study?

Randomized controlled trials (RCTs) have established the fact that sodium-glucose cotransporter-2 inhibitors (SGLT-2i) and glucagon-like peptide 1 receptor agonist (GLP-1 RA) have additional renal benefit beyond their glycemic and cardiovascular (CV) effects. Evidence from DAPA-CKD and EMPA-KIDNEY has suggested that SGLT-2i can reduce estimated glomerular filtration rate (eGFR) decline and prevent progression of chronic kidney disease (CKD). In FLOW trial with injectable semaglutide, major kidney disease events, a composite of the onset of kidney failure (dialysis, transplantation, or an eGFR of <15 mL/min/1.73 m^2), at least a 50% reduction in the eGFR from baseline, or death from kidney-related or CV causes are assessed as primary kidney outcome. The risk of a primary-outcome event was 24% lower in the semaglutide group than in the placebo group. Based on these evidences, ADA-KDIGO (American Diabetes Association–Kidney Disease: Improving Global Outcomes) 2022 consensus stated that SGLT-2i have to be added in addition to metformin irrespective of glycemic status of the patient for renal benefits in type 2 diabetes and CKD. GLP-1 RA is to be added as second line if glycemic control is not achieved.

Several possible explanations, including reduced intraglomerular pressure through tubuloglomerular feedback, improved tubular oxygenation, attenuated inflammation, and increased erythropoiesis stimulation, could explain the advantage of SGLT-2i over GLP-1 RA in terms of kidney protection.

What this Study Adds?

- This study concluded that SGLT-2i use demonstrated superior kidney outcomes compared with GLP-1 RA use, regardless of the presence of proteinuria.
- Even in individuals with preserved eGFR and no proteinuria (early-stage diabetic kidney disease), SGLT-2i may exhibit a superior kidney-protective effect compared with GLP-1 RAs.

Major Strength

- To date, no study has reported a conclusive comparison between the kidney-protective effects of SGLT-2i and those of GLP-1 RAs.
- Large-scale epidemiological dataset has been used and kidney outcomes with SGLT-2i and GLP-1 RA use have been directly compared in individuals through propensity-score matching.
- This database primarily consisted of employees and their families. The study population was relatively young (median age 52 years) and had a preserved eGFR (median eGFR 77.8 mL/min/1.73 m^2). Even in this relatively low-risk population with less advanced diabetes, SGLT-2i were superior to GLP-1 RAs in terms of kidney outcomes.
- Finding was consistent regardless of the baseline clinical characteristics.

Limitations

- As it is a retrospective and observational study, possibility of unmeasured residual confounding is present.
- Small sample size (510 GLP-1 RA users and 2,039 SGLT-2i users after propensity-score matching) and the short observational period (mean follow-up of 1.9 years after propensity-score matching) are also the major limitations of this study.

Clinical Implications

The study highlighted the superior kidney-protective outcome of SGLT-2i on reduction of CKD progression, compared to GLP-1 RA.

Knowledge Gaps and Scope for Future Research

Large sample size and long-term analyses are necessary to examine whether there are clinical differences between SGLT-2i and GLP-1 RAs in terms of kidney failure (renal outcome) after kidney replacement therapy.

---

12. Major Adverse Events in Youth-onset Type 1 and Type 2 Diabetes: The SEARCH and TODAY Studies

Ref: Mottl AK, Tryggestad JB, Isom S, Gubitosi-Klug RA, Henkin L, White NH, et al.; SEARCH for Diabetes in Youth Study Group; TODAY Study Group. Major adverse events in youth-onset type 1 and type 2 diabetes: The SEARCH and TODAY studies. Diabetes Res Clin Pract. 2024;210:111606.

ABSTRACT

Goals: To ascertain current incidence rates and risk factors for significant adverse events in type 1 diabetes (T1D) and type 2 diabetes (T2D) with a juvenile onset.

Techniques: Interviews with participants were done semiannually in TODAY (Treatment Options for Type 2 Diabetes in Adolescents and Youth) from 2014 to 2020 (T2D: n = 495) and once during in-person visits in SEARCH from 2018 to 2019 (T1D: n = 564; T2D: n = 149). Harmonized, preset, uniform criteria were used to judge the results.

Findings: A total of 10.9 ophthalmologic, 0 kidney, 11.1 nerve, 3.1 cardiac, 3.1 peripheral vascular, 1.6 cerebrovascular, and 15.6 gastrointestinal events were among the T1D participants' incidence rates (events per 10,000 person-years). 40.0 ophthalmologic, 6.2 renal, 21.2 nerve, 21.2 cardiac, 10.0 peripheral vascular, 5.0 cerebrovascular, and 42.8 gastrointestinal incidents were among the T2D subjects.

Youth with T2D experienced more difficulties than those with T1D, although having equal mean durations of diabetes: Microvascular complications were 2.5 times greater, macrovascular complications were 4.0 times higher, and gastrointestinal disease was 2.7 times worse. Univariate logistic regression analyses relation of microvascular events to T1D-associated mean arterial pressure (MAP), female sex, age of diagnosis, and hemoglobin A1c (HbA1c). Composite macrovascular events were only associated with MAP in youth-onset T2D, although composite microvascular events were favorably associated with MAP and negatively associated with body mass index (BMI).

Conclusion: End-organ events were rare in youth-onset diabetes, but they did happen before the age of 15 years. Compared to T1D, T2D had greater rates and distinct risk factors.

CRITICAL APPRAISAL

What was Known Prior to this Study?

As per the SEARCH for Diabetes in Youth Study, the prevalence of T2D in youth (10–19 years) doubled between 2002 and 2018 with annual increase of 2.0% and 5.3% per year, respectively for T1D and T2D. A Chinese study with young-onset (<40 years) T1D and T2D found that rates of major adverse cardiovascular events, peripheral vascular disease, and end-stage kidney disease (ESKD) were no longer different in T2D compared to T1D, after adjusting for body mass index (BMI), blood pressure, and lipids. As previous studies showed in adults with T2D, glycemic control has been implicated in the development of advanced microvascular disease, but significantly less important for macrovascular complications. In the Treatment Options for Type 2 Diabetes in Adolescents and Youth (TODAY) study diabetes-related complications were seen in 60% by 10 years and high hemoglobin A1c (HbA1c), lower insulin sensitivity, hypertension, and dyslipidemia are the predicting risk factors for microvascular complications. Regarding microvascular complications, retinopathy is much more common. One study that included both T1D and youth-onset T2D showed that ophthalmic complications are much common in youth-onset T2D compared to T1D with hazard ratio (HR) for proliferative diabetic retinopathy (PDR): 1.9 [95% confidence interval (CI) 1.1–3.1]. But it is not clear from previous studies whether differences exist between youth-onset T1D versus T2D in predicting micro- and macrovascular complications.

What this Study Adds?

- This analysis concluded that major adverse events begin to emerge in youth-onset T1D and T2D within 10–15 years of diagnosis.
- This study documents that although infrequent, severe vascular events [ESKD, blindness, myocardial infarctions (MIs)] take place in individuals <30 years.
- Compared to T1D, youth-onset T2D showed much more incidence rates of micro- and macrovascular complications.
- Blood pressure was the sole predictor for macrovascular complications in youth-onset T2D.

Major Strength

- No previous studies analyzed comprehensive rates of major adverse events early in the course of both youth-onset T1D and T2D.
- The combination of the SEARCH and TODAY cohorts allowed for evaluation of the two largest collections youth-onset T2D individuals.
- Participants were followed longitudinally over a minimum of 10 years.

- While TODAY was a clinical trial and SEARCH was an observational cohort study, pooling of data was justified by several factors. As for example, participants in each study are quite similar, with overlapping rates of preclinical complications. The criteria for the diagnosis of T2D is very similar between the two studies such that all youth in TODAY would meet the inclusion criteria set forth for T2D in SEARCH.

Limitations

- Ascertainment of events was based on relying on participant recall, which may potentially result in under-reporting of events.
- Adjudication was conducted via review of medical records. Some records were unavailable and others may have been missed, contributing to possible under-reporting.
- Some of the socioeconomic data was not available across the entire cohort, which could have impacts on complication rates.
- Due to the low number of events, statistical power was limited, therefore the factors which are identified as predictors for vascular events should be interpreted with caution.

Clinical Implications

- This study underscores the aggressive nature of youth-onset T2D.
- The differences in rates of micro- and macrovascular complications between T1D and T2D suggest that distinct pathogenetic mechanisms of vascular complications may exist in youth-onset T1D and T2D.
- Adequate blood pressure monitoring and treatment of hypertension is needed to prevent vascular complications in T2D.

Knowledge Gaps and Scope for Future Research

Given the small number of kidney events in this study, further data are needed to determine the true difference in the epidemiology of diabetic kidney disease in youth onset T1D versus T2D. Underlying pathogenic mechanisms regarding aggressive nature of youth-onset T2D is less understood. Further research is essential to devise novel drug targets and treatment approaches to minimize the devastating effects of youth onset T2D.

---

13. Effect of Proteinuria on the Rapid Kidney Function Decline in Chronic Kidney Disease Depends on the Underlying Disease: A Post Hoc Analysis of the BRIGHTEN Study

Ref: Gohda T, Murakoshi M, Suzuki Y, Kagimura T, Wada T, Narita I. Effect of proteinuria on the rapid kidney function decline in chronic kidney disease depends on the underlying disease: A post hoc analysis of the BRIGHTEN study. Diabetes Res Clin Pract. 2024;212:111682.

ABSTRACT

Goals: Especially in individuals with severe chronic kidney disease, it is unknown if proteinuria has an equal impact on the rapid deterioration of kidney function in diabetic kidney disease (DKD), non-DKD with diabetes (NDKD + DM), and nephrosclerosis without diabetes (NS–DM).

Methods: The current study comprised 1,038 individuals with chronic renal disease who took part in the BRIGHTEN study. The anticipated yearly reduction in glomerular filtration rate for each illness group was calculated using a linear mixed effect model.

Results: Compared to the NDKD + DM (27.9%) and NS–DM (27.0%) groups, the DKD group had a substantially greater prevalence of rapid decliners (rapid kidney function decline, defined as an eGFR loss of > 5 mL/min/1.73 m^2/year) (44.6%). In contrast, the DKD and NS–DM groups had the same prevalence of rapid decliners in the various urine total protein to creatinine ratio (UPCR) categories (<0.5, 0.5 to <1.0, 1.0 to <3.5, and ≥3.5 g/g). Furthermore, the NS–DM group's rapid decliners had a UPCR < 1.0 g/g prevalence that was more than twice as high as that of the DKD and NDKD + DM groups.

Conclusion: NS–DM patients with minimal proteinuria may be at more risk than first thought for a rapid deterioration in kidney function.

CRITICAL APPRAISAL

What was Known Prior to this Study?

Some of the previous studies have shown that nephrosclerosis (NS) has favorable outcome than diabetic kidney disease (DKD). It is also observed that non-DKD with diabetes (NDKD + DM) was associated with a better end-stage kidney disease (ESKD)-free survival compared with DKD. Higher albuminuria/proteinuria was reported to be associated with a steep estimated glomerular filtration rate (eGFR) decline or poor kidney outcome in both DKD and NS. Hunsicker et al. demonstrated that several factors such as higher arterial blood pressure, lower serum high-density lipoprotein cholesterol, and greater urinary proteinuria were associated with a rapid decline in the eGFR in CKD patients. Relative risk for the rate of decline in the eGFR or the rapid kidney function decline according to the proteinuria categories among DKD, NS without diabetes (NS–DM), and NDKD + DM have not been fully evaluated. To address this issue, this post hoc analysis of BRIGHTEN study was planned.

What this Study Adds?

- Kidney prognosis in NS–DM patients with a low level of proteinuria (0.5–1.0 g/g) may be worse than originally assumed.
- The effect of the urine total protein to creatinine ratio (UPCR) on rapid kidney function decline was comparable between the DKD and NS–DM groups if the UPCR category was the same.
- Rapid kidney function decline may be different and greater in NS–DM patients with low levels of proteinuria (0.5–1.0 g/g) compared with DKD or NDKD + DM patients with the same level of proteinuria.
- Approximately 30% of patients with a UPCR ≥ 3.5 g/g did not develop a rapid kidney function decline in the present study, indicating that proteinuria alone does not necessarily predict rapid kidney function decline.

Major Strength

- Previous studies have not fully evaluated the relative risk for the rate of decline in the eGFR (i.e., eGFR slope) or the rapid kidney function decline according to the proteinuria categories among DKD, NS–DM, and NDKD + DM, particularly in advanced CKD patients.
- To reduce misclassification between DKD and NS, NS–DM has been included separately.

Limitations

- Subtypes of glomerulonephritis and duration of diabetes were also almost unknown.
- To reduce misclassification between DKD and NS, this study has included NS–DM.
- NDKD includes a variety of kidney diseases rather than being a single disease.
- Only Japanese population were enrolled, and the mean eGFR in the study patients was 20.3 mL/min/1.73 m^2. Therefore, the results may not apply to other races.

Clinical Implications

- Prevalence of rapid decliners in the DKD group was much higher than that in the

NDKD + DM group, which highlights the importance of classifying these two diseases separately.
- Rate of an eGFR recovery of >0 mL/min/1.73 m²/year was significantly fewer in the DKD group as compared with the NDKD + DM and NS–DM groups, which indicates that once the eGFR begins to decline in patients with DKD, kidney function is less likely to recover than in those with NDKD + DM or NS–DM.
- Relatively low level of proteinuria of up to 0.5 g/g should be treated more aggressively in patients with NS–DM, because they are more likely to experience a rapid eGFR decline at low levels of proteinuria than patients with DKD or NDKD + DM.

Knowledge Gaps and Scope for Future Research

Further investigation is needed to determine the reason behind more rapid decline of eGFR in NS–DM, even if their proteinuria level is low than patients with DKD or NDKD + DM. Other biomarkers, such as circulating tumor necrosis factor receptors (TNFRs—TNFR1 and TNFR2) and kidney injury molecule-1 should be studied, which can predict rapid kidney function decline in CKD independent of the UPCR. Further investigation is necessary to determine whether the results of this study apply to CKD patients without anemia or those at earlier CKD stages (GFR 30–60 mL/min/1.73 m²).

14. Editorials: Diabetic Kidney Disease—Semaglutide Flows into the Mainstream

Ref: Herrington WG, Haynes R. Editorials: Diabetic Kidney Disease—Semaglutide Flows into the Mainstream. N Engl J Med. 2024;391(2):178-9.

ABSTRACT

In type 2 diabetes with chronic kidney disease (CKD), glucagon-like peptide 1 (GLP-1) receptor agonists are advised for blood sugar management. These agents also offer cardiovascular (CV) advantages and some reduction in albuminuria. The FLOW trial aimed to evaluate if semaglutide could decrease the risk of kidney failure and CV events in individuals with type 2 diabetes and CKD.

For this study, CKD was characterized by an estimated glomerular filtration rate (eGFR) of 50–75 mL/min/1.73 m² of body surface area with a urinary albumin to creatinine ratio (ACR) of >300 and <5,000, or an eGFR of 25 to <50 mL/min/1.73 m² with a urinary ACR of >100 and <5,000. The trial involved 3,533 participants with CKD, randomly allocated to receive either subcutaneous semaglutide (n = 1,767) or placebo (n = 1,766). The primary outcome was a composite of kidney failure, a sustained eGFR reduction of at least 50% from baseline, or death from kidney-related or CV causes.

During a median follow-up of 3.4 years, semaglutide demonstrated a 24% lower risk of primary outcome events compared to placebo. Secondary outcomes also favored semaglutide: The mean annual eGFR decline was 1.16 mL/min/1.73 m² less in the semaglutide group, the risk of major CV events was 18% lower (hazard ratio 0.82; 95% CI 0.68–0.98), and the risk of all-cause mortality was 20% lower (hazard ratio 0.80; 95% CI 0.67–0.95). The incidence of adverse events was also lower in the semaglutide group compared to placebo (49.6% vs. 53.8%).

In conclusion, the study found that semaglutide decreased the risk of clinically significant kidney outcomes and CV-related deaths in patients with type 2 diabetes and chronic kidney disease.

CRITICAL APPRAISAL

What was Known Prior to this Study?

As per ADA–KDIGO (American Diabetes Association–Kidney Disease: Improving Global Outcomes) consensus 2022, glucagon-like peptide 1 receptor agonist (GLP-1 RA) is advised in type 2 diabetes with chronic kidney disease (CKD) in addition to metformin and sodium-glucose cotransporter-2 inhibitor (SGLT-2i), if glycemic control is not achieved. Previous randomized controlled trials (RCTs) with cardiovascular (CV) outcomes like LEADER, SUSTAIN-6, REWIND have shown added benefits in the form of reduction of albuminuria as secondary outcomes.

However, patients with more advanced CKD have been underrepresented in previous trials, and the effect of GLP-1 RA on albuminuria reduction has not yet been shown to translate into a reduced risk of kidney failure. Possible mechanism behind this renal benefit is multifactorial. Intrinsic kidney and immune cells contain the GLP-1 receptor, and it is postulated that GLP-1 RAs reduce cellular expression of proinflammatory and profibrotic mediators.

What this Study Adds?

- There is lack of dedicated trials addressing clinically important kidney outcomes, such as kidney failure or a substantial decline in the eGFR.
- The reduction in the urinary albumin to creatinine ratio (ACR) ratio caused by semaglutide suggests that the drug does target glomerular dysfunction.
- As 95% of the FLOW participants were already on renin–angiotensin system inhibitor (RASi), it can be concluded from FLOW trial that the benefits of semaglutide went beyond those conferred by use of a RASi.
- Also 16% of the FLOW participants were already receiving SGLT-2i.
- FLOW trial also assessed eGFR slope, which is distinct from that of RASi, SGLT-2i, and finerenone. All the three medications cause a clear acute "dip" in eGFR on initiation, followed by a slowing of the decline in the eGFR over the long term, in contrast in the FLOW trial, semaglutide did not result in a difference in eGFR from placebo at 12 weeks, and then the eGFR slopes diverged.

Major Strength

The trial included large population and provides clear conclusions about benefits and risks of using semaglutide in type 2 diabetes with CKD patients. This study was not only designed for kidney failure outcomes, but it also assessed major CV events and death from any cause.

Limitations

- SGLT-2i and nonsteroidal mineralocorticoid receptor antagonists (MRAs) had not been approved for kidney protection when FLOW trial initiated. Therefore, the number of participants who were receiving these agents at baseline was modest, which limited the ability to assess the effects of combination therapy.
- The trial was also not adequately powered to detect differences within and between important subgroups. The trial was not powered to separately detect effects on kidney failure as well.
- Most participants were from white population, whereas kidney disease disproportionately affects especially Black and Indigenous population. So, the effects on kidney function may not be generalizable to other populations, such as those at lower risk.

Clinical Implications

Benefits observed in the FLOW trial, reflect the important clinical effects on kidney, cardiovascular, and survival outcomes among high-risk patients with a reassuring safety findings, and support a therapeutic role for semaglutide in this population. After the conclusion of FLOW trial, semaglutide should emerge as a first-line treatment for patients with type 2 diabetes with CKD and albuminuria in near future and hopefully it can mitigate the risk of CKD progression.

Knowledge Gaps and Scope for Future Research

In future, large renoprotection trials of GLP-1 RAs for patients without diabetes are much needed, as well as for persons with diabetes and minimal or modest albuminuria. No conclusion can be drawn from the FLOW trial regarding application of combination therapy (GLP-1 RA and SGLT-2i), as statistical power of this analysis was limited. Further analyses of these data are planned, and studies assessing approaches to combination therapy should be a priority.

---

15. A Phase 2 Randomized Trial of Survodutide in MASH and Fibrosis

Ref: A Phase 2 Randomized Trial of Survodutide in MASH and Fibrosis. N Engl J Med. 2024;391(4):311-9.

ABSTRACT

Background: For the treatment of metabolic dysfunction-associated steatohepatitis (MASH), dual agonism of the glucagon receptor and glucagon-like peptide 1 (GLP-1) receptor may be more beneficial than GLP-1 receptor agonism alone. It is unknown if survodutide, a dual agonist of the glucagon and GLP-1 receptors, is safe and effective for those with MASH with liver fibrosis.

Methods: Adults with biopsy-confirmed MASH with fibrosis stages F1 through F3 were randomized in a 1:1:1:1 ratio to receive once-weekly subcutaneous injections of survodutide at a dose of 2.4, 4.8, or 6.0 mg or a placebo in this 48-week phase 2 trial.

A 24-week rapid-dose-escalation phase and a 24-week maintenance phase comprised the trial's two stages. Histologic improvement (reduction) in MASH with no worsening of fibrosis was the main outcome. A minimum 30% reduction in liver fat content and a minimum one-stage improvement (reduction) in fibrosis as determined by biopsy were secondary endpoints.

Results: A minimum of one dosage of either survodutide or a placebo was administered to 293 randomly allocated subjects. In contrast to 14% of participants in the placebo group, 47% of participants in the survodutide 2.4-mg group, 62% of participants in the 4.8-mg group, and 43% of participants in the 6.0-mg group experienced improvement in MASH with no worsening of fibrosis ($p < 0.001$ for the quadratic dose–response curve as bestfitting model).

63% of participants in the survodutide 2.4-mg group, 67% of those in the 4.8-mg group, 57% of those in the 6.0-mg group, and 14% of those in the placebo group experienced a decrease in liver fat content of at least 30%. 34%, 36%, 34%, and 22% of participants experienced an improvement in fibrosis by at least one stage, respectively. Serious side events occurred in 8% of cases with survodutide and 7% of cases with a placebo; nausea (66% vs. 23%), diarrhea (49% vs. 23%), and vomiting (41% vs. 4%) were more common with survodutide than with a placebo.

Conclusion: In terms of improving MASH without exacerbating fibrosis, survodutide outperformed a placebo, which calls for additional research in phase 3 studies (Boehringer Ingelheim funded it; 1404-0043) ClinicalTrials.gov number, NCT04771273; EudraCT number, 2020-002723-11).

CRITICAL APPRAISAL

What was Known Prior to this Study?

Dual agonism of glucagon receptor and glucagon-like peptide 1 (GLP-1) receptor may confer clinical advantages over GLP-1 receptor monoagonist pharmacotherapies for MASH (metabolic dysfunction-associated steatohepatitis). In a phase 2 trial, treatment with the GLP-1 receptor monoagonist semaglutide resulted in a significantly higher percentage of patients with MASH resolution than placebo. Cotadutide, a once-daily glucagon receptor and GLP-1 receptor dual agonist, improved the nonalcoholic fatty liver disease (NAFLD) fibrosis score and levels of ALT, AST, and propeptide of type III collagen. The selective thyroid hormone receptor beta agonist resmetirom gained conditional approval from the Food and Drug Administration as the first pharmacotherapy for MASH with moderate-to-advanced liver fibrosis. In a phase 3 trial, resmetirom was superior to placebo in MASH resolution and improvement in fibrosis.

Survodutide is a dual agonist of glucagon receptor and GLP-1 receptor that is derived from glucagon and administered once weekly. In a phase 2 trial with obesity or overweight, survodutide treatment led to significant dose-dependent weight loss as compared with placebo.

What this Study Adds?

- Survodutide was superior to placebo with respect to improvement in MASH without worsening of fibrosis.
- Trial discontinuation due to adverse events occurred in 20% of the participants across all survodutide doses (with 16% due to gastrointestinal events).

Major Strength

- A screening biopsy was performed within 6 months before randomization and used as a baseline for histologic variables.
- Baseline and end-of-treatment values were derived from one central pathologist.

Limitations

- Relatively smaller sample size
- Relatively short duration of follow-up (48 weeks)

Clinical Implications

This finding supports the use of survodutide as a treatment for patients with MASH and liver fibrosis.

Knowledge Gaps and Scope for Future Research

This is a phase 2 study warranting further investigation in phase 3 trials. Larger and longer trials are needed to further assess the efficacy and safety of survodutide.

16. Tirzepatide for Metabolic Dysfunction–associated Steatohepatitis with Liver Fibrosis

Ref: Loomba R, Hartman ML, Lawitz EJ, Vuppalanchi R, Boursier J, Bugianesi E, et al.; SYNERGY-NASH Investigators. Tirzepatide for Metabolic Dysfunction–Associated Steatohepatitis with Liver Fibrosis. N Engl J Med. 2024;391(4):299-310.

ABSTRACT

History: The progressive liver condition known as metabolic dysfunction-associated steatohepatitis (MASH) is linked to complications and even mortality. In individuals with MASH with moderate or severe fibrosis, it is unknown if tirzepatide, an agonist of the glucose-dependent insulinotropic polypeptide (GIP) and glucagon-like peptide 1 (GLP-1) receptors, is safe and effective.

Methods: We recruited people with biopsy-confirmed MASH and stage F2 or F3 (moderate or severe) fibrosis for a phase 2, dose-finding, multicenter, double-blind, randomized, placebo-controlled study. For 52 weeks, participants were randomized to receive either a placebo or once-weekly subcutaneous tirzepatide (5 mg, 10 mg, or 15 mg). At 52 weeks, the main outcome was the remission of MASH without a worsening of fibrosis. An improvement (reduction) of at least one fibrosis stage without a deterioration of MASH was a crucial secondary end aim.

Findings: Of the 190 randomly assigned subjects, 157 had possible liver biopsy findings at week 52, with missing data imputed based on the hypothesis that the results would be similar to those in the placebo group. 10% of participants in the placebo group, 44% in the 5-mg tirzepatide group [difference vs. placebo, 34 percentage points; 95% confidence interval (CI) 17–50], 56% in the 10-mg tirzepatide group (difference, 46 percentage points; 95% CI 29–62), and 62% in the 15-mg tirzepatide group (difference, 53 percentage points; 95% CI 37–69) met the criteria for resolution of MASH without worsening of fibrosis ($p < 0.001$ for all three comparisons).

30% of participants in the placebo group, 55% in the 5-mg tirzepatide group (difference vs. placebo, 25 percentage points; 95% CI 5–46), 51% in the 10-mg tirzepatide group (difference, 22 percentage points; 95% CI 1–42), and 51% in the 15-mg tirzepatide group (difference, 21 percentage points; 95% CI 1–42) experienced an improvement of at least one fibrosis stage without worsening of MASH. Gastrointestinal problems were the most frequent adverse events in the tirzepatide groups, and the majority were mild to severe in severity.

Conclusion: In this phase 2 trial, tirzepatide medication for 52 weeks was more successful than a placebo in resolving MASH without exacerbating fibrosis in participants with MASH and moderate or severe fibrosis. To further evaluate tirzepatide's safety and effectiveness in treating MASH, larger and longer trials are required (SYNERGY-NASH ClinicalTrials.gov number: NCT04166773; funded by Eli Lilly).

CRITICAL APPRAISAL

What was Known Prior to this Study?

More than 10% weight loss has been seen to associated with higher incidences of resolution of MASH and regression of liver fibrosis. In previous studies, glucagon-like peptide 1 (GLP-1) receptor agonists have been shown to be efficacious for the resolution of metabolic dysfunction-associated steatohepatitis (MASH) but not for regression of fibrosis. Tirzepatide, a once-weekly glucose-dependent insulinotropic polypeptide (GIP) and GLP-1 receptor agonist, has been shown to cause substantial weight reduction in previous trials in type 2 diabetes mellitus with obesity. Previously in type 2 diabetes mellitus, tirzepatide resulted in a reduction in liver fat and improvement in biomarkers of MASH and fibrosis. Addition of GIP receptor to GLP-1 receptor agonism increases the degree of weight reduction as well as may have direct effects on white adipose tissue that may benefit patients with MASH. In subcutaneous white adipose tissue, GIP receptor activation increases blood flow, augmenting postprandial triglyceride uptake and improves insulin sensitivity. This study has been designed to assess the efficacy of tirzepatide in biopsy-confirmed MASH and moderate or severe fibrosis.

What this Study Adds?

- Previous trials have shown substantial reductions in body weight and liver fat with tirzepatide therapy; in addition this trial used histologic assessments to show that treatment with tirzepatide led to a higher incidence of MASH resolution.
- Tirzepatide treatment was associated with regression in fibrosis, the nonalcoholic fatty liver disease (NAFLD) activity score, and the subscores for the individual components of the NAFLD activity score, including steatosis, lobular inflammation, and hepatocellular ballooning.
- Changes were also observed in body weight; in blood markers of liver injury, including serum alanine transaminase (ALT), aspartate transaminase (AST),

gamma-glutamyl transferase (GGT), and cytokeratin 18; and in biomarkers of liver fat, inflammation, and fibrosis such as liver fat content, liver stiffness, the Pro-C3 level and the score on the Enhanced Liver Fibrosis test in participants receiving tirzepatide.
- The safety profile of tirzepatide in this trial involving persons with MASH was consistent with that observed in previous phase 3 clinical trials involving persons with type 2 diabetes mellitus and obesity.
- The incidence of nausea and diarrhea was higher in both the placebo group and the tirzepatide groups of the current trial than in the SURPASS-1 trial and the SURMOUNT-1 trial.
- There were no reports of drug-induced liver injury or pancreatitis in this trial with tirzepatide.

Major Strength
- The trial included adequate numbers of persons with and persons without type 2 diabetes mellitus.
- Liver biopsy results were evaluated in a blinded manner by two expert liver pathologists.
- The histologic inclusion criteria and endpoints have been endorsed by both the Food and Drug Administration and the European Medicines Agency.

Limitations
- Sample size was small, which did not provide adequate statistical power to evaluate the effect of tirzepatide on fibrosis.
- Trial duration was too short to assess the effect of tirzepatide on major adverse liver outcomes.
- The trial did not assess the safety and efficacy of tirzepatide in patients with MASH that had progressed to cirrhosis.
- The trial had good representation of Asian and Hispanic persons, but persons of African and Indian descent were underrepresented.

Clinical Implications
This study showed that tirzepatide can be used for resolution of MASH without worsening of fibrosis in addition to weight loss without increased risk of serious adverse events.

Knowledge Gaps and Scope for Future Research
As the study duration was short in this trial, larger and longer trials are needed to further assess the efficacy and safety of tirzepatide for the treatment of MASH. Treatment periods of longer than 52–72 weeks will help to show substantial treatment effects on fibrosis with pharmacologic agents that induce and maintain weight reduction.

17. Effects of Semaglutide on Chronic Kidney Disease in Patients with Type 2 Diabetes

Ref: Perkovic V, Tuttle KR, Rossing P, Mahaffey KW, Mann JFE, Bakris G, et al.; FLOW Trial Committees and Investigators. Effects of Semaglutide on Chronic Kidney Disease in Patients with Type 2 Diabetes. N Engl J Med. 2024;391(2):109-21.

ABSTRACT

Background: Individuals with chronic renal disease and type 2 diabetes are at a heightened risk of mortality, cardiovascular (CV) events, and kidney failure. It is unknown if semaglutide medication might lessen these risks.

Methods: Patients with type 2 diabetes and chronic kidney disease (CKD) [defined as having an estimated glomerular filtration rate (eGFR) of 50–75 mL/min/1.73 m² of body surface area and a urinary albumin-to-creatinine ratio (with albumin measured in milligrams and creatinine measured in grams) of >300 and <5,000 or an eGFR of 25 to <50 mL/min/1.73 m² and a urinary albumin-to-creatinine ratio of >100 and <5,000] were randomly assigned to receive subcutaneous semaglutide at a weekly dose of 1.0 mg or a placebo.

Major renal disease events, a composite of the start of kidney failure (dialysis, transplantation, or an eGFR of <15 mL/min/1.73 m^2), at least a 50% decrease in the baseline eGFR, or death from CV or kidney-related causes were the main outcomes. Hierarchical testing was done on predetermined confirmatory secondary outcomes.

Results: The median follow-up for the 3,533 randomly assigned individuals (1,767 in the semaglutide group and 1,766 in the placebo group) was 3.4 years following the recommendation to terminate the study early at a predetermined interim analysis.

Compared to the placebo group, the semaglutide group had a 24% decreased chance of a primary-outcome event [331 vs. 410 first events; hazard ratio 0.76; 95% confidence interval (CI) 0.66–0.88; $p = 0.0003$]. The findings were comparable for death from CV causes (hazard ratio 0.71; 95% CI 0.56–0.89) and a composite of the kidney-specific components of the primary outcome (hazard ratio 0.79; 95% CI 0.66–0.94).

Semaglutide was preferred by the results for all confirmatory secondary outcomes: The risk of major CV events was 18% lower (hazard ratio 0.82; 95% CI 0.68–0.98; $p = 0.029$), the risk of death from any cause was 20% lower (hazard ratio 0.80; 95% CI 0.67–0.95, $p = 0.01$), and the mean annual eGFR slope was less steep (indicating a slower decrease) by 1.16 mL/min/1.73 m^2 in the semaglutide group ($p < 0.001$). Compared to the placebo group, fewer patients in the semaglutide group experienced serious adverse events (49.6% vs. 53.8%).

Conclusion: In patients with type 2 diabetes and chronic renal disease, semaglutide decreased the risk of CV death and clinically significant kidney outcomes (Novo Nordisk provided funding for FLOW ClinicalTrials.gov number, NCT03819153).

CRITICAL APPRAISAL

What was Known Prior to this Study?

Type 2 diabetes is one of the leading causes of chronic kidney disease (CKD). A previous systematic review and meta-analysis reported that glucagon-like peptide 1 receptor agonists (GLP-1 RAs) significantly reduced the risk of major adverse cardiovascular events (MACE) and the individual components of MACE, and the risk of all-cause death, hospitalization for heart failure, and a composite kidney disease outcome. In ADA–KDIGO (American Diabetes Association–Kidney Disease: Improving Global Outcomes) consensus 2022, it is mentioned that GLP-1 RA is advised in type 2 diabetes with CKD in addition to metformin and sodium-glucose cotransporter-2 inhibitor (SGLT-2i), if glycemic control is not achieved. Previous randomized controlled trials (RCTs) with cardiovascular (CV) outcomes like LEADER, SUSTAIN-6, and REWIND have shown added benefits in the form of reduction of albuminuria as secondary outcomes. Previous dedicated trials addressing clinically important kidney outcomes, such as kidney failure or a substantial decline in the estimated glomerular filtration rate (eGFR), have been lacking. Also, there are uncertainties related to the effects of GLP-1 RAs on CV and kidney disease outcomes in people without diabetes. Therefore, this FLOW trial has been designed as primary kidney outcome trials with injectable semaglutide.

Semaglutide acts on intrinsic kidney and immune cells which express GLP-1 receptor, and thereby it reduces cellular expression of proinflammatory and profibrotic mediators.

What this Study Adds?

- Semaglutide at a dose of 1.0 mg once weekly significantly reduced the risk of major kidney disease events (the primary outcome) by 24%.
- Semaglutide also reduced the risk of major CV events and death from any cause.

Semaglutide also slows down the annual loss of kidney function by a mean of 1.16 mL/min/1.73 m².

Major Strength

- The trial was large and meticulous which provides clear conclusions about benefits and risks of semaglutide in type 2 diabetes and CKD.

Limitations

- SGLT-2i and nonsteroidal mineralocorticoid receptor antagonists (MRAs) had not been approved for kidney protection at the time the trial was initiated. Therefore, effects of GLP-1 RA over and above SGLT-2i have not been clearly identified.
- Most participants participated in the study belonged to White, whereas kidney disease disproportionately affects marginalized populations, especially Black.

Clinical Implications

- As the effect of semaglutide in reducing kidney disease progression is substantial, clinicians and patients need to consider the order and priority of use for semaglutide in CKD.
- Combination therapy is likely to be a part standard of care in near future, and we found no clear heterogeneity of effect among patients receiving SGLT-2i at baseline as compared with those who were not.

Knowledge Gaps and Scope for Future Research

Combination therapy with SGLT-2i and GLP-1 RA can become the standard of care in type 2 diabetes and CKD in near future. The statistical power of this analysis was limited. Therefore, a larger prospective RCT must be conducted to come to a conclusion regarding this.

18. Effect of SGLT2 Inhibitors on Heart Failure Outcomes and Cardiovascular Death Across the Cardiometabolic Disease Spectrum: A Systematic Review and Meta-analysis

Ref: Usman MS, Bhatt DL, Hameed I, Anker SD, Cheng AYY, Hernandez AF, et al. Effect of SGLT2 inhibitors on heart failure outcomes and cardiovascular death across the cardiometabolic disease spectrum: a systematic review and meta-analysis. Lancet Diabetes Endocrinol. 2024;12(7):447-61.

ABSTRACT

Context: Patients with heart failure, type 2 diabetes, chronic renal disease, atherosclerotic cardiovascular disease, and acute myocardial infarction have all been examined with sodium-glucose cotransporter-2 inhibitors (SGLT-2i). To examine composite outcomes in a single illness state, individual trials were powered. Our goal was to assess how SGLT-2i affected certain clinical outcomes in a variety of disease and demographic subgroups.

Techniques: In order to conduct primary and secondary analyses of large trials ($n > 1,000$) of SGLT-2i in patients with heart failure, type 2 diabetes, chronic kidney disease, and atherosclerotic cardiovascular disease (including acute myocardial infarction), we searched online databases (PubMed, Cochrane CENTRAL, and SCOPUS) through February 10, 2024.

All-cause mortality, total (first and recurring) hospitalization for heart failure, cardiovascular death, first hospitalization for heart failure, and the composite of first hospitalization for heart failure or cardiovascular death were among the outcomes examined. Random-effects models were used to pool effect sizes. The PROSPERO registration number for this study is CRD42024513836.

Results: Fifteen trials (n = 100,952) were included. In patients with heart failure {hazard ratio (HR) 0.71 [95% confidence interval (CI) 0.67–0.77]}, type 2 diabetes [0.72 (0.67–0.77)], chronic kidney disease [0.68 (0.61–0.77)], and atherosclerotic cardiovascular disease [0.72 (0.66–0.79)], SGLT-2i decreased the risk of first hospitalization for heart failure by 29%, 28%, and 32%, respectively, when compared to a placebo.

In patients with heart failure [HR 0.86 (95% CI 0.79–0.93)], type 2 diabetes [0.85 (0.79–0.91)], chronic kidney disease [0.89 (0.82–0.96)], and atherosclerotic cardiovascular disease [0.87 (0.78–0.97)], SGLT-2i decreased cardiovascular death by 14%, 11%, and 13%, respectively. In most of the 51 subgroups that were examined, the advantage of SGLT-2i on both initial hospitalization for heart failure and cardiovascular death was constant. Heart failure with intact ejection fraction (26% reduction in first hospitalization for heart failure; no effect on cardiovascular mortality) and acute myocardial infarction (22% reduction in first hospitalization for heart failure; no effect on cardiovascular death) featured notable exceptions.

Interpretation: Patients with heart failure, type 2 diabetes, chronic renal disease, and atherosclerotic cardiovascular disease saw fewer heart failure episodes and cardiovascular deaths when taking SGLT-2i. Within these populations, similar impacts held true for a large number of subgroups. This demonstrates that SGLT-2i can be used to treat a sizable population with cardiorenal–metabolic disorders.

CRITICAL APPRAISAL

What was Known Prior to this Study?

Sodium-glucose cotransporter-2 inhibitors (SGLT-2i) are largely known for their cardiovascular and renal benefit. Postulated mechanisms of SGLT-2i are lowering of blood pressure, increasing the hematocrit, and improving endothelial function, decreasing arterial stiffness, and are associated with favorable cardiac remodeling, mediated by the anti-inflammatory effects and by attenuation of NLRP3 inflammasome. Oxidative stress is another feature of heart failure, chronic kidney disease, type 2 diabetes, and atherosclerotic cardiovascular disease, which can be prevented by production of reactive oxygen species (ROS).

The EMPA REG OUTCOME is the CVOT trial for empagliflozin, which demonstrated a 35% decline in hospitalization for heart failure. Almost similar findings were observed with canagliflozin in CANVAS trial and with dapagliflozin in DECLARE TIMI trial. The DAPA-MI trial enrolled 4,017 patients with acute myocardial infarction without previous type 2 diabetes or chronic heart failure. After approximately 1 year of treatment with dapagliflozin, there were significant benefits with regard to improvement in cardiometabolic outcomes but no impact on the composite of cardiovascular death or hospitalization for heart failure compared with placebo. The EMPACT-MI trial enrolled a similar population (n = 6,522). Empagliflozin did not lead to a significantly lower risk of a first hospitalization for heart failure or death from any cause than placebo.

What this Study Adds?

- This study showed that SGLT-2i reduced the risk of first hospitalization for heart failure by 29% in patients with heart failure, 28% in patients with type 2 diabetes, 32% in patients with chronic kidney disease, and 28% in patients with atherosclerotic cardiovascular disease.
- The findings were consistent when subgroups with different demographics and combinations of diseases were analyzed separately.

Major Strength

Fifteen large-scale trials encompassing over 100,000 patients were included in this meta-analysis.

Limitations

- Each trial was powered to study composite outcomes in the overall population. Therefore, the effect of SGLT-2i on individual endpoints and especially cardiovascular death, was not powered.

- Although each trial represents a particular disease state, most patients have multiple long-term conditions.
- Despite a random effect model, certain methodological differences among the trials might limit interpretation (e.g., variations in the SGLT-2i used, differences in background therapy).
- Publication bias was indicated by Egger's regression test, which was probably due to the decision to exclude smaller studies.
- Data for some subgroup analyses were not available in all trials and their secondary analyses.

Clinical Implications

According to this data, there is need for widespread adoption of SGLT-2i in patients with heart failure, type 2 diabetes, chronic kidney disease, and atherosclerotic cardiovascular disease.

Knowledge Gaps and Scope for Future Research

There is a need for longer and larger prospective trials with different SGLT-2i, as the shorter follow-up can limit the ability to robustly assess cardiovascular death outcomes independently.

REFERENCES (Complications)

1. Gregg EW, Cheng YJ, Srinivasan M, Lin J, Geiss LS, Albright AL, et al. Trends in cause-specific mortality among adults with and without diagnosed diabetes in the USA: an epidemiological analysis of linked national survey and vital statistics data. Lancet. 2018;391:2430-40.
2. Pearson-Stuttard J, Bennett J, Cheng YJ, Vamos EP, Cross AJ, Ezzati M, et al. Trends in predominant causes of death in individuals with and without diabetes in England from 2001 to 2018: an epidemiological analysis of linked primary care records. Lancet Diabetes Endocrinol. 2021;9:165-73.
3. ElSayed NA, Aleppo G, Aroda VR, Bannuru RR, Brown NM, Bruemmer D, et al.; American Diabetes Association. 10. Cardiovascular disease and risk management: Standards of Care in Diabetes—2023. Diabetes Care. 2023;46(Suppl 1):S158-S190.
4. Chung YR, Ha KH, Lee K, Kim DJ. Effects of sodium glucose cotransporter-2 inhibitors and dipeptidyl peptidase-4 inhibitors on diabetic retinopathy and its progression: a real world Korean study. PLoS One. 2019;14(10):e0224549.
5. Cho EH, Park SJ, Han S, Song JH, Lee K, Chung YR. Potent oral hypoglycemic agents for microvascular complication: sodium glucose cotransporter 2 inhibitors for diabetic retinopathy. J Diabetes Res. 2018;2018:6807219.
6. Lin TY, Kang EY, Shao SC, Lai EC, Garg SJ, Chen KJ, et al. Risk of diabetic retinopathy between sodium-glucose cotransporter-2 inhibitors and glucagon-like peptide-1 receptor agonists. Diabetes Metab J. 2023;47:394-40.
7. Marso SP, Bain SC, Consoli A, Eliaschewitz FG, Jódar E, Leiter LA, et al.; SUSTAIN-6 Investigators. Semaglutide and cardiovascular outcomes in patients with type 2 diabetes. N Engl J Med. 2016;375(19):1834-44.
8. Marso SP, Daniels GH, Brown-Frandsen K, Kristensen P, Mann JF, Nauck MA, et al.; LEADER Steering Committee; LEADER Trial Investigators. Liraglutide and cardiovascular outcomes in type 2 diabetes. N Engl J Med. 2016;375(4):311-22.
9. Gaborit B, Julla JB, Besbes S, Proust M, Vincentelli C, Alos B, et al. Glucagon-like peptide 1 receptor agonists, diabetic retinopathy and angiogenesis: the AngioSafe type 2 diabetes study. J Clin Endocrinol Metab. 2020;105(4):e1549-60.
10. Heerspink HJL, Oshima M, Zhang H, Li J, Agarwal R, Capuano G, et al. Canagliflozin and Kidney-Related Adverse Events in Type 2 Diabetes and CKD: Findings From the Randomized CREDENCE Trial. Am J Kidney Dis. 2022;79(2):244-256.e1.
11. Wheeler DC, Stefánsson BV, Jongs N, Chertow GM, Greene T, Hou FF, et al.; DAPA-CKD Trial Committees and Investigators. Effects of dapagliflozin on major adverse kidney and cardiovascular events in patients with diabetic and non-diabetic chronic kidney disease: a prespecified analysis from the DAPA-CKD trial. Lancet Diabetes Endocrinol. 2021;9(1):22-31.
12. EMPA-KIDNEY Collaborative Group. Impact of primary kidney disease on the effects of empagliflozin in patients with chronic kidney disease: secondary analyses of the EMPA-KIDNEY trial. Lancet Diabetes Endocrinol. 2024;12(1):51-60.
13. Gerstein HC, Colhoun HM, Dagenais GR, Diaz R, Lakshmanan M, Pais P, et al.; REWIND Investigators. Dulaglutide and cardiovascular outcomes in type 2 diabetes (REWIND): a double-blind, randomised placebo-controlled trial. Lancet. 2019;394(10193):121-30.
14. Gragnano F, De Sio V, Calabrò P. FLOW trial stopped early due to evidence of renal protection with semaglutide. Eur Heart J Cardiovasc Pharmacother. 2024;10(1):7-9.
15. Frías JP, Guja C, Hardy E, Ahmed A, Dong F, Öhman P, et al. Exenatide once weekly plus dapagliflozin once daily versus exenatide or dapagliflozin alone in patients with type 2 diabetes inadequately controlled with metformin monotherapy (DURATION-8): a 28 week, multicentre, double-blind, phase 3, randomised controlled trial. Lancet Diabetes Endocrinol. 2016;4(12):1004-16.

16. Zinman B, Bhosekar V, Busch R, Holst I, Ludvik B, Thielke D, et al. Semaglutide once weekly as add-on to SGLT-2 inhibitor therapy in type 2 diabetes (SUSTAIN 9): a randomised, placebo-controlled trial. Lancet Diabetes Endocrinol. 2019;7(5):356-67.
17. Venketasubramanian N, Yoon BW, Pandian J, Navarro JC. Stroke epidemiology in south, east, and South-East Asia: a review. J Stroke. 2017;19(3):286-94.
18. Chen R, Ovbiagele B, Feng W. Diabetes and stroke: epidemiology, pathophysiology, pharmaceuticals and outcomes. Am J Med Sci. 2016;351(4):380-6.
19. Zinman B, Wanner C, Lachin JM, Fitchett D, Bluhmki E, Hantel S, et al.; EMPA-REG OUTCOME Investigators. Empagliflozin, cardiovascular outcomes, and mortality in type 2 diabetes. N Engl J Med. 2015;373(22):2117-28.
20. Anker SD, Butler J, Filippatos G, Ferreira JP, Bocchi E, Böhm M, et al.; EMPEROR-Preserved Trial Investigators. Empagliflozin in heart failure with a preserved ejection fraction. NEngl J Med. 2021;385(16):1451-61.
21. Neal B, Perkovic V, Mahaffey KW, de Zeeuw D, Fulcher G, Erondu N, et al.; CANVAS Program Collaborative Group. Canagliflozin and cardiovascular and renal events in type 2 diabetes. N Engl J Med. 2017;377(7):644-57.
22. Wiviott SD, Raz I, Bonaca MP, Mosenzon O, Kato ET, Cahn A, et al.; DECLARE–TIMI 58 Investigators. Dapagliflozin and cardiovascular outcomes in type 2 diabetes. N Engl J Med. 2019;380(4):347-57.
23. Crawley WT, Jungels CG, Stenmark KR, Fini MA. U-shaped association of uric acid to overall-cause mortality and its impact on clinical management of hyperuricemia. Redox Biol. 2022;51:102271.
24. Dominguez Rieg JA, Xue J, Rieg T. Tubular effects of sodium–glucose cotransporter 2 inhibitors: intended and unintended consequences. Curr Opin Nephrol Hypertens. 2020;29(5):523-30.
25. Zhao Y, Xu L, Tian D, Xia P, Zheng H, Wang L, et al. Effects of sodium-glucose co-transporter 2 (SGLT2) inhibitors on serum uric acid level: A meta-analysis of randomized controlled trials. Diabetes Obes Metab. 2018;20(2):458-62.
26. Hu X, Yang Y, Hu X, Jia X, Liu H, Wei M, et al. Effects of sodium-glucose cotransporter 2 inhibitors on serum uric acid in patients with type 2 diabetes mellitus: a systematic review and network meta-analysis. Diabetes Obes Metab. 2022;24(2):228-38.
27. Matthews DR, Li Q, Perkovic V, Mahaffey KW, de Zeeuw D, Fulcher G, et al. Effects of canagliflozin in amputation risk in type 2 diabetes: the CANVAS program. Diabetologia. 2019;62(6):926-38.
28. Wiviott SD, Raz I, Bonaca MP, Mosenzon O, Kato ET, Cahn A, et al.; DECLARE–TIMI 58 Investigators. Dapagliflozin and cardiovascular outcomes in type 2 diabetes. N Engl J Med. 2019;380:347-57.
29. American Diabetes Association. 10. Cardiovascular Disease and Risk Management: Standards of Medical Care in Diabetes—2019. Diabetes Care. 2019;42(Supplement_1):S103-S123.
30. ASCEND Study Collaborative Group, Bowman L, Mafham M, et al. Effects of aspirin for primary prevention in persons with diabetes mellitus. N Engl J Med. 2018;379(16):1529-39.
31. Arnett DK, Blumenthal RS, Albert MA, Buroker AB, Goldberger ZD, Hahn EJ, et al. 2019 ACC/AHA guideline on the primary prevention of cardiovascular disease: a report of the American College of Cardiology/American Heart Association Task Force on clinical practice guidelines. Circulation. 2019;140(11):e596-e646.
32. Visseren FLJ, Mach F, Smulders YM, Carballo D, Koskinas KC, Bäck M, et al.; ESC Scientific Document Group. 2021 ESC guidelines on cardiovascular disease prevention in clinical practice: developed by the task Force for cardiovascular disease prevention in clinical practice with representatives of the European Society of Cardiology and 12 medical societies with the special contribution of the European Association of Preventive Cardiology (EAPC). Eur Heart J. 2021;42(34):3227-337.
33. Belch J, MacCuish A, Campbell I, Cobbe S, Taylor R, Prescott R, et al.; Prevention of Progression of Arterial Disease and Diabetes Study Group; Diabetes Registry Group; Royal College of Physicians Edinburgh. The prevention of progression of arterial disease and diabetes (POPADAD) trial: factorial randomised placebo controlled trial of aspirin and antioxidants in patients with diabetes and asymptomatic peripheral arterial disease. BMJ. 2008;337:a1840.
34. Zheng SL, Roddick AJ. Association of aspirin use for primary prevention with cardiovascular events and bleeding events: a systematic review and meta-analysis. JAMA. 2019;321(3):277-87.
35. Waeber B, de la Sierra A, Ruilope LM. The ADVANCE trial: clarifying the role of perindopril/indapamide fixed-dose combination in the reduction of cardiovascular and renal events in patients with diabetes mellitus. Am J Cardiovasc Drugs. 2009;9(5):283-91.
36. Intensive blood-glucose control with sulphonylureas or insulin compared with conventional treatment and risk of complications in patients with type 2 diabetes (UKPDS 33). UK Prospective Diabetes Study (UKPDS) Group. Lancet. 1998 Sep 12;352(9131):837-53. Erratum in: Lancet 1999;354(9178):602.
37. Yeboah J, Byington B, Bertoni A. Association between mean systolic blood pressure and cardiovascular outcomes in diabetes mellitus: ACCORD trial. J Hum Hypertens. 2018;32(2):167-9.
38. Control Group; Turnbull FM, Abraira C, Anderson RJ, Byington RP, Chalmers JP, Duckworth WC, et al. Intensive glucose control and macrovascular outcomes in type 2 diabetes. Diabetologia. 2009;52(11):2288-98.
39. Gæde P, Oellgaard J, Carstensen B, Rossing P, Lund-Andersen H, Parving HH, et al. Years of life gained by multifactorial intervention in patients with type 2 diabetes mellitus and microalbuminuria: 21 years follow-up on the Steno-2 randomised trial. Diabetologia. 2016;59(11):2298-307.
40. Ceriello A, Ihnat MA, Thorpe JE. Clinical review 2: the "metabolic memory": is more than just tight glucose control necessary to prevent diabetic complications? J Clin Endocrinol Metab. 2009;94(2):410-5.

41. Bethel MA, Diaz R, Castellana N, Bhattacharya I, Gerstein HC, Lakshmanan MC. HbA1c change and diabetic retinopathy during GLP-1 receptor agonist cardiovascular outcome trials: a meta-analysis and meta-regression. Diabetes Care. 2021;44(1):290-6.
42. Astor BC, Matsushita K, Gansevoort RT, van der Velde M, Woodward M, Levey AS, et al. Lower estimated glomerular filtration rate and higher albuminuria are associated with mortality and end-stage renal disease. A collaborative meta-analysis of kidney disease population cohorts. Kidney Int. 2011;79(12):1331-40.
43. Mogensen CE. Microalbuminuria predicts clinical proteinuria and early mortality in maturity-onset diabetes. N Engl J Med. 1984;310(6):356-60.
44. Gerstein HC, Mann JF, Yi Q, Zinman B, Dinneen SF, Hoogwerf B, et al.; HOPE Study Investigators. Albuminuria and risk of cardiovascular events, death, and heart failure in diabetic and nondiabetic individuals. JAMA. 2001;286(4):421-6.
45. Klausen K, Borch-Johnsen K, Feldt-Rasmussen B, Jensen G, Clausen P, Scharling H, et al. Very low levels of microalbuminuria are associated with increased risk of coronary heart disease and death independently of renal function, hyper tension, and diabetes. Circulation. 2004;110(1):32-5.
46. Writing Group for the CKD Prognosis Consortium; Grams ME, Coresh J, Matsushita K, Ballew SH, Sang Y, Surapaneni A, et al. Estimated glomerular filtration rate, albuminuria, and adverse outcomes: an individual-participant data meta-analysis. JAMA. 2023;330(13):1266-77.
47. Gansevoort RT, Matsushita K, van der Velde M, Astor BC, Woodward M, Levey AS, et al.; Chronic Kidney Disease Prognosis Consortium. Lower estimated GFR and higher albuminuria are associated with adverse kidney outcomes. A collaborative meta-analysis of general and high-risk population cohorts. Kidney Int. 2011;80(1):93-104.
48. Kidney Disease: Improving Global Outcomes (KDIGO) Diabetes Work Group. KDIGO 2022 Clinical Practice Guideline for Diabetes Management in Chronic Kidney Disease. Kidney Int. 2022;102(5S):S1-S127.
49. Wagenknecht LE, Lawrence JM, Isom S, Jensen ET, Dabelea D, Liese AD, et al.; SEARCH for Diabetes in Youth study. Trends in incidence of youth-onset type 1 and type 2 diabetes in the USA, 2002–18: results from the population-based SEARCH for diabetes in youth study. Lancet Diabetes Endocrinol. 2023;11:242-50.
50. Luk AO, Lau ES, So WY, Ma RC, Kong AP, Ozaki R, et al. Prospective study on the incidences of cardiovascular-renal complications in Chinese patients with young- onset type 1 and type 2 diabetes. Diabetes Care. 2014;37:149-57.
51. TODAY Study Group; Bjornstad P, Drews KL, Caprio S, Gubitosi-Klug R, Nathan DM, Tesfaldet B, et al. Long-term complications in youth-onset type 2 diabetes. N Engl J Med. 2021;385:416-26.
52. Bai P, Barkmeier AJ, Hodge DO, Mohney BG. Ocular sequelae in a population-based cohort of youth diagnosed with diabetes during a 50-year period. JAMA Ophthalmol. 2022;140:51-7.
53. Furuichi K, Shimizu M, Okada H, Narita I, Wada T. Clinico-pathological features of kidney disease in diabetic cases. Clin Exp Nephrol. 2018;22:1046-51.
54. Ovrehus MA, Oldereid TS, Dadfar A, Bjorneklett R, Aasarod KI, Fogo AB, et al. Clinical phenotypes and long-term prognosis in white patients with biopsy-verified hypertensive nephrosclerosis. Kidney Int Rep. 2020;5:339-47.
55. Hamano T, Imaizumi T, Hasegawa T, Fujii N, Komaba H, Ando M, et al. Biopsy-proven CKD etiology and outcomes: the Chronic Kidney Disease Japan Cohort (CKD-JAC) study. Nephrol Dial Transplant. 2023;38:384-95.
56. Sumida K, Kovesdy CP. Disease Trajectories Before ESRD: Implications for Clinical Management. Semin Nephrol. 2017;37:132-43.
57. Hunsicker LG, Adler S, Caggiula A, England BK, Greene T, Kusek JW, et al. Predictors of the progression of renal disease in the Modification of Diet in Renal Disease Study. Kidney Int. 1997;51:1908-19.
58. de Boer IH, Khunti K, Sadusky T, Tuttle KR, Neumiller JJ, Rhee CM, et al. Diabetes Management in Chronic Kidney Disease: A Consensus Report by the American Diabetes Association (ADA) and Kidney Disease: Improving Global Outcomes (KDIGO). Diabetes Care. 2022;45(12):3075-90.
59. Alicic RZ, Cox EJ, Neumiller JJ, Tuttle KR. Incretin drugs in diabetic kidney disease: biological mechanisms and clinical evidence. Nat Rev Nephrol. 2021;17:227-44.
60. Tuttle KR, Wilson JM, Lin Y, Qian HR, Genovese F, Karsdal MA, et al. Indicators of kidney fibrosis in patients with type 2 diabetes and chronic kidney disease treated with dulaglutide. Am J Nephrol. 2023;54:74-82.
61. Newsome PN, Buchholtz K, Cusi K, Linder M, Okanoue T, Ratziu V, et al.; NN9931-4296 Investigators. A placebo-controlled trial of subcutaneous semaglutide in nonalcoholic steatohepatitis. N Engl J Med. 2021;384:1113-24.
62. Pocai A, Carrington PE, Adams JR, Wright M, Eiermann G, Zhu L, et al. Glucagon-like peptide 1/glucagon receptor dual agonism reverses obesity in mice. Diabetes. 2009;58:2258-66.
63. Harrison SA, Bashir MR, Guy CD, Zhou R, Moylan CA, Frias JP, et al. Resmetirom (MGL-3196) for the treatment of non-alcoholic steatohepatitis: a multicentre, randomised, double-blind, placebo-controlled, phase 2 trial. Lancet. 2019;394(10213):2012-24.
64. le Roux CW, Steen O, Lucas KJ, Startseva E, Unseld A, Hennige AM. Glucagon and GLP-1 receptor dual agonist survodutide for obesity: a randomised, double-blind, placebo-controlled, dose finding phase 2 trial. Lancet Diabetes Endocrinol. 2024;12:162-73.
65. Verrastro O, Panunzi S, Castagneto-Gissey L, De Gaetano A, Lembo E, Capristo E, et al. Bariatric-metabolic surgery versus lifestyle intervention plus best medical care in non-alcoholic steatohepatitis (BRAVES): a multicentre, open-label, randomised trial. Lancet. 2023;401:1786-97.
66. Armstrong MJ, Gaunt P, Aithal GP, Barton D, Hull D, Parker R, et al. Liraglutide safety and efficacy in patients with non-alcoholic steatohepatitis (LEAN): a multicentre, double-blind, randomised, placebo-controlled phase 2 study. Lancet. 2016;387:679-90.

67. Rosenstock J, Wysham C, Frías JP, Kaneko S, Lee CJ, Fernández Landó L, et al. Efficacy and safety of a novel dual GIP and GLP-1 receptor agonist tirzepatide in patients with type 2 diabetes (SURPASS-1): a double-blind, randomised, phase 3 trial. Lancet. 2021;398:143-55.
68. Garvey WT, Frias JP, Jastreboff AM, le Roux CW, Sattar N, Aizenberg D, et al.; SURMOUNT-2 investigators. Tirzepatide once weekly for the treatment of obesity in people with type 2 diabetes (SURMOUNT-2): a double-blind, randomised, multicentre, placebo-controlled, phase 3 trial. Lancet. 2023;402:613-26.
69. Hartman ML, Sanyal AJ, Loomba R, Wilson JM, Nikooienejad A, Bray R, et al. Effects of novel dual GIP and GLP-1 receptor agonist tirzepatide on biomarkers of nonalcoholic steatohepatitis in patients with type 2 diabetes. Diabetes Care. 2020;43:1352-5.
70. Samms RJ, Coghlan MP, Sloop KW. How may GIP enhance the therapeutic efficacy of GLP-1? Trends Endocrinol Metab. 2020;31:410-21.
71. Badve SV, Bilal A, Lee MMY, Sattar N, Gerstein HC, Ruff CT, et al. Effects of GLP-1 receptor agonists on kidney and cardiovascular disease outcomes: a meta-analysis of randomised controlled trials. Lancet Diabetes Endocrinol. 2025;13:15-28.
72. Juni RP, Al-Shama R, Kuster DWD, van der Velden J, Hamer HM, Vervloet MG, et al. Empagliflozin restores chronic kidney disease-induced impairment of endothelial regulation of cardiomyocyte relaxation and contraction. Kidney Int. 2021;99:1088-101.
73. Uthman L, Baartscheer A, Bleijlevens B, Schumacher CA, Fiolet JWT, Koeman A, et al. Class effects of SGLT2 inhibitors in mouse cardiomyocytes and hearts: inhibition of Na+/H+ exchanger, lowering of cytosolic Na+ and vasodilation. Diabetologia. 2018;61:722-6.
74. Mosenzon O, Wiviott SD, Heerspink HJL, Dwyer JP, Cahn A, Goodrich EL, et al. The Effect of Dapagliflozin on Albuminuria in DECLARE-TIMI 58. Diabetes Care. 2021;44(8):1805-15.
75. Peikert A, Vaduganathan M. Sodium Glucose Co-Transporter 2 Inhibition Following Acute Myocardial Infarction: The DAPA-MI and EMPACT-MI Trials. JACC Heart Fail. 2024;12(5):949-53.

Section 5: TYPE 1 DIABETES MELLITUS

Section Editor: Mainak Banerjee

1. Disparities in Continuous Glucose Monitor Use between Children with Type 1 Diabetes Living in Urban and Rural Areas

Ref: Tilden DR, French B, Datye KA, Jaser SS. Disparities in Continuous Glucose Monitor Use Between Children with Type 1 Diabetes Living in Urban and Rural Areas. Diabetes Care. 2024;47(3):346-52.

ABSTRACT

Objective: Although there is evidence linking the use of continuous glucose monitoring (CGM) to a lower hemoglobin A1c (HbA1c) in children with type 1 diabetes, the adoption of this technology is still lower among people who have trouble accessing healthcare, such as members of racial and ethnic minorities and those from lower socioeconomic backgrounds. The purpose of this study was to investigate how rural location affects the usage of CGM technology to inform decisions made by patients and providers.

Design and methods of research: In this retrospective study of electronic health record demographic and visits data from a single diabetes program from 1 January 2018 through 31 December 2021, we compared the odds of completing a visit with (+) and without (−) CGM interpretation between rural and urban commuting area (RUCA) designations.

Results: We found that children living in small rural towns had 31% lower odds [6.3% of CGM+ visits, 8.6% of CGM2 visits; adjusted odds ratio (aOR) 0.69, 95% CI 0.51–0.94] and children living in isolated rural towns had 49% lower odds (2.0% of CGM+ visits, 3.4% of CGM2 visits; aOR 0.51, 95% CI 0.28–0.92) of completing a CGM-billed clinic visit compared to those living in urban areas (70.0% of CGM+ visits, 67.2% of CGM2 visits). These findings were based on 13,645 visits completed by 2,008 patients with type 1 diabetes younger than the age of 18 years. Significant variations in CGM-billed visits by neighborhood deprivation, race/ethnicity, and insurance payor were also discovered.

Conclusion: For individuals with type 1 diabetes, geographic location poses a significant obstacle to receiving care. To improve the care of these patients, more work is required to identify and address the needs of rural families and children.

CRITICAL APPRAISAL

What was Known Prior to this Study?

Prior to this study, it was established that continuous glucose monitoring (CGM) use is associated with lower hemoglobin A1c (HbA1c) levels among children with type 1 diabetes. However, prior research indicated that uptake of CGM technology was lower among populations facing access barriers, particularly those from lower socioeconomic backgrounds and racial or ethnic minorities. Previous evaluations of CGM use among children and adolescents primarily relied on medical records or prescriptions, which did not accurately reflect actual device usage due to various barriers such as cost and stigma.

What this Study Adds?

This study enhances understanding of CGM use among pediatric patients with type 1 diabetes by examining the association between geographic location (rural vs. urban) and CGM usage rates. It reveals that children living in rural areas, particularly small and isolated towns, have significantly lower odds of completing visits with CGM data compared to their urban counterparts. The study uses CGM billing codes as the primary outcome, which more accurately captures real-world device usage and the barriers faced by these populations.

Major Strengths of the Study

- The study encompasses a large dataset from a single diabetes program that spans both urban and rural settings, improving the generalizability of the findings.
- The reliance on CGM billing codes ensures that the data reflects actual device usage rather than mere prescription rates, addressing previous methodological weaknesses.
- The study identifies the impact of socioeconomic factors and geographic location on CGM usage, contributing to the understanding of health disparities in diabetes care.
- It provides insights into the unique challenges faced by rural populations, highlighting the need for targeted interventions.

Limitations of the Study

- It is retrospective, which may introduce biases related to the data collection process.
- The dataset includes demographic information only from the end of the study period, potentially overlooking changes in patient location or migration patterns.
- The study spans the coronavirus disease 2019 (COVID-19) pandemic, which may have influenced diabetes care delivery and access, complicating the interpretation of results.
- It does not account for the variability in healthcare access and technology use outside the studied population.

Implications of the Finding for the Clinicians

The findings suggest that clinicians should be aware of the geographic disparities in CGM use among pediatric patients with type 1 diabetes. Understanding that rural and socioeconomically disadvantaged populations face unique barriers can inform clinical practices and guide the development of tailored interventions. Clinicians may need to advocate for improved access to diabetes technologies and support systems in rural areas to enhance patient outcomes.

Knowledge Gaps Identified and Scope for Future Research

The study highlights the need for further research into specific barriers faced by rural populations in accessing diabetes technology and healthcare. Future studies could explore:
- The effectiveness of interventions aimed at increasing CGM adoption in rural settings.
- The long-term impact of geographic and socioeconomic factors on diabetes management outcomes.
- The role of telemedicine and digital health solutions in bridging care gaps for rural patients.
- A comparative analysis of CGM outcomes across diverse populations to identify the best practices.

2. Longitudinal Assessment of Pancreas Volume by MRI Predicts Progression to Stage 3 Type 1 Diabetes

Ref: Virostko J, Wright JJ, Williams JM, Hilmes MA, Triolo TM, Broncucia H, et al. Longitudinal Assessment of Pancreas Volume by MRI Predicts Progression to Stage 3 Type 1 Diabetes. Diabetes Care. 2024;47(3):393-400.

ABSTRACT

Objective: In order to predict the progression of people with multiple diabetes-related autoantibodies to stage 3 type 1 diabetes (T1D), this multicenter prospective cohort study compared pancreas volume as determined by magnetic resonance imaging (MRI), metabolic scores obtained from oral glucose tolerance testing (OGTT), and a combination of pancreas volume and metabolic scores.

Research design and methods: A total of 65 individuals with various autoantibodies who were recruited in the type 1 diabetes TrialNet pathway to prevention project had pancreas MRIs. The Diabetes Prevention Trial–Type 1 Risk Score (DPTRS), the OGTT-derived Index60 score, the pancreatic volume index (PVI), and a combination of PVI and DPTRS were used to predict the progression to stage 3 T1D.

Results: A total of 11 patients who went on to advance to stage 3 T1D had significantly different PVI, Index60, and DPTRS at study entry than did the 54 participants who did not ($p < 0.005$). Metabolic tests did not connect with PVI among study subjects. In the 11 patients with stage 3 T1D, PVI decreased over time, but Index60 and DPTRS rose. When using measures at study entrance to predict progression to stage 3, the area under the receiver operating characteristic curve was 0.76 for PVI, 0.79 for Index60, 0.79 for DPTRS, and 0.91 for PVI plus DPTRS.

Conclusion: The results of this study indicate that measurements of pancreatic volume and metabolism represent distinct aspects of the risk of stage 3 type 1 diabetes, and that a combination of both measurements may offer a more accurate prediction than each one alone.

CRITICAL APPRAISAL

What was Known Prior to this Study?

Before this study, it was established that smaller pancreas size is associated with type 1 diabetes (T1D). Previous MRI studies indicated that smaller pancreas size could be detected at the onset of T1D and in autoantibody-positive individuals at risk for progression. However, the correlation between pancreas size and the progression to stage 3 T1D had not been thoroughly explored, leaving a gap in understanding how pancreas imaging could enhance predictions of T1D progression.

What this Study Adds?

This study demonstrates that small pancreas volume can predict faster progression to stage 3 T1D, indicating that pancreas imaging provides distinct information compared to traditional metabolic testing methods. The research introduces a prediction model combining both pancreas volume measurements and metabolic tests, which outperformed either method used alone. This suggests a novel approach to risk assessment in individuals with early-stage T1D.

Major Strengths of the Study

The study's strengths include:
- Use of longitudinal MRI assessments to track pancreas volume changes
- Inclusion of a well-defined cohort with multiple diabetes-associated autoantibodies
- Development of a prediction model integrating MRI and metabolic measures
- Demonstration that pancreas volume and metabolic measures reflect different disease aspects
- Potential for improving participant retention with a quicker and less invasive MRI procedure compared to traditional glucose tolerance testing

Limitations of the Study

- The cost and convenience of MRI may restrict its applicability as a widespread screening tool.
- Participants who progressed to stage 3 T1D had longer median follow-up times, which may introduce bias.
- The study sample size, while adequate, may limit the generalizability of the findings.

- MRI's inability to correlate pancreas volume directly with metabolic measures could indicate oversimplification of disease mechanisms.

Implications of the Findings for Clinicians

The findings suggest that clinicians could incorporate pancreas imaging as a predictive tool in monitoring patients at risk for T1D progression. This could enhance early interventions during the presymptomatic stages of the disease. Additionally, the study underscores the need for integrating MRI assessments into therapeutic trials aimed at delaying or preventing the onset of stage 3 T1D.

Knowledge Gaps Identified and Scope for Future Research

Future research could focus on:
- Expanding the cohort size and diversity to enhance generalizability
- Investigating the underlying mechanisms linking pancreas size and progression to T1D
- Exploring the utility of MRI in broader populations at risk, including various age groups and genetic backgrounds
- Assessing the long-term outcomes of using pancreas imaging in clinical practice for T1D management
- Developing standardized protocols for MRI usage in routine clinical settings

3. Low-dose Antithymocyte Globulin: A Pragmatic Approach to Treating Stage 2 Type 1 Diabetes

Ref: Foster TP, Jacobsen LM, Bruggeman B, Salmon C, Hosford J, Chen A, et al. Low-Dose Antithymocyte Globulin: A Pragmatic Approach to Treating Stage 2 Type 1 Diabetes. Diabetes Care. 2024;47(2):285-9.

ABSTRACT

Objective: In new-onset stage 3 type 1 diabetes, low-dose antithymocyte globulin (ATG) (2.5 mg/kg) lowers HbA1c and preserves C-peptide; however, its ability to postpone the progression from stage 2 to stage 3 has not been assessed.

Research design and methods: Off-label, low-dose ATG was administered to six children ($n = 6$) with stage 2 type 1 diabetes, ages 5–14. For 18–48 months, HbA1c, C-peptide, continuous glucose monitoring, insulin needs, and adverse effects were monitored.

Results: Three participants (50%) acquired stage 3 diabetes within 1–2 months of medication, while three subjects remained free of the disease after 1.5, 3, and 4 years of follow-up. At 18 months after treatment, even disease progressors showed robust C-peptide 90 minutes after mixed meal (1.3 ng/dL, 2.3 ng/dL, and 1.4 ng/dL), time in range (93%, 88%, and 98%), low insulin requirements (0.17, 0.18, and 0.34 units/kg/day), and near-normal HbA1c [5.1% (32 mmol/mol), 5.6% (38 mmol/mol), and 5.3% (34 mmol/mol)].

Conclusion: These findings provide credence to further prospective research assessing ATG in type 1 diabetic patients in stage 2.

CRITICAL APPRAISAL

What was Known Prior to this Study?

Prior to this study, it was established that low-dose antithymocyte globulin (ATG) at a dosage of 2.5 mg/kg was effective in preserving C-peptide levels and reducing HbA1c in patients with new-onset stage 3 type 1 diabetes. However, its efficacy in delaying the progression from stage 2 to 3 diabetes had not been evaluated. Teplizumab was the only immunotherapeutic with demonstrated capacity to delay progression from stage 2 to 3 on a large scale, although multiple immunotherapeutics had shown potential for preserving C-peptide in later stages.

What this Study Adds?

This study contributes new evidence regarding the use of off-label low-dose ATG in children with stage 2 type 1 diabetes. It reports that 50% of the participants remained diabetes-free for 1.5–4 years post-treatment, indicating that low-dose ATG may be beneficial in delaying the progression to stage 3 diabetes. Furthermore, even those who progressed maintained favorable metabolic profiles and low insulin requirements.

Major Strengths of the Study

- It explores an innovative treatment approach for a high-risk population.
- It provides long-term follow-up data (18–48 months) for patients receiving low-dose ATG.
- The findings indicate that half of the treated children maintained near-normal metabolic markers.
- It reports real-world clinical outcomes, reflecting pragmatic use of ATG.
- The cohort was small but focused, allowing for detailed individual follow-up.
- The study highlights the economic and logistical advantages of low-dose ATG treatment.
- It opens avenues for further research into combination therapies and patient responsiveness.
- Acknowledges the need for more extensive, powered studies to validate findings.

Limitations of the Study

Several limitations were identified in this study:
- The sample size was small ($n = 6$), limiting the statistical power and generalizability of the findings.
- It lacked a control group, which makes it difficult to draw definitive conclusions about the efficacy of low-dose ATG.
- The observational nature of the study means results may be influenced by confounding variables.
- The treatment was off-label, raising ethical considerations regarding its application without comprehensive prior evidence.
- Follow-up duration varied among participants, complicating the assessment of long-term effects.

Implications of the Finding for the Clinicians

The findings suggest that clinicians may consider low-dose ATG as a potential therapeutic option for managing stage 2 type 1 diabetes in children, particularly for those at high risk of progression. The study supports the need for careful patient selection and monitoring, as well as consideration of the treatment's economic and logistical feasibility. Clinicians should remain cautious given the off-label status and aim to integrate findings into broader clinical trials.

Knowledge Gaps Identified and Scope for Future Research

- There is need for larger, randomized controlled trials to confirm the efficacy of low-dose ATG in delaying progression from stage 2 to 3 diabetes.
- Research should explore which specific patient populations are most responsive to ATG therapy.
- Investigations into the mechanisms of action and potential side effects of low-dose ATG are warranted.
- Future studies could examine the combination of ATG with other therapies to enhance treatment efficacy.
- There is a need to assess long-term safety and outcomes beyond the initial follow-up periods.

4. Exploring Factors that Influence Postexercise Glycemia in Youth with Type 1 Diabetes in the Real World: The Type 1 Diabetes Exercise Initiative Pediatric (T1DEXIP) Study

Ref: Sherr JL, Bergford S, Gal RL, Clements MA, Patton SR, Calhoun P, et al. Exploring Factors That Influence Postexercise Glycemia in Youth with Type 1 Diabetes in the Real World: The Type 1 Diabetes Exercise Initiative Pediatric (T1DEXIP) Study. Diabetes Care. 2024;47(5):849-57.

ABSTRACT

Objective: Data from the Type 1 Diabetes Exercise Initiative Pediatric (T1DEXIP) study were evaluated to look at variables that might affect glycemia in order to investigate 24-hour postexercise glycemia and hypoglycemia risk.

Research design and methods: This was an observational study conducted in the real world, and participants self-reported their food intake, insulin dosage, and physical activity (they were multiple day injectors). We gathered heart rate, accessible pump data, and continuous glucose data.

Results: A total of 3,319 activities were recorded over ~10 days by 251 teenagers (42% female), with a mean ± SD age of 14 ± 2 years and a hemoglobin A1c (HbA1c) of 7.1 ± 1.3% (54 ± 14.2 mmol/mol). Those with shorter illness duration and lower HbA1c showed trends toward lower mean glucose after exercise; no difference by insulin administration mechanism was found. Greater glucose declines during exercise, immediately following activity ($p < 0.001$), and 12–16 hours later ($p = 0.02$) were associated with lower postexercise mean glucose levels. 14% of nights after exercise had hypoglycemia, compared to 12% after days of inactivity. More hypoglycemia happened on nights after exercise on days with longer individual exercise sessions and on days with an average total activity of $60 minutes per day (17% vs. 8% of nights, $p = 0.01$). Individuals with a longer history of the condition, a lower HbA1c, traditional pump use, and a period below range of ≥4% during the previous 24 hours also had higher incidence of nocturnal hypoglycemia.

Conclusion: Nights with higher average activity durations had increased rates of nocturnal hypoglycemia in this extensive real-world pediatric exercise investigation. In order to effectively support exercise in young people with diabetes, it may be possible to design new guidelines, decision support tools, and improved insulin delivery algorithms by characterizing participant and event-level characteristics that affect glucose throughout the postexercise recovery phase.

CRITICAL APPRAISAL

What was Known Prior to this Study?

Prior to this study, existing research primarily focused on the physiological effects of exercise in controlled environments rather than the real-world impacts on glycemia for youth with type 1 diabetes. Studies indicated that exercise could lead to hypoglycemia post-activity, but the specific dynamics of physical activity in everyday settings, including variations in exercise type, intensity, and timing, were not well understood. Additionally, there was limited insight into how different insulin delivery methods affected glycemic responses during recovery from exercise.

What this Study Adds?

This study adds significant real-world data on the impact of various types of physical activity on post-exercise glycemia in youth with type 1 diabetes. It collected information from 3,319 exercise sessions over 10 days, providing insights into the frequency and types of activities engaged in by participants. The findings highlight the potential for hybrid closed-loop (HCL) therapy to mitigate post-exercise dysglycemia and document the actual experiences of adolescents managing their diabetes during typical daily activities, emphasizing the variability in responses based on individual circumstances.

Major Strengths of the Study

- Extensive data collection from 3,319 exercise sessions
- Inclusion of a diverse range of physical activities
- Utilization of real-world scenarios instead of controlled laboratory settings
- Evaluation of multiple insulin delivery modalities (HCL and MDI)
- Insight into the post-exercise recovery period concerning glycemia
- Analysis of both participant-level and exercise event-level factors influencing glycemic responses.
- Contribution to understanding the relationship between exercise and hypoglycemia risk.
- A focus on youth aged 12–17, filling a gap in pediatric diabetes research.

Limitations of the Study

- The cohort predominantly consisted of White non-Hispanic participants, limiting generalizability.
- Participants were required to have a minimum activity level, excluding less active individuals.
- Data on behavioral modifications (insulin adjustments and carbohydrate intake) were collected only after the study, not in real-time.
- The lack of objective measures for exercise intensity may affect the accuracy of the findings.
- Relatively low rates of hypoglycemia in the participant group may not represent all youth with diabetes.
- Family dynamics and support systems were not assessed, which could influence outcomes.

Implications of the Finding for the Clinicians

Clinicians can utilize the findings to better advise youth with type 1 diabetes on managing their glucose levels during and after physical activity. Understanding that HCL therapy may help prevent post-exercise dysglycemia allows healthcare providers to tailor recommendations based on individual activity patterns. The study underscores the importance of monitoring glycemic responses in real-life settings, encouraging proactive adjustments in insulin delivery and carbohydrate intake during physical activities.

Knowledge Gaps Identified and Scope for Future Research?

The study identifies several knowledge gaps, including the need for further exploration of the intersection between family dynamics, insulin delivery methods, and behavioral strategies in managing diabetes during physical activity. Future research should aim to include a more diverse population, investigate the effects of varying exercise intensities, and examine the long-term impacts of physical activity on glycemic control in youth with type 1 diabetes. Additionally, real-time data collection on behavioral modifications during exercise could enhance understanding of effective management strategies.

5. A Randomized Comparison of Postprandial Glucose Excursion Using Inhaled Insulin versus Rapid-acting Analog Insulin in Adults with Type 1 Diabetes Using Multiple Daily Injections of Insulin or Automated Insulin Delivery

Ref: Hirsch IB, Beck RW, Marak MC, Calhoun P, Mottalib A, Salhin A, et al. A Randomized Comparison of Postprandial Glucose Excursion Using Inhaled Insulin Versus Rapid-Acting Analog Insulin in Adults With Type 1 Diabetes Using Multiple Daily Injections of Insulin or Automated Insulin Delivery. Diabetes Care. 2024;47(9):1682-7.

ABSTRACT

Goal: To evaluate the effects of subcutaneous rapid-acting analog (RAA) insulin or inhaled technosphere insulin (TI) on postprandial glucose excursions after a bolus.

Research design and methods: 122 persons with type 1 diabetes who were receiving automated insulin delivery (AID), multiple daily injections (MDI), or a nonautomated pump were randomly assigned to bolus with either TI ($n = 61$) or their regular RAA insulin ($n = 61$) after completing a meal challenge.

Results: TI and RAA had smaller treatment group differences in the area under the curve for glucose >180 mg/dL over 2 hours (adjusted difference –12 mg/dL; 95% CI –22 to –2; $p = 0.02$) for the main outcome. TI resulted in a shorter time to peak glucose ($p = 0.006$), a smaller glucose excursion ($p = 0.01$), and a lower peak glucose ($p = 0.01$). There was one person in each group with blood glucose levels below 70 mg/dL.

Conclusion: In a group comprising both AID and MDI users, post-meal glucose excursion was lower with TI than with RAA insulin.

CRITICAL APPRAISAL

What was Known Prior to this Study?

Prior to this study, it was established that managing postprandial hyperglycemia in individuals with type 1 diabetes is challenging, particularly when using subcutaneous rapid-acting analog (RAA) insulin. Previous research suggested that inhaled insulin [technosphere insulin (TI)] could provide a more effective alternative, potentially allowing for dosing at meal onset rather than before. Earlier studies indicated that TI might lead to reduced glucose excursions compared to RAA insulin, yet the comparative effectiveness was not definitively established in a randomized controlled setting involving both multiple daily injections (MDI) and automated insulin delivery (AID) systems.

What this Study Adds?

This study contributes to the body of knowledge by demonstrating that TI significantly reduces postprandial glucose excursions compared to RAA insulin in adults with type 1 diabetes. Specifically, it showed that the area under the curve for glucose above 180 mg/dL was lower with TI, alongside smaller glucose excursions and a shorter time to peak glucose. The findings support the hypothesis that TI can be an effective alternative for managing post-meal hyperglycemia.

Major Strengths of the Study

- Multicenter randomized trial design enhances the reliability of results.
- Inclusion of diverse subjects utilizing both MDI and AID systems, increasing generalizability.
- Standardized meal protocol ensured consistency in testing conditions.
- Comparison of insulin types under real-world dosing conditions (TI at meal start vs. RAA before meals).

- Robust statistical analysis supporting the validity of findings.
- Demonstration of low occurrence of hypoglycemia events in both treatment groups.

Limitations of the Study
- Lack of continuous glucose monitoring (CGM) data for some participants during the meal challenge, which may affect data completeness.
- Potential variability in individual responses to insulin types is not fully explored due to limited sample size.
- The study did not assess longer-term effects beyond the immediate postprandial period.

Implications of the Finding for the Clinicians

Clinicians may consider incorporating TI as a viable option for patients struggling with postprandial hyperglycemia. The ability to administer TI at the start of meals could simplify insulin management and potentially improve glycemic control. This study encourages healthcare providers to reevaluate insulin regimens, particularly for patients using AID systems, and may lead to more personalized treatment strategies.

Knowledge Gaps Identified and Scope for Future Research
- The long-term effects and safety of TI in various patient populations need further investigation.
- More research is warranted to understand the pharmacodynamic interactions between TI and different insulin delivery systems.
- Future studies could explore patient adherence and satisfaction with inhaled insulin compared to traditional methods.
- Additional investigation is needed to determine the optimal dosing strategies for TI across different meal types and sizes.

6. Comparing the Glycaemic Outcomes between Real-time Continuous Glucose Monitoring (rt-CGM) and Intermittently Scanned Continuous Glucose Monitoring (isCGM) among Adults and Children with Type 1 Diabetes: A Systematic Review and Meta-analysis of Randomised Controlled Trials

Ref: Zhou Y, Sardana D, Kuroko S, Haszard JJ, de Block MI, Weng J, et al. Comparing the glycaemic outcomes between real-time continuous glucose monitoring (rt-CGM) And intermittently scanned continuous glucose monitoring (isCGM) among adults and children with type 1 diabetes: A systematic review and meta-analysis of randomized controlled trials. Diabetic Med. 2024;41(3):e15280.

ABSTRACT

Objective: In order to compare the effects of intermittently scanned continuous glucose monitoring (isCGM) and real-time continuous glucose monitoring (rtCGM) on important glycemic metrics [co-primary outcomes HbA1c and time-in-range (TIR) 70–180 mg/dL, 3.9–10.0 mmol/L] in individuals with type 1 diabetes (T1D), a systematic review and meta-analysis of randomized controlled trials (RCTs) will be carried out.

Methods: We searched the Cochrane Central Register of clinical trials, Medline, PubMed, Scopus, and Web of Science. RCTs, T1D populations of any age and insulin regimen, comparing any kind of rtCGM with isCGM (up until now, only the first generation had been tested), and disclosing the glycemic results were the requirements for inclusion. Following the intervention, glucose results were retrieved and presented as mean differences and 95% confidence intervals between the two comparators. A random-effect meta-analysis was used to aggregate the results. The Cochrane RoB2 tool was used to evaluate the risk of bias. The GRADE method was used to evaluate the quality of the evidence.

Results: Five RCTs with 446 participants (354 adults; 92 children and adolescents) and four parallel and one crossover designs (four with CGM use <8 weeks) satisfied the inclusion criteria. A beneficial effect on time-below-range <70 mg/dL (3.9 mmol/L) was also observed, with rtCGM improving absolute TIR by +7.0% (95% CI 5.8%–8.3%, I2 = 0%, $p < 0.01$) when compared to isCGM, according to the meta-analysis. Regarding HbA1c, there were no variations seen.

Conclusion: This meta-analysis shows that rtCGM is better than isCGM for individuals with T1D, mainly because it raises TIR and improves hypo- and hyperglycemia.

CRITICAL APPRAISAL

What was Known Prior to this Study?

Previous research established that real-time continuous glucose monitoring (rtCGM) and intermittently scanned continuous glucose monitoring (isCGM) are valuable tools for managing type 1 diabetes. However, head-to-head comparisons of their efficacy on glycemic metrics, such as time in range (TIR) and HbA1c, had been limited to individual randomized controlled trials (RCTs). No systematic review or meta-analysis had consolidated these findings to evaluate their overall effectiveness comprehensively.

What this Study Adds?

This systematic review and meta-analysis synthesized data from five RCTs comparing rtCGM and isCGM, involving 446 participants. The findings demonstrated that rtCGM significantly improves TIR (+7.0%) and reduces time in hyperglycemia and hypoglycemia compared to isCGM. These benefits were particularly notable in adults. However, no significant differences were observed in HbA1c reductions between the two technologies.

Major Strengths of the Study

The study's strengths include its rigorous adherence to PRISMA guidelines, the use of the Cochrane RoB2 tool for bias assessment, and the application of the GRADE framework to evaluate evidence quality. The meta-analysis comprehensively analyzed primary and secondary outcomes, offering robust insights into the comparative efficacy of rtCGM and isCGM. The inclusion of both adult and pediatric populations ensured broader applicability of findings.

Limitations of the Study

The meta-analysis was limited by the small number of included studies and participants, reducing statistical power. Heterogeneity in study design, population characteristics, and intervention durations further complicated the interpretation of some outcomes. Additionally, the analysis focused primarily on first-generation isCGM, limiting the relevance of findings for newer device iterations with enhanced features.

Implications of the Finding for Clinicians

The study supports the use of rtCGM over isCGM for optimizing glycemic control in patients with type 1 diabetes, particularly for increasing TIR and minimizing hyperglycemia and hypoglycemia. Clinicians can consider rtCGM as the preferred technology for patients at high risk of glucose excursions. However, the lack of HbA1c differences suggests that rtCGM's advantages are most relevant for immediate glucose management rather than long-term glycemic outcomes.

Knowledge Gaps Identified and Scope for Future Research

Future research should focus on evaluating second- and third-generation isCGM devices to determine if they close the gap in efficacy with rtCGM. Larger, more diverse cohorts are needed to validate findings across different populations and settings. Additionally, studies should explore the cost-effectiveness and patient-reported outcomes associated with these technologies to guide equitable access and reimbursement policies.

7. A First-in-Human, Open-label Phase 1b and a Randomised, Double-blind Phase 2a Clinical Trial in Recent-onset Type 1 Diabetes with AG019 as Monotherapy and in Combination with Teplizumab

Ref: Mathieu C, Wiedeman A, Cerosaletti K, Long SA, Serti E, Cooney L, et al. A first-in-human, open-label Phase 1b and a randomised, double-blind Phase 2a clinical trial in recent-onset type 1 diabetes with AG019 as monotherapy and in combination with teplizumab. Diabetologia. 2024;67(1):27-41.

ABSTRACT

Objectives and hypotheses: We postulated that antigen-specific tolerance in type 1 diabetes would result from the presentation of islet beta cell antigen in the gut in conjunction with a tolerizing cytokine. Oral AG019, food-grade *Lactococcus lactis* bacterium genetically engineered to express human proinsulin and human IL-10, was used as a monotherapy in a parallel open-label Phase 1b research. AG019 was also used in a parallel, randomized, double-blind Phase 2a study in combination with teplizumab.

Techniques: Participants were adults (18–42 years old) and adolescents (12–17 years old) with type 1 diabetes who had been diagnosed within 150 days and had a stimulated peak C-peptide level >0.2 nmol/L and documented evidence of at least one autoantibody. Interactive response technology was used to assign participants to interventions. 42 patients with newly diagnosed type 1 diabetes, ages 12–42, received treatment from us; 24 received open-label Phase 1b monotherapy and 18 received Phase 2a combination therapy. All participants in the Phase 2a study, with the exception of the unblinded statistician and the members of the Data Safety Monitoring Board, were blinded to group assignment following the treatment of the first two open-label subjects. Based on data gathered up to 6 months after the start of treatment, the main objective was safety and tolerability as measured by the frequency of treatment-emergent adverse events. Pharmacokinetics, as determined by the discovery of AG019 in blood and feces, and pharmacodynamic activity were the secondary objectives. Insulin use, HbA1c levels, stimulated C-peptide levels during a mixed meal tolerance test, and antigen-specific CD4+ and CD8+ T cell responses utilizing an activation-induced marker assay and pooled tetramers were among the metabolic and immunological endpoints.

Results: Analysis was done on data from 18 Phase 2a participants and 24 Phase 1b participants. None of the subjects stopped taking AG019 because of treatment-emergent adverse events, and no significant adverse events were documented. There was no evidence of systemic exposure to proinsulin, human IL-10, or AG019 bacteria. Metabolic indicators in individuals treated with AG019 monotherapy were stable for either 6 months (C-peptide, insulin usage) or 12 months (HbA1c) after the start of treatment. All assessed metabolic indicators stabilized or improved in patients receiving AG019/teplizumab combination therapy for up to 12 months, and at 6 months, CD8+ T cells with a partially fatigued phenotype showed a substantial increase. Preproinsulin-specific CD4+ and CD8+ T cells were shown to be circulating both before and after treatment. Following monotherapy or combination therapy, the frequency of preproinsulin-specific CD8+ T cells decreased.

Conclusion/Interpretation: AG019 administered orally was safe and well tolerated both as a stand-alone treatment and in conjunction with teplizumab. AG019 might have other biological effects, such as modifications to preproinsulin-specific T cells, and was not demonstrated to disrupt the safety profile of teplizumab. In type 1 diabetes, these early findings lend support to ongoing research using this medication both by itself and in conjunction with teplizumab or other systemic immunotherapies.

CRITICAL APPRAISAL

What was Known Prior to this Study?

Preclinical data and early trials demonstrated that antigen-specific immune tolerance could be a promising therapeutic approach for type 1 diabetes. *Lactococcus lactis*, genetically engineered to deliver proinsulin and IL-10, had shown efficacy in reversing diabetes in animal models, while teplizumab was known to modulate T cell activity in recent-onset type 1 diabetes. However, the safety and combined effects of AG019 (oral antigen delivery) and teplizumab had not been studied in humans.

What this Study Adds?

This study provides the first human data demonstrating the safety and preliminary efficacy of AG019, both as a monotherapy and in combination with teplizumab. The combination therapy showed improvements in metabolic markers, including stabilization of C-peptide levels and reductions in HbA1c, while also inducing antigen-specific regulatory T cells (Tregs) and reducing autoreactive CD8+ T cells.

Major Strengths of the Study

The study is innovative in its use of a novel antigen-specific immune therapy delivered via the gut, providing a potentially less invasive and more targeted alternative to systemic immunosuppressants. Its design includes both monotherapy and combination therapy arms, allowing for the evaluation of synergistic effects. Safety assessments were thorough, and the study incorporated both metabolic and immunological endpoints, offering insights into the biological mechanisms of action.

Limitations of the Study

The small sample size and limited duration of follow-up restrict the generalizability and robustness of the findings. There was no comparison group for teplizumab monotherapy, limiting the ability to isolate the effects of AG019. The adolescent cohort was underpowered due to enrollment challenges, and functional assays for antigen-specific T cells were not conducted.

Implications of the Finding for Clinicians

The findings suggest that antigen-specific therapies, especially in combination with immune modulators such as teplizumab, could stabilize β-cell function in recent-onset type 1 diabetes. Clinicians may consider such combination therapies as a future strategy for preserving β-cell function and delaying disease progression, particularly in early-stage patients.

Knowledge Gaps Identified and Scope for Future Research

Future studies should explore the long-term safety and efficacy of AG019 and its potential for sustained β-cell preservation. Larger and more diverse cohorts are needed to validate these findings and assess their applicability across different populations. Investigations into the functional activity of induced Tregs and the mechanisms underlying immune tolerance are warranted. Additionally, trials should examine the use of AG019 in earlier stages of type 1 diabetes or in combination with other immune-modulating therapies.

8. Progression of Type 1 Diabetes is Associated with High Levels of Soluble PD-1 in Islet Autoantibody-positive Children

Ref: Bruzzaniti S, Piemonte E, Bruzzese D, Lepore MT, Strollo R, Izzo L, et al. Progression of type 1 diabetes is associated with high levels of soluble PD-1 in islet autoantibody-positive children. Diabetologia. 2024;67(4):714-23.

ABSTRACT

Objectives and hypotheses: The autoimmune disease known as type 1 diabetes is typified by autoreactive T lymphocytes that destroy beta cells in the pancreas. There are certain immunological indicators that can be utilized as target molecules to stop the development of type 1 diabetes, despite the fact that islet autoantibodies (AAb) are a sign of the disease's progression. Although soluble immune checkpoint molecules (sICM) are essential for reducing excessive lymphocyte responses, little is known about how they relate to type 1 diabetes. In order to find molecules linked to the progression of type 1 diabetes, we examined the sICM levels in children who tested positive for AAb (AAb+) in this long-term study.

Techniques: Using sera from two cohorts, we examined the levels of 14 sICM in children with AAb+ ($n = 57$), children with recent-onset type 1 diabetes ($n = 79$), and healthy children ($n = 44$). AAb+ children were monitored and classified according to whether they developed type 1 diabetes (AAbP) or not (AAbNP) (if they did not develop disease in later years and lost islet autoimmunity). In children with AAbP, sICM were also quantified in the sample collected during the visit nearest to the commencement of the condition.

Findings: When compared to children in good health and those with newly diagnosed type 1 diabetes, we discovered that children with AAb+ exhibited a different sICM profile. Furthermore, sICM concentrations were higher in AAb+ children who developed type 1 diabetes (AAbP) than in non-progressors (AAbNP). Additionally, AAbP children's sICM levels dropped around the beginning of the condition. High levels of soluble programmed cell death protein 1 (sPD-1) are linked to the advancement of type 1 diabetes, according to the use of Cox regression models (HR 1.71; 95% CI 1.16, 2.51; $p = 0.007$).

Conclusion and interpretation: In addition to identifying sPD-1 as a pathophysiologically significant molecule linked to the evolution of the illness, this work also uncovers a dysregulated sICM profile during the preclinical stage of type 1 diabetes, suggesting a possible target for early therapies in autoimmune diabetes.

CRITICAL APPRAISAL

What was Known Prior to this Study?

Prior research highlighted the role of islet autoantibodies (AAb) as indicators of type 1 diabetes progression but did not identify specific immune biomarkers for early intervention. Previous studies noted the dysregulation of soluble immune checkpoint molecules (sICM) in autoimmune conditions, suggesting their potential role in type 1 diabetes, although limited exploration of sICM in this context existed.

What this Study Adds?

This study identifies a distinct sICM profile in islet autoantibody-positive (AAb+) children, demonstrating that those who progressed to type 1 diabetes (AAbP) had higher levels of soluble programmed cell death protein 1 (sPD-1) compared to non-progressors (AAbNP). It establishes sPD-1 as a significant biomarker associated with the progression of type 1 diabetes, offering insights into immune mechanisms at the preclinical stage and highlighting a potential target for early intervention.

Major Strengths of the Study

- Utilization of a longitudinal design to track changes in sICM levels over time
- Inclusion of participants from two distinct cohorts, enhancing the robustness of findings
- Identification of a specific biomarker (sPD-1) linked to disease progression
- Application of Cox regression models to provide statistical validation of results
- Comprehensive measurement of 14 different sICM molecules
- Clear distinction between progressors and non-progressors, allowing for focused analysis.
- Contribution to understanding the immune dysregulation involved in type 1 diabetes
- Potential for clinical application in early intervention strategies

Limitations of the Study

- The sample size may limit the generalizability of the findings.
- The study primarily focuses on a specific demographic (children), which may not reflect broader populations.
- The temporal relationship between sICM levels and disease progression needs further exploration.
- Lack of long-term follow-up data beyond the initial disease onset for further validation
- Potential confounding factors in immune response not fully accounted for in the analysis

Implications of the Findings for Clinicians

The identification of sPD-1 as a biomarker for type 1 diabetes progression suggests that clinicians could monitor sICM levels in high-risk populations. This could aid in early diagnosis and intervention strategies, potentially delaying or preventing the onset of type 1 diabetes. Understanding the immune mechanisms involved may also inform future therapeutic approaches targeting autoimmune responses.

Knowledge Gaps Identified and Scope for Future Research

Future research should explore:
- The mechanistic pathways through which sPD-1 influences type 1 diabetes progression.
- The role of other sICM molecules in the disease process
- Longitudinal studies involving larger and more diverse populations to validate findings
- Investigation of potential interventions targeting sPD-1 and other sICM to assess their effectiveness in preventing type 1 diabetes.
- The implications of sICM profiles in adults or other age groups are at risk for type 1 diabetes.

9. Autoimmune Comorbidity in Type 1 Diabetes and its Association with Metabolic Control and Mortality Risk in Young People: A Population-based Study

Ref: Samuelsson J, Bertilsson R, Bülow E, Carlsson S, Åkesson S, Eliasson B, et al. Autoimmune comorbidity in type 1 diabetes and its association with metabolic control and mortality risk in young people: a population-based study. Diabetologia. 2024;67(4):679-89.

ABSTRACT

Objective: The purpose of this register-based study was to characterize autoimmune comorbidity in children and young adults with type 1 diabetes from the time of onset and to find out if this comorbidity was linked to a different HbA1c or mortality risk when compared to children and young adults with type 1 diabetes who did not have autoimmune comorbidity.

Methods: 15,188 people with type 1 diabetes who were registered before the age of 18 in the Swedish National Diabetes Register between 2000 and 2019 were included. Every person with type 1 diabetes was matched with five randomly chosen control individuals from the Swedish population (Statistics Sweden) [n =74,210 (346 individuals with type 1 diabetes were not found in the Statistics Sweden register at the time of type 1 diabetes diagnosis, so they could not be matched to control individuals)]. ICD-10 codes for autoimmune disorders were obtained from the National Patient Register, and deceased people were identified using the Cause of Death Register.

Findings: The mean ± SD age at type 1 diabetes onset was 9.5 ± 4.4 years, and the mean duration of the disease at the end of follow-up was 8.8 ± 5.7 years, for the entire type 1 diabetes cohort. Compared to 4.0% of the control group, 19.2% of people with type 1 diabetes had a diagnosis of at least one autoimmune illness. Within 19 years of the onset of type 1 diabetes, the HRs for comorbidities were as follows: 1.1 (95% CI 0.8, 1.3) for inflammatory bowel disease, 1.0 (95% CI 0.7, 1.2) for systemic connective tissue disorder, 1.3 (95% CI 1.1, 1.6) for psoriasis, 4.1 (95% CI 3.2, 5.3) for vitiligo, 1.7 (95% CI 1.4, 2.2) for rheumatic joint disease, 1.0 (95% CI 0.8, 1.3) for psoriasis, 1.4, 1.8 (95% CI 0.9, 3.6) for multiple sclerosis, 3.7 (95% CI 1.6, 8.7) for inflammatory liver disease, 19.6 (95% CI 4.2, 92.3) for atrophic gastritis, and 95% CI 8.4, 40.0) for Addison's disease. HbA1c and mortality risk were not statistically significantly impacted by autoimmune illness or type 1 diabetes.

Conclusion and interpretation: It is the first comprehensive study that we are aware of that tracks the beginning of a wide range of autoimmune disorders in young people with type 1 diabetes at the same time. According to this population-based, nationwide survey, childhood autoimmune disorders, particularly thyroid and celiac disease, were already highly prevalent. Neither metabolic control nor mortality risk was statistically impacted by the presence of autoimmune comorbidities.

CRITICAL APPRAISAL

What was Known Prior to this Study?

Prior research indicated a notable prevalence of autoimmune diseases (AIDs) among individuals with type 1 diabetes, particularly in children and young adults. Autoimmune diseases such as coeliac disease and thyroid disorders have been frequently observed as comorbidities in this population. Previous studies suggested that these comorbidities might influence metabolic control and mortality risk. However, the exact relationship between autoimmune comorbidity and these clinical factors in young people with type 1 diabetes remained inadequately explored.

What this Study Adds?

This study contributes new insights by demonstrating that while autoimmune comorbidities are prevalent in a young population with type 1 diabetes, they do not significantly affect HbA1c levels or mortality risk. Specifically, the study found a high prevalence of coeliac disease and thyroid disorders but concluded that the presence of these autoimmune conditions does not correlate with impaired metabolic control or increased mortality in this demographic.

Major Strengths of the Study

- Large sample size of 15,188 individuals with type 1 diabetes and 74,210 matched controls.
- Utilization of a national diabetes register which ensures high data quality and coverage.
- Comprehensive analysis of autoimmune comorbidity from the onset of type 1 diabetes.

- Population-based design enhances the external validity of the findings.
- Inclusion of a control group allows for a comparative analysis.
- Well-defined methodology for data collection and analysis, utilizing ICD-10 codes for autoimmune diseases.

Limitations of the Study
- Dependence on the accuracy of registrations in the National Diabetes Register, which may introduce biases due to incorrect documentation.
- Lack of access to family history of autoimmune diseases, which could influence the findings.
- No control over the tests conducted for diagnosis of autoimmune diseases, potentially affecting the comprehensiveness of data.
- The study's retrospective design limits the ability to establish causation between autoimmune comorbidities and clinical outcomes.

Implications of the Finding for the Clinicians
Clinicians should be aware that while autoimmune comorbidities are common in young patients with type 1 diabetes, these conditions may not necessarily result in poorer metabolic control or increased mortality risk. This understanding can help inform clinical practice, guiding healthcare providers in monitoring and managing these patients without undue alarm regarding the implications of comorbid autoimmune conditions.

Knowledge Gaps Identified and Scope for Future Research
Future research should focus on:
- A detailed exploration of each autoimmune disease associated with elevated risk in the type 1 diabetes population.
- Longitudinal studies to assess long-term complications related to autoimmune comorbidities.
- Investigation into the genetic factors, such as human leukocyte antigen (HLA) genotyping, that may contribute to the development of autoimmune diseases in this population.
- Understanding the impact of different interventions on managing both type 1 diabetes and autoimmune comorbidities.

10. The Association of Chronic Complications with Time in Tight Range and Time in Range in People with Type 1 Diabetes: A Retrospective Cross-sectional Real-world Study

Ref: De Meulemeester J, Charleer S, Visser MM, De Block C, Mathieu C, Gillard P. The association of chronic complications with time in tight range and time in range in people with type 1 diabetes: a retrospective cross-sectional real-world study. Diabetologia. 2024;67(8):1527-35.

ABSTRACT

Objectives and hypotheses: This study sought to determine whether time in tight range (TITR: 3.9–7.8 mmol/L) and time in range (TIR: 3.9–10.0 mmol/L) were associated with chronic problems in individuals with type 1 diabetes.

Techniques: In 808 individuals with type 1 diabetes, the prevalence of macrovascular problems and microvascular consequences [diabetic retinopathy, diabetic nephropathy, and diabetic peripheral neuropathy (DPN)] as determined by sensor-measured TITR/TIR was examined cross-sectionally. The relationship between TITR/TIR and the presence of complications was assessed using binary logistic regression without, with, and with adjustment for HbA1c and other confounding factors [sex, age, duration of diabetes, body mass index (BMI), blood pressure, lipid profile, smoking, and use of statins and renin–angiotensin–aldosterone system inhibitors].

Findings: The average TIR was 52.5 ± 15.0%, and the average TITR was 33.9 ± 12.8%. In all, 16.3% experienced any macrovascular consequence and 46.0% experienced any microvascular complication (34.5% diabetic retinopathy, 23.8% diabetic nephropathy, and 16.0% DPN). As TITR/TIR quartiles increased, the prevalence of cerebrovascular accidents (CVAs), diabetic retinopathy, diabetic nephropathy, and any microvascular consequence reduced (all p trend <0.05). For every 10% rise in TITR, the incidence of diabetic retinopathy (OR 0.757; 95% CI 0.670, 0.856; $p < 0.001$), background diabetic retinopathy, and any microvascular consequence decreased (OR 0.762; 95% CI 0.679, 0.855; $p < 0.001$). Diabetic nephropathy (OR 0.799; 95% CI 0.699, 0.915; $p < 0.001$), severe diabetic retinopathy (OR 0.854; 95% CI 0.731, 0.998; $p = 0.048$), DPN (OR 0.837; 95% CI 0.717, 0.977; $p = 0.026$), and cerebrovascular accident (OR 0.651; 95% CI 0.470, 0.902; $p = 0.010$). After controlling for HbA1c, TITR continued to be independently associated with any microvascular complication (OR 0.867; 95% CI 0.762, 0.988; $p = 0.032$), diabetic retinopathy (OR 0.837; 95% CI 0.731, 0.959; $p = 0.010$), background diabetic retinopathy (OR 0.831; 95% CI 0.705, 0.979; $p = 0.027$), and CVA (OR 0.619; 95% CI 0.426, 0.899; $p = 0.012$). After adjusting for HbA1c and other confounding variables, similar outcomes were seen.

Conclusion and interpretation: In individuals with type 1 diabetes, TITR and TIR are inversely correlated with the occurrence of microvascular problems and cerebrovascular accidents. This research lends legitimacy to the use of TITR and TIR as important metrics in glycemic management, even if the study was not intended to prove a causal association.

CRITICAL APPRAISAL

What was Known Prior to this Study?

Prior to this study, the association between various glycemic management metrics and chronic complications in type 1 diabetes remained unclear. Recent guidelines had recommended the inclusion of time in tight range (TITR) as a metric, defined as the percentage of time spent in normoglycemia (3.9–7.8 mmol/L). Despite this recommendation, there was no concrete evidence directly linking TITR to the development of complications. Studies had shown contradictory findings regarding the relationship between time in range (TIR) and cardiovascular disease (CVD) outcomes, indicating a gap in understanding the clinical validity of these metrics.

What this Study Adds?

This study provides new insights by demonstrating a robust, independent association between CGM-measured TITR and the presence of microvascular complications as well as cerebrovascular accidents (CVA) in individuals with type 1 diabetes. It highlights that both TITR and TIR are inversely associated with the occurrence of these complications, thereby validating their use as key measures in glycemic management. Additionally, it underscores the importance of maintaining blood glucose levels within the normal range to minimize chronic complications.

Major Strengths of the Study

- It is the first to evaluate the association between TITR and chronic complications systematically.
- A large sample size of 808 adults with type 1 diabetes enhances the reliability of the findings.
- The use of binary logistic regression allows for a comprehensive assessment of the relationship between TITR/TIR and complications, adjusting for multiple confounding factors.

- The study provides substantial evidence supporting the clinical validity of TITR, which may help guide therapeutic goals in diabetes management.
- Findings contribute to the ongoing discussion regarding optimal glycemic targets for reducing complications.

Limitations of the Study

- The cross-sectional design prevents the establishment of causal relationships between TITR/TIR and the presence of complications, raising concerns about potential reverse causality.
- The findings may not generalize to all populations, as the study was conducted in a specific cohort of adults with type 1 diabetes.
- The methodology did not differentiate between types of cerebrovascular accidents, which may influence the interpretation of results.
- A low number of participants with macrovascular complications limited the ability to draw definitive conclusions regarding those outcomes.
- Ethical considerations prevent conducting a longitudinal study similar to the Diabetes Control and Complications Trial (DCCT), which could provide more robust data on long-term effects.

Implications of the Finding for the Clinicians

The findings suggest that clinicians should prioritize maintaining TITR and TIR in managing patients with type 1 diabetes to reduce the risk of chronic complications, particularly microvascular issues and CVA. The study supports the integration of TITR as a critical metric in clinical practice, potentially influencing therapeutic decisions and setting glycemic targets. It also highlights the need for a multifactorial approach that includes assessing other risk factors in addition to glycemic metrics for effective management of cardiovascular and renal complications.

Knowledge Gaps Identified and Scope for Future Research

- Longitudinal studies to establish causal relationships between glycemic metrics and chronic complications.
- Investigations into the impact of newer diabetes medications, such as sodium-glucose cotransporter-2 inhibitors and glucagon-like peptide-1 receptor agonists, on complications in type 1 diabetes
- Further exploration of the mechanisms linking TITR/TIR with different types of complications, particularly macrovascular outcomes
- Studies to assess the applicability of these findings across diverse populations and settings.

11. Safety and Efficacy of Teplizumab in the Treatment of Type 1 Diabetes Mellitus: An Updated Systematic Review and Meta-analysis of Randomized Controlled Trials

Ref: Grando Alves G, Cunha L, Henkes Machado R, Lins de Menezes V. Safety and efficacy of teplizumab in the treatment of type 1 diabetes mellitus: An updated systematic review and meta-analysis of randomized controlled trials. Diabetes Obes Metab. 2024;26(7):2652-61.

ABSTRACT

Goal: To present the most recent data on teplizumab's safety and effectiveness in treating Stage 3 type 1 diabetes mellitus (T1DM).

Materials and methods: Randomized controlled trials (RCTs) comparing teplizumab to placebo for type 1 diabetes (T1DM) that reported any of the following outcomes were found using the PubMed, Embase, and Cochrane databases: (1) C-peptide area under the curve (AUC); (2) glycated hemoglobin (HbA1c) levels; (3) insulin requirements; and (4) adverse events. I2 statistics were used to investigate heterogeneity. A p-value of <0.05 was considered statistically significant. The pooled mean difference (MD) was used to compare the continuous endpoints, and risk ratios with 95% CIs were used to evaluate the binary endpoints. Review Manager Web was used to conduct statistical analyses.

Results: A total of 1,052 patients (754 receiving teplizumab) were enrolled in eight RCTs. Teplizumab significantly decreased HbA1c levels at 6 (MD −0.57%, 95% CI −1.07, −0.08) and 12 months (MD −0.31%, 95% CI −0.59, −0.02), and significantly decreased insulin requirements at 6 (MD −0.12 U/kg, 95% CI −0.16, −0.08), 12 (MD −0.11 U/kg, 95% CI −0.15, −0.07), 18 (MD −0.17 U/kg, 95% CI −0.26, −0.09), and 24 months (MD 0.16 nmol/L, 95% CI 0.02, 0.31).

Conclusion: Teplizumab reduces insulin utilization and HbA1c levels while increasing the AUC of C-peptide levels without increasing the risk of significant side events.

CRITICAL APPRAISAL

What was Known Prior to this Study?

Prior to this study, the safety and efficacy of teplizumab as an immunotherapy for type 1 diabetes mellitus (T1DM) were based on earlier research suggesting it could delay the onset of Stage 3 T1DM in patients with Stage 2. Previous studies highlighted teplizumab's mechanism of action targeting CD3 on T cells and indicated its potential to preserve beta-cell function. However, concerns arose due to the presence of duplicate outcome data in earlier meta-analyses, which raised questions about the reliability of results regarding its efficacy and safety profile.

What this Study Adds?

This study provides an updated systematic review and meta-analysis of randomized controlled trials (RCTs) specifically evaluating teplizumab in patients with Stage 3 T1DM. Key additions include the following:
- A significant increase in C-peptide levels, indicating improved beta-cell function.
- A concomitant reduction in insulin requirements, sustained for at least 2 years.
- A decrease in HbA1c levels for a minimum of 1 year, suggesting better glycemic control.
- A favorable safety profile with no significant difference in serious adverse events compared to placebo.

Major Strengths of the Study

- Comprehensive analysis involving eight RCTs with a total of 1,052 patients
- High certainty in findings related to HbA1c levels and insulin dosage, based on GRADE assessments.
- Clear documentation of safety outcomes, indicating that adverse effects were primarily minor and manageable.
- The systematic approach aligned with PRISMA (Preferred Reporting Items for Systematic Reviews and Meta-Analyses) guidelines, ensuring methodological rigor.

Limitations of the Study

- Concerns regarding significant heterogeneity in C-peptide level analyses, leading to a moderate level of certainty for these findings.
- The possibility that adverse effects such as cytokine release syndrome, while statistically significant, had a low incidence.
- The absence of long-term follow-up data beyond 2 years, which limits understanding of prolonged safety and efficacy.
- Potential biases from included studies, such as selective reporting and patient population variations.

Implications of the Finding for Clinicians

The findings suggest that teplizumab is a promising therapeutic option for managing Stage 3 T1DM, with implications including:
- Encouraging clinicians to consider teplizumab for patients to improve glycemic control and reduce insulin dependency.
- The need for shared decision-making with patients regarding the balance of efficacy and safety, especially in pediatric populations.
- Potential to influence treatment guidelines and clinical practice standards for T1DM management.

Knowledge Gaps Identified and Scope for Future Research

The study highlights several knowledge gaps, including:
- The need for further research on long-term safety and efficacy beyond 2 years.
- Exploration of the impact of baseline patient characteristics on the efficacy of teplizumab.
- Investigation into the effects of teplizumab in diverse populations and settings.
- Further studies to assess the economic implications and cost-effectiveness of teplizumab treatment for T1DM.

12. Mortality in Type 1 Diabetes Mellitus: A Single Centre Experience from the ICMR–Youth Onset Diabetes Registry in India

Ref: Madhu SV, Shukla P, Kaur T, Dhaliwal RS. Mortality in type 1 diabetes mellitus: A single centre experience from the ICMR - Youth onset diabetes registry in India. Diabetes Res Clin Pract. 2024;217:111868.

ABSTRACT

Introduction: Youth-onset diabetes is becoming more common worldwide, and its associated complications and mortality rate are also increasing. The goal of the current study was to investigate the mortality and reasons of death among young diabetic patients who were admitted to a North Indian tertiary care facility.

Methods: We examined the mortality and causes of death of 1,088 young diabetic patients who were enrolled at the University College of Medical Sciences in Delhi between 2006 and 2019. When available, information on the death was gathered from hospital records, home visits, or phone calls. The cause of death was ascertained using WHO ICD-10/11, and a verbal autopsy was conducted in accordance with the ICMR questionnaire.

Results: 105 deaths (11.6%) occurred among 898 youth-onset type 1 diabetes mellitus (T1D) patients with a mean follow-up of 6.4 years. 75.6% of deaths had a HbA1c >10%, and 43% had diabetes that started at age 15 or younger. Of those diagnosed, 24.2% died within 2 years and 53.6% died within 3 years. The most frequent causes were infections, ketoacidosis, and chronic kidney disease.

Conclusion: In a North Indian tertiary care hospital, we observed increased mortality and inadequate glycemic management among patients with juvenile-onset T1D.

CRITICAL APPRAISAL

What was Known Prior to this Study?

Prior to this study, there was a recognized increase in the prevalence of youth onset diabetes globally, including type 1 diabetes (T1D). The burden of complications and mortality associated with youth onset diabetes was acknowledged, yet studies specifically addressing mortality rates in this demographic, especially in India, were scarce. Existing literature indicated high mortality rates in T1D patients, primarily due to acute complications shortly after diagnosis and chronic complications as patients aged.

What this Study Adds?

This study provides critical insights into mortality and causes of death among youth onset T1D patients in India, revealing a high mortality rate of 11.6% over a mean follow-up of 6.4 years. It establishes that renal complications and infections were the leading causes of death, significantly higher than previously reported. Additionally, nearly half of the deaths occurred during the COVID-19 pandemic, suggesting a possible exacerbation of mortality rates during this period.

Major Strengths of the Study

- A comprehensive analysis of a large cohort (898 patients) with a significant follow-up duration
- Utilization of a validated verbal autopsy questionnaire to ascertain causes of death, providing a robust dataset
- Examination of factors contributing to mortality, such as glycemic control and comorbid conditions, offering a nuanced understanding of patient outcomes
- Contribution to the limited literature on youth onset diabetes mortality in India, filling a critical knowledge gap

Limitations of the study

- Mortality data was not based on death certificates, potentially compromising the accuracy of cause of death determination.
- Contact challenges during the COVID-19 pandemic may have led to an underestimation of mortality due to incomplete data collection.
- Lack of access to all patients for follow-up assessments may skew results and limit generalizability.

Implications of the Findings for Clinicians

The findings underscore the urgent need for improved management strategies for youth onset T1D patients, particularly regarding:
- Enhanced glycemic control measures to mitigate complications and mortality
- Increased awareness of the significant mortality risk associated with renal complications and infections
- Development of targeted interventions to address psychosocial factors affecting treatment adherence and regular follow-up

Knowledge Gaps Identified and Scope for Future Research

- There is a need for further research on the long-term impacts of diabetes management strategies on mortality rates in youth onset T1D.
- Exploration of psychosocial factors contributing to poor glycemic control and adherence to treatment.
- Investigation into the effects of the COVID-19 pandemic on diabetes management and patient outcomes.
- Comparative studies with other regions or countries to better understand the context of youth onset diabetes mortality.

13. Islet-after-kidney Transplantation versus Kidney Alone in Kidney Transplant Recipients with Type 1 Diabetes (KAIAK): A Population-based Target Trial Emulation in France

Ref: Maanaoui M, Lenain R, Foucher Y, Buron F, Blancho G, Antoine C, et al. Islet-After-Kidney Transplantation Versus Kidney Alone in Kidney Transplant Recipients with Type 1 Diabetes (KAIAK): A Population-based Target Trial Emulation in France. Lancet Diabetes Endocrinol. 2024;12:716-24.

ABSTRACT

Context: Although there is little concrete proof of its impact on hard clinical endpoints, islet transplantation has been linked to improved metabolic management and quality of life compared to insulin therapy alone. In kidney transplant recipients with type 1 diabetes, we sought to evaluate the impact of islet transplantation on patient-graft survival.

Techniques: All patients with type 1 diabetes who got a kidney transplant in France throughout the research period and were found through the CRISTAL countrywide registry were included in this retrospective cohort analysis. Recipients from transplant centers that did not offer islet transplantation during the study period, recipients who had a functioning pancreas during the follow-up period, recipients who had received more than two kidney transplants, recipients who were HLA-sensitized, recipients who had received less than a year of follow-up following kidney transplantation. Misclassified recipients included those with type 2 diabetes, those over 65, those who received kidney grafts from donors of donation after circulatory death, those who had hepatitis or HIV, those who had cancer, and those who received combination liver-kidney transplants. In order to ensure patient comparability at the time of islet transplantation, patients who additionally got islet-after-kidney (IAK) transplantation were compared with controls who received kidney transplantation alone using a 1:2 matching method based on time-dependent propensity scores. Patient-graft survival, a composite outcome that can be characterized by death, re-transplantation, or dialysis recurrence, was the main outcome.

Results: Of the 2,391 individuals with type 1 diabetes who got kidney transplants between January 1, 2000, and December 31, 2017, 47 also received islet transplants. 62 patients were eliminated because of missing data, and 2002 patients were not eligible for islet transplantation. In the target trial emulation study, 327 suitable participants from 15 centers were included. A successful match was made between 80 patients who got kidney transplantation alone and 40 patients who received IAK transplantation. Compared to 36 (45%) of 80 patients in the kidney transplantation alone group, 13 (33%) of 40 patients in the IAK transplantation group either died or went back to dialysis. When compared to kidney transplantation alone, we discovered that islet transplantation significantly improved patient-graft outcomes mostly due to a protective impact on the risk of mortality (HR 0.41, 0.13–0.91; $p = 0.042$), with a hazard ratio (HR) of 0.44 (95% CI 0.23–0.88; $p = 0.022$). IAK and death-censored graft survival did not significantly correlate (0.73, 0.30–1.89; $p = 0.36$).

Interpretation: Due primarily to a protective effect on the risk of death, IAK transplantation was linked to a considerably higher patient-graft survival in kidney transplant recipients with type 1 diabetes when compared to kidney transplantation alone. Since reimbursement for islet transplantation is only offered in a few number of nations worldwide, these findings may provide strong evidence in favor of promoting greater access to islet transplantation for patients with type 1 diabetes receiving kidney transplants.

CRITICAL APPRAISAL

What was Known Prior to this Study?
Prior to this study, islet transplantation was recognized as an effective method for improving metabolic control in diabetes management, particularly in type 1 diabetes. However, there was a significant lack of long-term mortality data comparing outcomes of islet transplantation with control cohorts, especially among patients who had undergone kidney transplantation. Two earlier studies suggested a potential advantage of islet transplantation in enhancing long-term graft and patient survival, but these studies were limited by discrepancies in baseline characteristics among the groups compared.

What this Study Adds?
This study presents new insights into the effectiveness of islet-after-kidney (IAK) transplantation compared to kidney transplantation alone in patients with type 1 diabetes. It provides robust long-term data demonstrating that IAK transplantation is associated with a significant reduction in all-cause mortality and improved renal function over a follow-up period of 27 years. The study utilized a comprehensive target emulation trial design to closely mimic randomized controlled trial conditions, thereby enhancing the reliability of the findings.

Major Strengths of the Study
- Comprehensive data collection from a nationwide registry, ensuring a representative sample.
- Utilization of a target trial design to eliminate biases associated with observational studies.
- Long follow-up period allowing for assessment of long-term outcomes.
- Advanced statistical methods, including propensity score matching and bootstrapping, to enhance the validity of results.
- Inclusion of relevant clinical endpoints such as kidney graft failure and mortality.
- Clear definition of inclusion and exclusion criteria to minimize confounding factors.
- Demonstration of significant clinical benefits associated with IAK transplantation.
- Contribution to the understanding of metabolic control in the context of diabetes and kidney transplantation.

Limitations of the Study
The study has several limitations:
- The retrospective nature of the cohort analysis may introduce biases inherent to observational studies.
- Potential residual confounding due to unmeasured variables or incomplete data.
- Limitations in subgroup analysis due to the outcome-focused nature of propensity score matching.
- The findings may not be generalizable to populations outside of France or to patients with different underlying conditions.
- Difficulties in capturing long-term complications related to both diabetes and transplantation.

Implications of the Finding for the Clinicians
Clinicians can utilize the findings to support the case for IAK transplantation in eligible type 1 diabetes patients undergoing kidney transplantation. Key implications include the following:
- Enhanced patient counseling regarding the potential long-term benefits of IAK transplantation.
- Re-evaluation of treatment protocols to include islet transplantation as a viable option for improving patient outcomes.
- Increased awareness of the importance of metabolic control in preventing complications post-transplant.
- Consideration of patient selection criteria based on the study's insights to optimize outcomes.

Knowledge Gaps Identified and Scope for Future Research
- The need for more granular data on the specific mechanisms by which islet

transplantation improves long-term outcomes.
- Exploration of the effects of islet transplantation in diverse populations and across varying clinical contexts.
- Longitudinal studies to assess the impact of islet transplantation on quality of life and psychological outcomes in patients.
- Investigation into the economic implications of islet transplantation versus kidney transplantation alone.
- Research focused on the optimal timing and criteria for islet transplantation in relation to kidney transplantation to maximize benefits.

14. Prediction of Progression to Type 1 Diabetes with Dynamic Biomarkers and Risk Scores

Ref: Joglekar MV, Kaur S, Pociot F, Hardikar AA. Prediction of progression to type 1 diabetes with dynamic biomarkers and risk scores. Lancet Diabetes Endocrinol. 2024;12(7):483-92.

ABSTRACT

Finding indicators of functional β-cell depletion is a crucial step in type 1 diabetes risk classification. A popular method for predicting the likelihood of type 1 diabetes is the use of genetic risk scores (GRS), which are produced by profiling a variety of single nucleotide polymorphisms. To identify those at high risk of type 1 diabetes, type 1 diabetes screening studies have used a combination of biochemical (autoantibody) and GRS screening approaches. One drawback of these screening methods is that autoantibodies are not the best biomarker of the development of early-stage type 1 diabetes because they signal the start of β-cell loss. In contrast, GRS is a static biomarker that provides a single risk score for the duration of a person's life. The difficulties and possibilities of both static and dynamic biomarkers in predicting the development of type 1 diabetes are examined in this personal view. We talk about potential future avenues in which more recent dynamic risk scores (DRS) could be used to predict the risk of type 1 diabetes, evaluate the effectiveness of novel medications to delay or prevent the disease, and perhaps replace or improve the predictive power provided by static biomarkers such as GRS.

CRITICAL APPRAISAL

What was Known Prior to this Study?

Prior to this study, it was established that GRS derived from single nucleotide polymorphisms (SNPs) were commonly used for predicting type 1 diabetes (T1D) risk. Screening methodologies primarily focused on the presence of autoantibodies, serving as early indicators of β-cell loss, but were limited in their predictive capabilities regarding disease progression. Previous research highlighted the need for improved biomarkers to differentiate between autoimmune and non-autoimmune T1D subtypes and indicated that static biomarkers such as GRS might not adequately capture the dynamic nature of disease progression influenced by environmental factors.

What this Study Adds?

This study introduces the concept of dynamic risk scores (DRS) as an advancement over static GRS in predicting the risk of progression to type 1 diabetes. It emphasizes the importance of identifying dynamic biomarkers that can respond to environmental triggers and accurately reflect changes in risk over time. The authors argue that integrating DRS with emerging therapeutics could enhance early intervention strategies, potentially delaying the onset of T1D, especially in high-risk populations.

Major Strengths of the Review
- Proposes the innovative use of DRS for T1D risk assessment.
- Highlights the necessity of identifying a variety of dynamic biomarkers (e.g., cell-free DNA, lipids, microRNAs).
- Discusses the clinical utility of DRS in monitoring risk changes due to environmental factors or treatments.
- Acknowledges the importance of ethnic variability in biomarker assessment.
- Addresses the limitations of current screening methods and suggests practical solutions.
- Suggests the potential for DRS to enhance treatment efficacy assessments.

Limitations of the Review
- Dynamic risk scores are still in the conceptual phase and require extensive validation through clinical trials.
- The complexity of identifying and standardizing dynamic biomarkers remains a significant challenge.
- Current methodologies for assessing genetic markers may have technical limitations, particularly with multi-ethnic populations.
- The review does not specify the precise biomarkers to be used within the DRS framework, leaving gaps in implementation.
- There is a need for more research to fully understand environmental exposures that contribute to T1D development.
- The reliance on existing GRS may limit the exploration of novel dynamic markers.
- The interactions among different biomarkers and their contributions to disease risk are not fully understood.

Implications of the Finding for the Clinicians
Clinicians can leverage the findings of this study to enhance early identification and monitoring of individuals at risk for type 1 diabetes. The implementation of DRS could facilitate timely interventions with immune-modulatory therapies, particularly in young patients. This approach may improve patient outcomes by delaying the onset of clinical diabetes and potentially reducing long-term complications associated with early diagnosis.

Knowledge Gaps Identified and Scope for Future Research
Future research should focus on:
- Identifying reliable dynamic biomarkers that can be easily integrated into clinical practice.
- Understanding the role of environmental factors (e.g., diet, infections) in influencing T1D risk.
- Exploring the interaction between genetic predisposition and environmental triggers.
- Conducting large-scale studies to validate the predictive accuracy of DRS across diverse populations.
- Investigating the efficacy of new therapies in modifying disease progression based on dynamic risk assessment.

Section 6: GESTATIONAL DIABETES MELLITUS AND PREGNANCY IN DIABETES MELLITUS

Section Editor: Indira Maisnam

1. Perinatal Outcomes Associated with Metformin Use during Pregnancy in Women with Pregestational Type 2 Diabetes Mellitus

Ref: Yland JJ, Huybrechts KF, Wesselink AK, Straub L, Chiu YH, Seely EW, et al. Perinatal Outcomes Associated With Metformin Use During Pregnancy in Women With Pregestational Type 2 Diabetes Mellitus. Diabetes Care. 2024;47(9):1688-95.

ABSTRACT

Goal: To evaluate the perinatal outcomes of women with type 2 diabetes mellitus who were treated with metformin plus insulin before pregnancy versus those who stopped taking the medication, we modeled a modified randomized trial [metformin in women with type 2 diabetes in pregnancy (MiTy)].

Design and methods of research: Two healthcare claims databases (US, 2000–2020) were used in this investigation. Eligible participants were type 2 diabetic mellitus pregnant women aged 18–45 years who were receiving metformin with insulin at the time of conception. Preterm birth, birth injury, neonatal respiratory distress, neonatal hypoglycemia, and hospitalization to the intensive care unit were the main outcomes.

Preeclampsia, maternal hypoglycemia, cesarean birth, newborns large for gestational age, infants small for gestational age (SGA), sepsis, hyperbilirubinemia, gestational hypertension, and the elements of the primary composite outcome were all considered secondary outcomes. Potential baseline confounders, such as comorbidities, demographic traits, and indicators of the course of diabetes, were taken into account.

Results: 72% of the 2,983 eligible individuals stopped using metformin while pregnant. A number of comorbidities were more common among continuers, and the average age at conception was 32 years. For those who continued, the composite outcome risk was 46%, while for those who stopped, it was 48%. At a 95% confidence interval (CI) of 0.81 and 1.03, the adjusted risk ratio was 0.92.

With the exception of SGA, which was higher in continuers only in the group with commercial insurance, risks were comparable across treatments and databases for the majority of secondary outcomes.

Conclusion: The results of the metformin in women with type 2 diabetes mellitus in pregnancy (MiTy) randomized study aligned with our findings. An elevated risk of a newborn composite poor outcome was not linked to continued use of metformin during pregnancy. However, more research is needed to rule out a potential metformin-associated risk of SGA.

CRITICAL APPRAISAL

What was Known Prior to the Study?

Metformin therapy is recommended in the management of gestational diabetes. Regarding pregestational diabetes, two randomized trials have assessed the safety of metformin in pregestational type 2 diabetes mellitus.

Metformin in women with type 2 diabetes in pregnancy (MiTy) trial showed there was no difference among composite perinatal outcomes [pregnancy loss, preterm birth, moderate to severe respiratory distress, neonatal hypoglycemia, and neonatal intensive care unit (NICU) admission for >24 hours] when metformin was added to insulin compared to placebo.

What Does this Study Add?

All the data regarding the use of metformin in pregestational diabetes was obtained in controlled settings as a part of the trials. There was no real-world data regarding this indication. The current study through the trial framework design on databases fills this gap.

Major Strengths of the Study

A large population was studied affirming the findings of clinical trials in the real-world setting. Both groups were matched in baseline characteristics including the use of both insulin and metformin at baseline. Baseline hyperglycemia, diabetes complications, and maternal adiposity were also adjusted to reduce bias.

Limitations of the Study

Being an observational study, there was a risk of bias due to confounding factors such as obesity and the degree of baseline hyperglycemia. There was heterogeneity amongst those covered with public insurance compared to those having commercial insurance. Outcome misclassification was possible since validated algorithms were available for only two outcomes (preeclampsia and preterm birth).

Implications of the Findings for the Clinicians

Metformin can be used in pregnant women with pregestational type 2 diabetes mellitus. It may reduce the insulin requirements and thus the adverse complications associated with it. However, the possible risk of small for gestational age (SGA) should be discussed before initiating therapy.

Knowledge Gaps Identified and Scope for Future Research

Mechanisms by which metformin affects the developing fetus resulting in small gestational age babies and factors affecting it need to be explored.

2. Earlier Detection of Gestational Diabetes Impacts on Medication Requirements, Neonatal and Maternal Outcomes

Ref: Tirado-Aguilar OA, Martinez-Cruz N, Arce-Sanchez L, Borboa-Olivares H, Reyes-Muñoz E, Espino-y-Sosa S, et al. Earlier detection of gestational diabetes impacts on medication requirements, neonatal and maternal outcomes. Diabetes Obes Metab. 2024;26:3110-8.

ABSTRACT

Goal: Maternal and newborn outcomes are significantly impacted by gestational diabetes (GD), a global health concern. This study examines the relationship between unfavorable newborn outcomes, the need for medication, and early gestational diabetes (eGD) diagnosis (<24 weeks).

Materials and procedures: A 75 g oral glucose tolerance test was administered to a group of 369 expectant mothers. T-tests, χ2 tests, and logistic regression were used to analyze maternal factors, medication prescriptions, and neonatal outcomes. Significant was defined as a $p < 0.05$.

Findings eGD raised the risk of respiratory distress syndrome [odds ratio (OR) 4.75, $p = 0.034$] and newborn hypoglycemia (OR 18.57, $p = 0.013$).

Women with eGD needed more often specialized nutritional advice + metformin to achieve glycemic control ($p = 0.027$), while the most common treatment for those diagnosed after 24 weeks was a prescription for nutritional therapy from a qualified nutritionist. Maternal hyperglycemia during the postpartum period at 2 hours of the oral glucose tolerance test [OR 1.03, 95% confidence interval (CI) 1.02–1.13, $p = 0.024$] and a higher need for nutritional therapy prescription + metformin (OR 2.26, 95% CI 1.25–4.09, $p = 0.007$) were linked to eGD.

Conclusion: Since an earlier presentation is linked to a higher risk of unfavorable newborn and maternal outcomes, prompt diagnosis and individualized treatment of GD are important.

CRITICAL APPRAISAL

What was Known Prior to the Study?

Early gestational diabetes (GD) has an increased risk of adverse neonatal outcomes like large for gestational age, Erb's palsy, and shoulder dystocia. Other studies have also reported an increased risk of neonatal hypoglycemia and Simmons et al. also showed an association with respiratory complications. Moreover, fetal abdominal fat was found to be higher at 20–24 weeks of pregnancy even before the diagnosis of gestational diabetes. This suggests the commencement of the pathophysiological process in early pregnancy.

What Does this Study Add?

Early GD is more common at a higher body mass index (BMI) compared to conventional GD. It confirms the increased risk of neonatal hypoglycemia and respiratory distress syndrome in early GD compared to conventional GD. There was a higher requirement of metformin in the early gestational diabetes (eGD) group suggesting the possibility of higher insulin resistance. Women with eGD are more likely to remain dysglycemic in the early postpartum period (6 weeks) compared to cGD (gestational diabetes diagnosed after 24 weeks).

Major Strengths of the Study

A well-formed single-center cohort ensured consistent approaches for the diagnosis, management of GD, and detection of complications. A unified maternal endocrinology group managed all GD cases including nutritional and medical therapy as per American Diabetes Association (ADA) targets thereby reducing the possible risk of variations in management and improving internal validity.

Limitations of the Study

The study failed to provide data on treatment adherence, and the influence of exercise on maternal and neonatal outcomes. There was no data on insulin usage, glycemic profiles, and ambulatory profiles which could have helped determine the impact of glycemic optimization on the outcomes. Moreover, the cause of small for gestational age (SGA) (overzealous diet control vs. GD itself) could not be determined due to a lack of accurate data on dietary adherence. Being an observational study, it limits the findings to associations and causality cannot be determined. The cutoffs suggested by the International Association of the Diabetes and Pregnancy Study Groups (IADPSG) were used for the diagnosis of GD, which might not be accurate in predicting the outcomes in the Latin American population.

Implications of the Findings for the Clinicians

Since early GD can impact neonatal outcomes, especially in obese and elderly women, it would be reasonable to do a screening for GD in early pregnancy and begin the appropriate nutritional and pharmacotherapy is required.

Knowledge Gaps Identified and Scope for Future Research

Well-designed prospective studies are needed to understand the effect of early gestational diabetes on neonatal outcomes. Research is required to distinguish pathophysiology between early and conventional GD and to evaluate the efficacy of early interventions on neonatal outcomes as well as long-term impacts on fetal development.

3. Prevalence of Gestational Diabetes Mellitus Risk Factors in Singleton Pregnancies Obtained by Assisted Reproductive Technology: An Observational, Retrospective, Real-world Study from a Pregnancy Registry

Ref: Vergani M, Conti M, Lari A, Mion E, Bertuzzi F, Pintaudi B. Prevalence of gestational diabetes mellitus risk factors in singleton pregnancies obtained by assisted reproductive technology: An observational, retrospective, real-world study from a pregnancy registry. Diabetes Res Clinic Pract. 2024;210:111654.

ABSTRACT

Aim: A number of research has demonstrated that the onset of gestational diabetes mellitus (GDM) may be impacted by assisted reproductive technology (ART). Estimating the prevalence of GDM risk variables in a group of women who had a singleton pregnancy achieved with ART and complicated by GDM was the goal of this study. Results for mothers and newborns were investigated.

Methods: We retrospectively gathered information on pregnancies of women who were treated at a specialist facility for diabetes and pregnancy care after obtaining ART for a singleton pregnancy and having GDM complicated it. Maternal-fetal outcomes, the prevalence of GDM risk variables, and their combinations were assessed.

Results: There were 50 women in our cohort overall, with a mean age of 40.4 ± 4.7 years and a mean body mass index (BMI) of 26.3 ± 6.2 kg/m^2 before pregnancy.

The most common traditional risk factors for GDM were being over 35 (94%) having a family history of diabetes (44%), being overweight (29%), and being obese (19%). When risk factors were combined, five groups were found to have 1, 2, 3, 4, or 5 risk factors, with corresponding prevalences of 28, 46, 20, 4, and 2%. When examining the characteristics of the aforementioned groups, it was found that there was a statistically significant difference in pre-pregnancy weight ($p < 0.0001$) and prepregnancy BMI ($p < 0.0001$) across the five groups, with the number of risk factors rising with each group. Only neonatal hypoglycemia ($p = 0.03$) varied significantly between the groups in terms of neonatal outcomes, with higher percentages among women who had more combined risk factors.

Conclusion: Traditional risk factors for GDM prevalence in singleton ART pregnancies complicated by GDM.

CRITICAL APPRAISAL

What was Known Prior to the Study?

Pregnancy-related complications are more common in singleton pregnancies achieved by assisted reproductive techniques. Various studies have shown a higher risk of gestational diabetes in such cases. Later age of conception, obesity, previous history of gestational diabetes mellitus (GDM), and family history of type 2 diabetes mellitus increase the chances of developing gestational diabetes. The former two factors are also more prevalent in women opting for assisted reproductive technology (ART).

What this Study Add?

This study shows the prevalence of various traditional risk factors for gestational diabetes among women with gestational diabetes conceiving through ART. It also assesses the proportion of women having multiple risk factors and the association of neonatal outcomes in this population. A higher age at conception and a positive family history of diabetes are likely the strongest predictors of developing GDM.

Major Strengths of the Study

Comprehensive data collection done at a single center gave a detailed account of all the neonatal outcomes.

Limitations of the Study

There was no control group of women who conceived spontaneously. Hence it is not possible to assess the difference between the prevalence of risk factors among the two groups. There was no data regarding the category of ART used, which may have possibly affected the risk of GDM. For example, metanalysis indicates that the risk of gestational diabetes is higher when using the in vitro technique compared to intracytoplasmic sperm injection (ICSI). There was no data on the prevalence of polycystic ovary syndrome (PCOS) as a cause of infertility, which may predispose to altered glucose metabolism in pregnancy. A proportion of women with gestational diabetes have persistent hyperglycemia even after pregnancy, especially with high pregnancy body mass index (BMI). This association was also not explored in the current study.

Implications of the Findings for the Clinicians

Women planning to use ART are usually at a higher risk of developing gestational diabetes. They should be counseled for a healthy lifestyle to reduce weight and optimize BMI before conceiving. This would reduce the risk of gestational diabetes and its possible adverse neonatal outcomes, most notably neonatal hypoglycemia.

Knowledge Gaps Identified and Scope for Future Research

The cumulative risk of gestational diabetes in the presence of multiple risk factors and stratification into high and low-risk women require further research.

---

4. Comparing the Different Phenotypes of Diabetes in Pregnancy: Are Outcomes Worse for Women with Young-onset Type 2 Diabetes Mellitus Compared to Type 1 Diabetes?

Ref: Zhen XM, Ross G, Gauld A, Nettel-Aguirre A, Noonan S, Constantino M, et al. Comparing the different phenotypes of diabetes in pregnancy: Are outcomes worse for women with young-onset type 2 diabetes mellitus compared to type 1 diabetes? Diabetes Res Clin Pract. 2024;217:111848.

ABSTRACT

Goal: Young-onset type 2 diabetes mellitus (YT2DM), an aggressive phenotype linked to a higher vascular risk profile than type 1 diabetes mellitus (T1DM), is becoming more prevalent during pregnancy. To identify places where different treatment advice could be required, we compared pregnancy outcomes.

Techniques: The 259 singleton pregnancies with pregestational T1DM ($n = 124$) or YT2DM ($n = 135$) diagnosed at <40 years were included in this retrospective single-center analysis (2010–2019). Preterm delivery, large for gestational age (LGA) babies, and preeclampsia were the main outcomes.

Findings: The YT2DM group was older, more obese, had a more apparent sociodemographic disadvantage, and had worse pregnancy readiness scores. The T1DM cohort also had a high prevalence of overweight and obesity (46% afflicted). The T1DM cohort had significantly higher mean glycated hemoglobin (HbA1c) values in the second and third trimesters. The rates of premature delivery and preeclampsia were comparable among the groups. The YT2DM cohort had a significantly decreased incidence of neonatal respiratory distress, neonatal hypoglycemia, neonatal intensive care unit (NICU) admission, and LGA infants ($p < 0.05$ for all).

Conclusion: Despite greater rates of obesity, YT2DM seems to be the lower-risk cohort during pregnancy as compared to T1DM. There are gaps in meeting glycemic goals for both subtypes, but T1DM in particular. More clarification is needed about the relative effects of rising BMI in pregnancies impacted by T1DM.

CRITICAL APPRAISAL

What was Known Prior to this Study?

From 2000 to 2010, the prevalence of pregestational diabetes (including type 2 diabetes mellitus) increased by 37%. With rising rates of diabetes in pregnancy, there is an increase in the adverse neonatal outcomes thereby associated. Young-onset type 2 diabetes mellitus (diagnosis < 40 years) has an accelerated presentation in terms of vascular complications and cardiometabolic derangements compared to type 1 diabetes mellitus (T1DM) outside pregnancy.

What Does this Study Add?

The study shows the baseline phenotypic differences between the young-onset type 2 diabetes mellitus and T1DM with respect to pregnancy, the former conceiving at a later age and having a higher pre-pregnancy body mass index (BMI). The poorer glycemic status of T1D in pregnancy is also highlighted as is the higher prevalence of LGA, neonatal hypoglycemia, and respiratory distress. These results point toward a high-risk profile of T1DM compared to YT2DM in pregnancy in terms of neonatal outcomes. Despite an expected greater risk of vascular complications in YT2DM, this is not observed during pregnancy as evidenced by the similar rates of gestational hypertension, preeclampsia, and preterm deliveries in both groups.

Major Strengths of the Study

Single-center study design ensured uniform healthcare practices. Comprehensive data was collected in a standardized manner. Multiple confounding factors such as age, duration of diabetes, and gestational weight gain were adjusted for during the analysis of maternal and neonatal outcomes.

Limitations of the Study

Being a single-center study, the results may not be generalizable to other geographical areas with different ethnicities. The majority (~70%) of T1D were Whites, whereas 53% of YT2DM were Asians, hence groups were not matched with respect to ethnicity. T1D women had a higher proportion of planned pregnancies and periconceptional folate use compared to YT2DM; considering these factors being addressed, there might be a further lower risk of adverse maternal and neonatal outcomes in the latter cohort increasing the difference between them.

Implications of the Findings for the Clinicians

Pregnant women with T1DM should receive special attention to optimize their glycemic status and weight gain to reduce adverse neonatal and maternal outcomes. Women with type 2 diabetes mellitus should receive thorough preconceptional counseling and appropriate lifestyle and pharmacotherapy to optimize pregnancy outcomes.

Knowledge Gaps Identified and Scope for Future Research

The contribution of increasing BMI in pregnancies affected by T1DM needs to be addressed.

5. Comparing Advanced Hybrid Closed Loop Therapy and Standard Insulin Therapy in Pregnant Women with Type 1 Diabetes (Cristal): A Parallel-group, Open-label, Randomised Controlled Trial

Ref: Benhalima K, Beunen K, Van Wilder N, Ballaux D, Vanhaverbeke G, Taes Y, et al. Comparing advanced hybrid closed loop therapy and standard insulin therapy in pregnant women with type 1 diabetes (CRISTAL): a parallel-group, open-label, randomised controlled trial. Lancet Diabetes Endocrinol. 2024;12(6):390-403.

ABSTRACT

Context: For pregnant women with type 1 diabetes, advanced hybrid closed loop (AHCL) therapy can help with glycemic management. However, as AHCL systems, including the MiniMed™ 780G, are not yet authorized for use in pregnant women, information regarding their effectiveness and safety is required. Our goal was to find out if pregnant women with type 1 diabetes may have better glycemic control and fewer hypoglycemia using the MiniMed™ 780G.

Techniques: Twelve hospitals (eleven in Belgium and one in the Netherlands) with secondary and tertiary care specialized endocrinology centers participated in the double-arm, parallel-group, open-label, randomized controlled study known as CRISTAL.

At a median gestational age of 10.1 (IQR 8.6–11.6) weeks, pregnant women with type 1 diabetes aged 18–45 years were randomized (1:1) to receive either normal insulin therapy (standard of care) or AHCL therapy (MiniMed 780G). Central randomization was used, with minimization based on the center, insulin administration technique, and baseline glycated hemoglobin (HbA1c). Group assignment was not concealed from study teams or participants. The main result was the percentage of time spent in the target glucose range (3.5–7.8 mmol/L) that is particular to pregnancy, as determined by continuous glucose monitoring (CGM) at 14–17, 20–23, 26–29, and 33–36 weeks. Overnight time within the goal range and overall and overnight time below the glucose range (<3.5 mmol/L) were important secondary outcomes. An intention-to-treat approach was used for the analyses. ClinicalTrials.gov has this trial registered (NCT04520971).

Results: 95 of the 101 patients who had screening between January 15, 2021, and September 30, 2022, were randomized to receive either regular insulin therapy ($n = 49$) or advanced hybrid closed loop (AHCL) therapy ($n = 46$). The trial was finished by 46 individuals receiving regular insulin medication and 43 patients receiving AHCL therapy. The mean HbA1c was 6.5% [standard deviation (SD) 0.6] at baseline, and 91 (95.8%) of the individuals utilized insulin pumps. Over four time periods, the AHCL therapy group's mean percentage of time spent in the target range was 66.5% (SD 10.0), while the standard insulin therapy groups were 63.2% (12.4) [adjusted mean difference 1.88% points [95% confidence interval (CI) −0.82 to 4.58, $p = 0.17$].

Advanced hybrid closed loop therapy decreased overnight [adjusted mean difference −1.86 percentage points (95% CI −2.90 to −0.81), $p = 0.0005$] and time below range overall (adjusted mean difference −1.34% points [95% CI −2.19 to −0.49], $p = 0.0020$) compared to standard insulin therapy. Overnight time in the target range was higher [adjusted mean difference 6.58% points (95% CI 2.31–10.85), $p = 0.0026$]. Higher levels of treatment satisfaction were reported by participants assigned to AHCL therapy. With AHCL treatment, there were no unexpected safety incidents.

Interpretation: AHCL therapy enhanced nighttime time in the target range, decreased time below range, and increased treatment satisfaction in pregnant women who had tighter glycemic control at the beginning of the treatment, but it did not improve total time in the target range. These findings imply that the MiniMed 780G is safe to use during pregnancy and offers a few extra advantages over conventional insulin therapy; still, it will be crucial to improve the algorithm to better suit the needs of pregnant women.

CRITICAL APPRAISAL

What Does this Study Add?
It is the first large, parallel-group, open-label, multicenter randomized controlled trial (RCT) that evaluated the utility of MiniMed 780G compared to standard insulin therapy in pregnant women with type 1 diabetes. In women with tightly controlled glycemic status in early pregnancy, advanced hybrid closed loop (AHCL) therapy resulted in a similar proportion of time spent in the target glucose range (3.5–7.8 mmol/L) compared with standard insulin therapy, with higher overnight time in the target range, less time below glucose range < 3.5 mmol/L overall and overnight, reduced hypoglycemia unawareness, reduced glycemic variability. This was accompanied by improved treatment satisfaction.

Major Strengths of the Study
The randomized controlled design of the trial and inclusion of women with tightly controlled diabetes could help assess the minor excursions in glycemic status. Any form of insulin therapy and all types of continuous glucose monitoring (CGM) was permitted in the standard insulin therapy group to allow for a representative population. To avoid bias by measuring glycemic outcomes with different types of CGM, the same was used CGM in both groups at prespecified time points.

Limitations of the Study
Being an open-label trial, the treatment allocation could not be masked from participants and the research team. Women requiring a total daily dose of insulin > 1.5 U/kg were excluded. Hence the performance of the device in higher insulin resistance states was not studied. Whether the benefits in terms of overnight hyperglycemia were clinically meaningful cannot be commented on since the study was not powered to detect differences in perinatal outcomes. The population was largely homogeneous (the majority of women were on an insulin pump at baseline, almost 90% were White, and more than two-thirds were highly educated). Therefore, the generalizability of the results to other populations is questionable. Additionally, the study was not powered for outcomes such as treatment satisfaction and risk of hypoglycemia (as these were all exploratory outcomes). Moreover, as randomization occurred on average at 10 weeks, data on early pregnancy were scarce.

Implications of the Findings for the Clinicians
It is safe to continue MiniMed 780G in women with type 1 diabetes who conceive.

Knowledge Gaps Identified and Scope for Future Research
Whether the use of AHCL (MiniMed 780G) can improve perinatal and neonatal outcomes remains to be determined.

---

6. Early Pregnancy HbA1c as the First Screening Test for Gestational Diabetes: Results from Three Prospective Cohorts

Ref: Saravanan P, Deepa M, Ahmed Z, Ram U, Surapaneni T, Kallur SD, et al. Early pregnancy HbA1c as the first screening test for gestational diabetes: results from three prospective cohorts. Lancet Diabetes Endocrinol. 2024;12(8):535-44.

ABSTRACT

Context: Low-income and middle-income countries (LMICs) are thought to account for over 90% of instances of gestational diabetes. An oral glucose tolerance test (OGTT) between weeks 24 and 28 of pregnancy is advised by the majority of current guidelines. Due to the OGTTs' demanding nature, particularly in LMICs, a significant percentage of women do not get checked. Our goal was to create a straightforward and efficient method of screening for gestational diabetes.

Techniques: A prospective cohort study called STRiDE (Stanford Translational Research Integrated Database Environment) was established in seven locations in western Kenya and seven in south India. It comprised pregnant women between the ages of 18 and 50 years who were <16 weeks along (<20 weeks in Kenya), as determined by dated ultrasonography. In two LMICs (India and Kenya) and a multiethnic population from the PRiDE (PRegnancy and Infant DEvelopment) study in the UK, we evaluated the effectiveness of early pregnancy glycated hemoglobin (HbA1c) (venous and capillary point-of-care), either by itself or in combination with age, body mass index (BMI), and family history of diabetes, in predicting gestational diabetes at 24–28 weeks' gestation. Evaluating if an early pregnancy composite risk score can lessen the requirement for OGTTs was a crucial secondary goal. A diagnosis of gestational diabetes was made using current World Health Organization (WHO) criteria.

Results: We enrolled 4,104 participants in Kenya and 3,070 individuals in India between February 15, 2016, and December 13, 2019. The PRiDE cohort had 4,320 participants. The prevalence of gestational diabetes by OGTT at 24–28 weeks was 14.5% in the UK, 3.0% in Kenya, and 19.2% in India. The incidence of gestational diabetes at 24–28 weeks' gestation was independently correlated with early pregnancy HbA1c. India's adjusted risk ratio was 1.60 [95% confidence interval (CI) 1.19–2.16], Kenya's was 3.49 (2.8–4.34), and the UK's was 4.72 (3.82–5.82).

The greatest predictors of testing positive for gestational diabetes were composite risk score models that integrated age, BMI, and family history of diabetes with venous or point-of-care HbA1c. The need for OGTTs could be decreased by 50–64% with a population-specific, two-threshold screening approach that uses the early pregnancy composite risk score to rule in and rule out gestational diabetes. India's thresholds for the HbA1c-alone model were 5.4% (rule in) and 4.9% (rule out), Kenya's were 6.0% (rule in) and 5.2% (rule out), and the UKs were 5.6% (rule in) and 5.2% (rule out).

Interpretation: In order to significantly lessen the requirement for OGTTs, early pregnancy HbA1c provides a straightforward screening test for gestational diabetes, enabling those who are most at risk to get early care. In LMICs, point-of-care HbA1c can also be used for this.

CRITICAL APPRAISAL

What was Known before this Study?

The oral glucose tolerance test (OGTT) performed at 24-28 weeks' gestation is currently considered the gold-standard approach for screening and diagnosis of gestational diabetes. However, it is tedious as it requires women to attend a facility with appropriate laboratory infrastructure, in a fasting state. This is even more difficult in rural settings in India, Kenya, and other low-income and middle-income countries (LMICs). Moreover, there is evidence of fetal adipose tissue accumulation in gestational diabetes mellitus (GDM) even before the diagnosis is established. Hence, WHO has recommended developing a simple and effective screening strategy in early pregnancy as a priority. A retrospective study in the US showed that glycated hemoglobin (HbA1c) along with other risk factors might be of value in predicting GDM.

What Does this Study Add?

This study showed that early pregnancy HbA1c, on its own or as a composite risk score with common risk factors, can be used to predict about 50% of gestational diabetes at 24–28 weeks' gestation. The risk ratios of developing gestational diabetes were different in different populations, highlighting the need for population-specific thresholds. Using two thresholds for rule-in and rule-out gestational diabetes helps with risk stratification in early pregnancy. The need for OGTTs can be reduced by 50–64% in different populations by using venous or point-of-care HbA1c. Data regarding population-specific diabetes risk was also obtained.

Major Strengths of the Study

A large population cohort of diverse ethnic and socioeconomic backgrounds was studied which would fairly represent low- and middle-income countries. The cohorts were representative of local populations in terms of age, body mass index (BMI), and socioeconomic status (SES). The role of composite risk score was prospectively studied by comparison with the OGTT (the current standard). The models for scoring were cross-validated by the bootstrapping approach.

Limitations of the Study

Women with severe anemia and hemoglobinopathies were excluded which are highly prevalent in LMICs. Considering this aspect, the applicability of the screening needs to be further evaluated. The higher cost of point-of-care HbA1c might also be a factor to consider in these countries despite being simple.

Implications of the Findings for the Clinicians

In LMICs, first-trimester HbA1c-based screening and risk assessment should be considered if feasible; with a caveat that it may require further testing at 24–28 weeks. Once ruled in, early intervention for GDM should be offered to keep in view the possible improved pregnancy outcomes.

Knowledge Gaps Identified and Scope for Future Research

Whether the two-step screening strategy results in improved pregnancy and neonatal outcomes is not known, which requires randomized controlled trials.

Section 7: DRUGS AND THERAPEUTICS

Section Editor: Sunetra Mondal

1. Comparative Effects of Randomized Second-line Therapy for Type 2 Diabetes on a Composite Outcome Incorporating Glycemic Control, Body Weight, and Hypoglycemia: An Analysis of the Glycemia Reduction Approaches in Diabetes: A Comparative Effectiveness Study (GRADE)

Ref: Kirkman MS, Tripputi M, Krause-Steinrauf H, Bebu I, AbouAssi H, Burch H, et al. Comparative Effects of Randomized Second-line Therapy for Type 2 Diabetes on a Composite Outcome Incorporating Glycemic Control, Body Weight, and Hypoglycemia: An Analysis of the Glycemia Reduction Approaches in Diabetes: A Comparative Effectiveness Study (GRADE). Diabetes Care. 2024;47(4):594-602.

ABSTRACT

Objective: The glycemic control of four randomized therapy added to metformin was shown to vary over time in the Glycemia Reduction Approaches in Diabetes: A Comparative Effectiveness Study (GRADE) (5,047 individuals, mean follow-up 5.0 years). Hypoglycemia and weight gain are significant consequences for individuals with type 2 diabetes. We examined how the four randomized GRADE drugs affected a composite outcome that included weight gain, hypoglycemia, and glycemic worsening.

Research design and methods: Time to first occurrence of any of the following was the composite outcome: ≥5% weight gain; severe or recurrent nonsevere hypoglycemia; or a verified hemoglobin A1c (HbA1c) >7.5%. Individual elements of the composite outcome, subgroup effects and possible mediators, and treatment satisfaction were all examined in secondary analyses. The Kaplan–Meier estimator was used to estimate cumulative incidence. Pairwise group variations in outcome risk were evaluated using Cox proportional hazards models.

Results: All pairwise comparisons were statistically significant, and liraglutide had the lowest risk of achieving the composite outcome [events per 100 participants per treatment year (PTYs)], followed by sitagliptin (26 per 100 PTYs), glargine (29 per 100 PTYs), and glimepiride (40 per 100 PTYs).

The risk of glycemic worsening was lowest with glargine, followed by glimepiride, liraglutide, and sitagliptin; the risk of weight gain and hypoglycemia were in the same order. There was no discernible variation in the risk of the composite outcome among the predetermined covariates. Treatment satisfaction was somewhat but significantly lower for participants who achieved the composite outcome.

Conclusion: The group receiving glimepiride had the highest risk of achieving a composite outcome that included weight gain, hypoglycemia, and glycemic worsening, whereas the group receiving liraglutide had the lowest risk among people treated with typical second-line medication classes for type 2 diabetes. These results could help guide treatment decisions for type 2 diabetes.

CRITICAL APPRAISAL

What was Known Prior to this Study?

The differential effects of the multiple second-line antidiabetic agents as add-on to metformin individually on hemoglobin A1c (HbA1c), body weight, hypoglycemia, and in the current years on the cardiovascular and renal risk is now well known. In a prior Glycemia Reduction Approaches in Diabetes: A Comparative Effectiveness Study (GRADE) trial, significant differences in glycemic control were demonstrated over time for four commonly used second line therapies.

What this Study Adds?

This study analyzed a composite of multiple end points incorporating glycemic deterioration, weight gain and hypoglycemia, and found differential effects of four common second-line antidiabetic agents—liraglutide, sitagliptin, glimepiride, and glargine as add-ons to metformin. The lowest risk of the composite outcome and of the individual components weight gain and hypoglycemia was seen with liraglutide followed by sitagliptin glargine and lastly, glimepiride. However, glycemic deterioration was lowest with glargine, followed by liraglutide, glimepiride, and sitagliptin. The results did not differ when subgroup analysis was done by age, body mass index (BMI), ethnicity or duration of diabetes. Those in the glimepiride group had significantly increased risk of reaching the hypoglycemia outcome compared to other groups after addition of rescue insulin.

Major Strengths of the Study

It was a large study of >5,000 patients with type 2 diabetes (T2D) of <10 years' duration, followed a rigorous trial design with multiple prespecified outcomes assessments over a long follow-up period and high rates of participant retention. These allowed for robust data analyses, including in several subgroups. The composite outcome included characteristics important to patients as well as clinicians. Patient-reported outcomes such as treatment satisfaction were also focused.

Limitations of the Study

The GRADE study was conducted before the widespread use of sodium-glucose cotransporter-2 inhibitor (SGLT-2i) and weekly glucagon-like peptide-1 receptor agonists (GLP-1-RAs). The medications and healthcare were provided free of charge and included repeated counseling on weight management and hypoglycemia prevention, which might be different from the real-world. Cardiovascular outcomes were not studied.

Implications of the Findings for the Clinicians

The differential effects of some common anti-diabetes drugs, when added to metformin, on a composite outcome incorporating glycemic deterioration, weight gain, and hypoglycemia can guide the choice of second- and third-line therapy for patients with T2D beyond just glycemic control. Incorporating patient satisfaction can aid in an approach to informed person-centric management of T2D.

Addition of rescue insulin increases the rates of weight gain, even when added to a baseline of weight-neutral or weight loss–promoting medications, mandating education and support for lifestyle efforts to avoid weight gain in those on insulin. Hypoglycemia risk is quite high if sulfonylureas are continued when insulin is initiated, even if basal insulin. The addition of prandial or rapid-acting insulins to glargine can lead to increased risk of hypoglycemia with relatively little effect on HbA1c%.

Knowledge Gaps Identified and Scope for Future Research

Future similar studies focusing on composite outcome inclusive of the cardiorenal events and including SGLT-2i as one of the arms are necessary. Also, the effects of rescue insulin to those on combination oral antidiabetic drugs (OADs) need to be highlighted.

2. Impact of Canagliflozin on Kidney and Cardiovascular Outcomes by Type 2 Diabetes Duration: A Pooled Analysis of the CANVAS Program and CREDENCE Trials

Ref: Tobe SW, Mavrakanas TA, Bajaj HS, Levin A, Tangri N, Slee A, et al. Impact of Canagliflozin on Kidney and Cardiovascular Outcomes by Type 2 Diabetes Duration: A Pooled Analysis of the CANVAS Program and CREDENCE Trials. Diabetes Care. 2024;47(3):501-7.

ABSTRACT

Objective: The purpose of the study was to determine whether the length of time a person has type 2 diabetes affects how the sodium-glucose cotransporter-2 inhibitor canagliflozin affects their renal and cardiovascular (CV) outcomes.

Design and methods of research: The effects of canagliflozin on kidney and CV outcomes, including the progression and regression of albuminuria over 5-year intervals of disease duration, were assessed using Cox proportional hazards and hazard ratios in this post hoc analysis of the Canagliflozin Cardiovascular Assessment Study (CANVAS) Program ($n = 10,142$) and Evaluation of the Effects of Canagliflozin on Renal and Cardiovascular Outcomes in Participants With Diabetic Nephropathy (CREDENCE) trial ($n = 4,401$).

Results: Canagliflozin showed varying degrees of benefit across the course of diabetes, with no variation in the incidence of significant adverse CV events, hospitalization for heart failure or CV death, renal failure requiring treatment, or doubling serum creatinine. Additionally, across all diabetes duration categories, canagliflozin increased albuminuria regression and decreased albuminuria progression without interacting.

Conclusion: According to our research, people with type 2 diabetes who get canagliflozin earlier on consistently see improvements in their heart health.

CRITICAL APPRAISAL

What was Known Prior to this Study?

Canagliflozin, like other sodium-glucose cotransporter-2 inhibitor (SGLT-2i), have shown benefits in reduction of cardiac events as well as renal adverse outcomes such as worsening of estimated glomerular filtration rate (eGFR), progression of albuminuria, new-onset nephropathy, or progression to end-stage renal disease (ESRD) in patients with type 2 diabetes mellitus (T2DM) in dedicated trials such as the Canagliflozin Cardiovascular Assessment Study (CANVAS) Program, and the Evaluation of the Effects of Canagliflozin on Renal and Cardiovascular Outcomes in Participants With Diabetic Nephropathy (CREDENCE) trials. The effects of duration of T2DM on these benefits were not clear.

What this Study Adds?

The authors did an integrated, pooled, and patient-level data meta-analysis using data from the CANVAS Program and CREDENCE trials to assess whether the duration of T2DM (by 5-year intervals) has a role in modulating the effects of canagliflozin on cardiovascular (CV) and kidney outcomes, focusing on the progression and regression of albuminuria in patients with high CV risk and/or chronic kidney disease (CKD).

They found that the benefits with canagliflozin were seen in T2DM irrespective of the duration, across all time intervals. There was no heterogeneity with respect to reduction in CV or renal events, including the progression and regression of albuminuria as early as within the first 5 years of diabetes.

Major Strengths of the Study

Being a post hoc analysis of three large randomized controlled trials (RCTs), the study had a large sample size including participants with heterogeneous baseline risk of cardiovascular disease (CVD) and different stages of diabetic kidney disease (DKD).

Limitations of the Study

Being a post hoc analysis, the study was not designed with adequate statistical power for subgroup analysis according to diabetes duration.

Additionally, participants in these trials had moderate- to high-risk CV disease and/or CKD, thus limiting the generalizability of the study to the standard population.

Implications of the Findings for the Clinicians

The cardiorenal benefits of canagliflozin in T2DM are seen in both recent onset T2DM and T2DM of prolonged duration. It may not be prudent for clinicians to wait for rising albuminuria or declining kidney function as an indication to initiate SGLT-2i therapy. Rather, early initiation of SGLT-2i is warranted in people with T2DM at highest risk of developing CKD or CV events.

Knowledge Gaps Identified and Scope for Future Research

The effect of duration of T2DM on the cardiorenal benefits of canagliflozin remains unknown in those without high risk of CVD or those without established diabetic kidney disease (DKD). A large proportion of individuals with recent onset T2DM will not be having high CV/renal risk or established atherosclerotic cardiovascular disease (ASCVD)/DKD. Additionally, the effect of canagliflozin as an add-on to angiotensin-converting enzyme inhibitor (ACEi)/angiotensin receptor blocker (ARB) and the role of other SGLT-2i apart from canagliflozin in early onset T2DM remain to be seen. Majority of the population was obese with mean body mass index (BMI) exceeding 30 and the mean age was around 60 years, thus the effects in nonobese and young T2DM in the early years after diagnosis remain to be explored.

3. Occurrence of Gastrointestinal Adverse Events Upon GLP-1 Receptor Agonist Initiation with Concomitant Metformin Use: A Post Hoc Analysis of LEADER, STEP 2, SUSTAIN-6, and PIONEER 6

Ref: Klein KR, Clemmensen KKB, Fong E, Olsen S, Abrahamsen T, Lingvay I. Occurrence of Gastrointestinal Adverse Events Upon GLP-1 Receptor Agonist Initiation With Concomitant Metformin Use: A Post Hoc Analysis of LEADER, STEP 2, SUSTAIN-6, and PIONEER 6. Diabetes Care. 2024;47(2):280-4.

ABSTRACT

Goal: To evaluate how concurrent metformin use affects gastrointestinal side effects after starting and titrating a glucagon-like peptide 1 receptor agonist (GLP-1 RA).

Design and methods of research: We compared the incidence of gastrointestinal adverse events during GLP-1RA initiation and titration in participants with and without concurrent metformin use using data from four clinical trials of liraglutide and semaglutide [Liraglutide Effect and Action in Diabetes: Evaluation of Cardiovascular Outcome Results (LEADER), Semaglutide Treatment Effect in

People with Obesity (STEP 2), Trial to Evaluate Cardiovascular and Other Long-Term Outcomes With Semaglutide in Subjects With Type 2 Diabetes (SUSTAIN-6), and Peptide Innovation for Early Diabetes Treatment (PIONEER) 6].

Results: 12,928 (76%) of the 16,996 patients received metformin treatment. The frequency or severity of gastrointestinal adverse events during the monitoring period was not increased by concurrent metformin use. Metformin use was not associated with a higher rate of study product discontinuation among participants who had gastrointestinal side effects. Compared to metformin users, a numerically larger proportion of metformin nonusers had gastrointestinal side effects and stopped taking the study medication within treatment arms (GLP-1 RA and placebo).

Conclusion: Taking metformin concurrently has no effect on stopping GLP-1 RA or increasing the likelihood of gastrointestinal complaints during GLP-1 RA beginning.

CRITICAL APPRAISAL

What was Known Prior to this Study?

Gastrointestinal (GI) symptoms are well-known and common adverse effects of glucagon-like peptide 1 receptor agonists (GLP-1 RAs) as well as of metformin. Although often transient and of mild-to-moderate severity, GI adverse effects account for most cases of discontinuation of GLP-1 RAs in clinical trials as well as in real world. The mechanisms for GI intolerance with metformin are different, but it is reasonable to have a concern that metformin use might be a factor exacerbating GLP-1 RA–induced GI symptoms. However, whether or not the concomitant use of metformin and GLP-1 RA have any synergistic role in worsening the GI symptoms were yet unknown prior to this study.

What this Study Adds?

The authors used data from four randomized controlled trials (RCTs) involving GLP-1 RAs—namely the Liraglutide Effect and Action in Diabetes: Evaluation of Cardiovascular Outcome Results (LEADER), Semaglutide Treatment Effect in People with Obesity (STEP 2), Trial to Evaluate Cardiovascular and Other Long-Term Outcomes With Semaglutide in Subjects With Type 2 Diabetes (SUSTAIN-6), and Peptide Innovation for Early Diabetes Treatment (PIONEER) 6 to assess whether the concomitant use of metformin during the initiation and titration of GLP-1 RA led to worsening of GI symptoms. They found that the concomitant use of metformin had no role in the incidence or severity of GI adverse events seen with GLP-1 RA initiation or titration. The proportion of participants randomized to a GLP-1 RA who experienced GI adverse events and/or withdrew from the study arm due to GI adverse effects were similar in those with and without baseline metformin use. Interestingly, in each of the RCTs, proportion of participants experiencing GI adverse effects was higher in those without concomitant metformin use, in both the GLP-1 RA and the placebo arms. Also, a higher percentage of participants who did not receive metformin had discontinued the study product for GI problems in both treatment arms.

Major Strengths of the Study

The post hoc analysis included a huge number of participants using modern day GLP-1 RAs, unlike a prior meta-analysis which included some studies of patients using short acting GLP-1 RAs with metformin. Metformin users were compared to nonusers both at initiation and phases of up titration of GLP-1 RAs. Subgroup analysis according to chronic kidney disease (CKD) and body mass index (BMI) was also conducted.

Limitations of the Study

It was a post hoc analysis limiting its statistical power to demonstrate the objective. The number of serious GI adverse effects leading to drug discontinuation was very less in all the trials. Although nonsignificant, but the fact that metformin nonusers had greater changes of GI adverse effects or drug discontinuation for the same could be attributed to other factors like increased baseline susceptibility to GI symptoms for which metformin was not used in them at the first place. Also, metformin nonusers might reflect a group of people who were sicker population with a greater symptom burden contraindicating metformin use. The authors did not evaluate the effects of simultaneous initiation of metformin and GLP-1 RA.

Implications of the Findings for the Clinicians

The use of concomitant metformin during the initiation or phases of uptitration of GLP-1 RA initiation did not worsen the GI side effects. Thus, it is not necessary to discontinue metformin prior to or during GLP-1 RA use in an attempt to annihilate GI symptoms.

Knowledge Gaps Identified and Scope for Future Research

Semaglutide users had numerically higher percentage of GI adverse events among metformin nonusers, but there indeed was a statistically significant increase in GI adverse events in participants treated with metformin in the liraglutide trials which could be due to differences in pharmacokinetics between liraglutide and semaglutide and demanding more trials in this area.

4. Early-onset Type 2 Diabetes and Tirzepatide Treatment: A Post Hoc Analysis from the SURPASS Clinical Trial Program

Ref: Zeitler P, Galindo RJ, Davies MJ, Bergman BK, Thieu VT, Nicolay C, et al. Early-Onset Type 2 Diabetes and Tirzepatide Treatment: A Post Hoc Analysis From the SURPASS Clinical Trial Program. Diabetes Care. 2024;47(6):1056-64.

ABSTRACT

Objective: We assessed tirzepatide's effects on glycemic control, body weight (BW), and cardiometabolic indicators, as well as the baseline characteristics of SURPASS program participants with early-onset type 2 diabetes (T2D).

Design and methods of research: At week 40 [A Study of Tirzepatide (LY3298176) in Participants With Type 2 Diabetes Not Controlled With Diet and Exercise Alone (SURPASS-1) and A Study of Tirzepatide (LY3298176) Versus Semaglutide Once Weekly as Add-on Therapy to Metformin in Participants With Type 2 Diabetes (SURPASS-2)] or week 52 [A Study of Tirzepatide (LY3298176) Versus Insulin Degludec in Participants With Type 2 Diabetes (SURPASS-3)], this post hoc analysis compared baseline characteristics and changes in mean hemoglobin A1c (HbA1c), BW, lipids, and blood pressure (BP) in 3,792 participants with early-onset versus later-onset T2D.

Data from individuals receiving allocated treatment without rescue medicine in the event of persistent hyperglycemia were analyzed by the study.

Outcomes: Those with early-onset T2D were younger at baseline in SURPASS-2, had a longer duration of diabetes (9 vs. 7 years, $p < 0.001$), higher glycemic levels (8.5% vs. 8.2%, $p < 0.001$), higher BW (97 vs. 93 kg, $p < 0.001$), higher BMI (35 vs. 34 kg/m^2, $p < 0.001$), and a similarly abnormal lipid profile (e.g., triglycerides 167 vs. 156 mg/dL). Similar improvements were seen in both subgroups with tirzepatide at week 40 in terms of HbA1c (22.6% vs. 22.4%), BW (214 vs. 213 kg), waist circumference (WC) (210 vs. 210 cm), triglycerides (226% vs. 224%), high-density lipoprotein (HDL) (7% vs. 7%), and systolic BP (26 vs. 27 mm Hg).

Conclusion: Participants with early-onset T2D from the SURPASS program had worse overall metabolic health and higher glucose levels at baseline than those with later-onset T2D, despite being younger. Regardless of age upon T2D diagnosis, tirzepatide was found to produce comparable improvements in HbA1c, BW, and cardiometabolic indicators in this post hoc research. To ascertain tirzepatide's long-term effects in early-onset T2D, more research is required.

CRITICAL APPRAISAL

Why was this Study Undertaken?

Early-onset type 2 diabetes (T2D) diagnosed before the age of 40 years, is known to be associated with high risk for cardiovascular (CV) complications. Tirzepatide is a once weekly glucose-dependent insulinotropic polypeptide (GIP) and glucagon-like peptide 1 (GLP-1) receptor agonist which has received approval in the US for the treatment of T2D and obesity. It has been studies in the SURPASS clinical trial program in which it has shown robust improvements in glycemic levels with 81–97% achieving hemoglobin A1c (HbA1c) < 7% and 23–62% achieving normoglycemia with HbA1c < 5.7%, substantial reductions in body weight (BW) (7–14%) as also improvement in anthropometric parameters like waist circumference and in cardiometabolic markers, including blood pressure (BP) and lipid profile. The authors assessed the baseline characteristics of participants with early-onset T2D and the effect of tirzepatide on glycemic parameters, BW, and cardiometabolic markers from the SURPASS group of trials.

What this Study Adds?

Though younger, the participants with early-onset type 2 diabetes mellitus (T2DM) had poorer glycemic control and glycemia, worse anthropometric parameters including high BW and a worse metabolic profile including dyslipidemia compared to later-onset T2D. The responses were dose dependent, with the highest proportion reaching HbA1c <7% or <5.7% being achieved with tirzepatide 15 mg. The improvement in glycemic status, BW, lipids, and BP seen with tirzepatide were seen irrespective of the age of diagnosis of T2DM.

Major Strengths of the Study

The authors included data from a large number of participants with early-onset T2DM with detailed baseline metabolic profile and this was the first study to highlight the effects of tirzepatide in this cohort.

Limitations

It was a post hoc data analysis from the SURPASS clinical trial program. There is lack of longitudinal or follow-up data leaving unresolved questions about the long term durability of the effects.

Implications of the Findings for the Clinicians

Despite being younger, participants with early-onset T2DM were found to have higher glucose levels and poorer overall metabolic health. The metabolic benefits of tirzepatide were seen irrespective of the age of diagnosis of T2DM and should be considered early in the disease course.

Knowledge Gaps Identified and Scope for Future Research

Further research is required to assess the long-term efficacy and safety of tirzepatide in young onset T2DM.

5. Efficacy and Safety of LX9211 for Relief of Diabetic Peripheral Neuropathic Pain (RELIEF-DPN 1): Results of a Double-blind, Randomized, Placebo-controlled, Proof-of-concept Study

Ref: Pop-Busui R, Patel A, Sang CN, Banks PL, Pierce PF, Sun F, et al. Efficacy and Safety of LX9211 for Relief of Diabetic Peripheral Neuropathic Pain (RELIEF-DPN 1): Results of a Double-Blind, Randomized, Placebo-Controlled, Proof-of-Concept Study. Diabetes Care. 2024;47(8):1325-32.

ABSTRACT

Purpose: To assess LX9211's ability to lessen diabetic peripheral neuropathy-related discomfort.

Design and methods of research: 319 patients with diabetic peripheral neuropathic pain (DPNP) were randomly assigned (1:1:1) to receive LX9211 10 mg ($n = 106$), LX9211 20 mg ($n = 106$), or a matching placebo ($n = 107$) once daily for 6 weeks in this double-blind, multicenter, proof-of-concept study. An 11-point numerical rating system was used to grade DPNP every day. The change in the average daily pain score from baseline to week 6 was the main outcome measure. Using mixed-model repeated-measures analysis, the differences between each LX9211 group and the placebo were assessed.

Results: High-dose LX9211 showed improvement in pain severity compared to placebo (21.27 vs. 20.72 points, respectively), but the between-group LS mean difference did not reach the prespecified statistical significance [20.55 (0.254), 95% confidence interval (CI) 21.06 to 20.05, $p = 0.030$]. For those on low-dose LX9211, the primary efficacy end point was achieved: 21.39 vs. 20.72 points for placebo, least squares mean (SE) difference 20.67 (0.249), 95% CI 21.16 to 20.18, $p = 0.007$. Benefits of the treatment were seen in week 1 and continued beyond that. Additionally, LX9211 results showed improvements in a number of secondary outcomes reported by patients. Headache, nausea, and dizziness were the most frequent adverse events (AEs).

Serious AEs were rare [2 (1.9%), 0, and 1 (0.9%), respectively], and more participants treated with LX9211 [20 mg, n = 28 (26.4%); 10 mg, 17 (16.0%)] than placebo [3 (2.8%)] stopped the study medication early because of AEs.

Conclusion: These early results of LX9211 improving DPNP lend credence to more research in larger trials.

CRITICAL APPRAISAL

What was Known Prior to this Study?

Diabetic peripheral neuropathy (DPN) is one of the most common complications of type 2 diabetes mellitus (T2DM) which affects approximately 50% of individuals with T2DM. Up to 30–40% of DPN experience neuropathic pain. Most currently available therapies for diabetic peripheral neuropathic pain (DPNP) used as monotherapy or in combination can provide only modest relief of pain and fewer than half of individuals being able to achieve 50% reduction in their pain severity. LX9211 is a nonopioid orally administered selective inhibitor of adapter protein-2-associated kinase 1 (AAK1) that showed good safety and efficacy in phase 1 and multiple ascending dose trials, demanding the need for further evaluation in trials.

What this Study Adds?

RELIEF-DPN 1, a phase 2 double-blind, randomized, multicenter, proof-of-concept study was conducted to evaluate the primary efficacy end point of low-dose LX9211 (10 mg daily) in DPNP. Low-dose LX9211 was seen to reduce pain at week 6, and to improve other patient-reported outcomes with minimal adverse effects. High-dose LX9211 (20 mg) showed numerical pain reduction which was statistically not significant, likely due to high incidence of treatment emergent adverse events (TEAEs) leading to treatment discontinuation. A proportion of the participants were already on baseline DPNP medication (mostly gabapentin) and treatment with LX9211 reduced neuropathic pain irrespective of the presence of baseline DPNP medication, though the reduction was numerically greater in the absence of baseline DPNP medication.

Major Strengths of the Study

The trial provides promising results of a molecule LX9211 breakthrough in the clinical management of a debilitating condition for which currently there are limited effective treatment option with only modest pain relief.

Limitations of the Study

It was a phase 2 proof-of-concept study with a relatively short treatment duration and enrolment of participants only from the US. Less than 40% of the participants were on baseline other DPNP medications, predominantly gabapentin and a small proportion on pregabalin and duloxetine while none were on other commonly used agents for DPNP.

Implications of the Findings for the Clinicians

LX9211 is a promising new therapeutic agent in DPNP but further investigation is required prior to widespread clinical use of the molecule.

Knowledge Gaps Identified and Scope for Future Research

Further advanced clinical trials for LX9211 for DPNP are required. Newer avenues and receptors for opioid and nonopioid analgesia must be studied.

---

6. Glucose-lowering Drugs and Liver-related Outcomes Among Individuals with Type 2 Diabetes: A Systematic Review of Longitudinal Population-based Studies

Ref: Khanmohammadi S, Habibzadeh A, Kamrul-Hasan ABM, Schuermans A, Kuchay MS. Glucose-lowering drugs and liver-related outcomes among individuals with type 2 diabetes: A systematic review of longitudinal population-based studies. Diabet Med. 2024;41(11):e15437.

ABSTRACT

Goals: Although there is a dearth of data from randomized controlled trials about the long-term impact of glucose-lowering drugs (GLDs) on liver-related outcomes, population-based studies have assessed the relationships between GLDs and liver-related outcomes in people with type 2 diabetes (T2D). Our goal was to perform a comprehensive analysis of population-based research assessing how GLDs affect liver-related outcomes in individuals with T2D.

Methods: From the beginning to February 23, 2024, the PubMed, Web of Science, and Embase databases were thoroughly searched for population-based studies examining the relationships between GLDs and liver-related outcomes in people with T2D and no liver disease other than nonalcoholic fatty liver disease (NAFLD). Glucagon-like peptide-1 receptor agonists (GLP-1 RAs), insulin, sodium-glucose cotransporter-2 inhibitors (SGLT-2is), thiazolidinediones (TZDs), and dipeptidyl peptidase-4 inhibitors (DPP-4is) were among the GLDs.

Findings: About 10 cohort studies with 1,274,641 participants satisfied the requirements for inclusion. 8.9–76 months were the median follow-up time. When compared to other drugs, SGLT-2is were linked to the greatest decrease in the incidence of NAFLD, cirrhosis, and composite liver-related events of all the GLDs that were being studied. Although TZDs were not substantially linked to a lower incidence of hepatocellular carcinoma, they were linked to a decreased risk of cirrhosis and NAFLD. Reduced liver-related mortality was significantly correlated with GLP-1-RAs.

Conclusion: In T2D patients with NAFLD, observational data from population-based research indicates that GLDs, such as SGLT-2is, are linked to positive long-term liver-related outcomes.

To validate these results, more research is required, such as randomized controlled trials with long-term follow-up.

CRITICAL APPRAISAL

What was Known Prior to this Study?

Type 2 diabetes mellitus (T2DM) increases the risk of developing metabolic dysfunction-associated steatotic liver disease (MASLD), previously nonalcoholic fatty liver disease (NAFLD), and vice versa, its progression to more severe forms and liver fibrosis. The coexistence of T2DM and MASLD increases the risk of cardiovascular and other complications by multiple times. There is lack of randomized controlled trials on the long-term effects of antihyperglycemic agents on liver-related outcomes. However, epidemiologic or population-based studies have studied their effects on liver-related outcomes in T2DM.

What this Study Adds?

This is a systematic review of 10 population-based studies which investigated the effects of different antihyperglycemic agents on liver-related outcomes in T2DM, comprising 1,274,641 participants, followed up for a period of 8.9–76 months. They concluded that while sodium-glucose cotransporter-2 inhibitors (SGLT-2is) led to the strongest reduction in the incidence of NAFLD, progression to cirrhosis, and composite liver-related events, thiazolidinediones (TZDs) also reduced the risk of developing NAFLD and cirrhosis but did not significantly lower the incidence of hepatocellular carcinoma (HCC). Glucagon-like peptide-1 receptor agonists (GLP-1 RAs) was significantly associated with reduced liver-related mortality.

Major Strengths of the Study

It was the first comprehensive systematic review of population-based cohort studies on the role of antidiabetic agents on multiple liver outcomes. Data from studies involving large number of studies was pooled, and various classes of antidiabetic medications including dipeptidyl peptidase-4 inhibitor (DPP-4i), SGLT-2is, GLP-1 RAs, thiazolidinediones, insulin, and sulfonylureas were studied. The follow-up period for most of these studies was longer than the usual 6 months follow-up used in most randomized controlled trials (RCTs), allowing for the analysis of mortality and other outcomes.

Limitations of the Study

The studies included were nonrandomized and the potential benefits seen with some of the drugs might be because they were being compared against a medication that is associated with higher risk. Heterogeneous study population incorporating those with and without NAFLD and variable duration of diabetes mellitus (DM) need to be considered. Liver-related outcomes including regression, progression, or cirrhosis were defined differently. There were discrepancies when the same agent was used in different studies. Other confounders included the heterogeneous data sources (single center vs. multicenter vs. databases), different study populations, and inclusion of observational studies with multiple variables.

Implications of the Findings for the Clinicians

In population-based studies, three classes of antidiabetic agents have been shown to improve liver-related outcomes. GLP-1 RAs could reduce liver-related mortality, SGLT-2is showed the greatest reduction in the incidence of NAFLD incidence, its progression to cirrhosis, and composite liver-related events. TZDs have been found to be effective in reducing NAFLD and cirrhosis risk but not in reduction of HCC incidence.

Knowledge Gaps Identified and Scope for Future Research

Dedicated RCTs, placebo controlled studies, and long-term prospective studies are needed to remove the role of confounders and establish the effect of individual antidiabetic agents on liver-related outcomes.

---

7. Dose-response Effects on HbA1c and Bodyweight Reduction of Survodutide, a Dual Glucagon/GLP-1 Receptor Agonist, Compared with Placebo and Open-label Semaglutide in People with Type 2 Diabetes: A Randomised Clinical Trial

Ref: Blüher M, Rosenstock J, Hoefler J, Manuel R, Hennige AM. Dose-response effects on HbA1c and bodyweight reduction of survodutide, a dual glucagon/GLP-1 receptor agonist, compared with placebo and open-label semaglutide in people with type 2 diabetes: a randomised clinical trial. Diabetologia. 2024;67(3):470-82.

ABSTRACT

Objectives and hypotheses: The purpose of this study was to evaluate the dose-response effects on bodyweight reduction and hemoglobin A1c (HbA1c) levels of survodutide (BI 456906), a subcutaneous glucagon receptor/glucagon-like peptide-1 receptor dual agonist.

Techniques: This multicenter, Phase II, randomized, double-blind, parallel-group, placebo-controlled study was carried out in clinical research centers and evaluated survodutide in participants aged 18–75 years who had type 2 diabetes, a body mass index (BMI) of 25–50 kg/m^2, a HbA1c level of 53–86 mmol/mol (7.0–10.0%), and were taking metformin. Using interactive response technology, participants were randomized to receive either semaglutide (up to 1.0 mg qw), a placebo, or survodutide {up to 0.3, 0.9, 1.8, or 2.7 mg once weekly [qw; dose group (DG) 1–4 respectively] or 1.2 or 1.8 mg twice weekly [DG 5 and 6 respectively]}.

The semaglutide arm was open-label, and all trial participants and those engaged in its conduct and analysis were blinded. After 16 weeks of treatment, the main outcome was the absolute change in HbA1c from baseline. After 16 weeks of treatment, the primary secondary objective was the relative change in bodyweight from baseline.

Findings: DG1, $n = 50$; DG2, $n = 50$; DG3, $n = 52$; DG4, $n = 50$; DG5, $n = 51$; DG6, $n = 50$; semaglutide, $n = 50$; placebo, $n = 60$ were among the 413 participants that were randomly assigned. 411 treated subjects (DG6, $n = 49$; placebo, $n = 59$) made up the complete analytic set. Adjusted mean [95% confidence interval (CI)] HbA1c decreased from baseline [mean ± SD 64.7 ± 9.2 mmol/mol (8.07 ± 0.84%) after 16 weeks' treatment: DG1 ($n = 41$), −9.92 mmol/mol {−12.27, −7.56; −0.91% (−1.12, −0.69)}; DG2 ($n = 46$), −15.95 mmol/mol {−18.27, −13.63; −1.46% (−1.67, −1.25)}; DG3 ($n = 36$), −18.72 mmol/mol {−21.15, −16.29; −1.71% (−1.94, −1.49)}; DG4 ($n = 33$), −17.01 mmol/mol {−19.59, −14.43; −1.56%

(−1.79, −1.32)}; DG5 (n = 44), −17.84 mmol/mol {−20.18, −15.51; −1.63% (−1.85, −1.42)}; DG6 (n = 36), −18.38 mmol/mol {−20.90, −15.87; −1.68% (−1.91, −1.45)}].

With low-dose semaglutide [−16.07 mmol/mol (−1.47%); n = 45] and survodutide [DG2: −15.95 mmol/mol (−1.46%); n = 46], the mean decrease in HbA1c was comparable. Survodutide ≥1.8 mg qw resulted in larger bodyweight reductions than semaglutide [−5.3% (−6.6, −4.1); n = 45]; mean (95% CI) bodyweight fell dose-dependently up to −8.7% (−10.1, −7.3; DG6, n = 37). 52.5% of people getting a placebo, 52.0% receiving semaglutide, and 77.8% of persons receiving survodutide experienced adverse events (AEs), primarily gastrointestinal.

Conclusion and interpretation: After 16 weeks of treatment, survodutide decreased body weight and HbA1c levels in individuals with type 2 diabetes. Slower dose increases may help reduce gastrointestinal AEs linked to the dose.

CRITICAL APPRAISAL

What was Known Prior to this Study?

Glucagon-like peptide-1 receptor (GLP-1R) agonists, such as liraglutide and semaglutide, are in use clinically for the management of type 2 diabetes mellitus (T2DM) and obesity and are known to cause gastrointestinal (GI) adverse events though otherwise well tolerated. Dual agonists such as the glucose-dependent insulinotropic polypeptide receptor (GIPR)/GLP-1R agonist tirzepatide and glucagon receptor (GCGR)/GLP-1R dual agonists have shown the potential to more effectively lower hemoglobin A1c (HbA1c) and bodyweight than sole agonists of the GLP-1R. GCGR agonism, via receptors in the liver, can lead to increased energy expenditure at doses that do not activate the sympathetic nervous system, as well as stimulate lipolysis while suppressing hepatic fat accumulation. Survodutide (BI 456906) is one such novel subcutaneous GCGR/GLP-1R dual agonist with addition of a C18 fatty acid into the acylated peptide to extend its half-life and allow for its weekly administration. Several preclinical studies in murine models have showed its benefits and were generally well tolerated in Phase I studies without unexpected safety or tolerability concerns in healthy volunteers and people with overweight/obesity. The current Phase II study was conducted to assess the effects of multiple rising doses survodutide on HbA1c, bodyweight in T2DM as well as its tolerability and safety compared to placebo and weekly semaglutide.

What this Study Adds?

Survodutide was found to lead to dose-dependent reduction in HbA1c after 16 weeks by up to 1.7%. The efficacy of low-dose survodutide was comparable to open label semaglutide use (HbA1c% lowering −1.46% vs. −1.47% for semaglutide). Survodutide at doses ≥1.8 mg caused greater bodyweight reductions than semaglutide. The maximum reductions in HbA1c and bodyweight observed in this study (1.71% and −8.4 kg, respectively) exceeded all prior studies with GLP-1 RAs and also of another dual GCGR/GLP-1R agonism cotadutide within a short span of 16 weeks. Treatment related adverse events were mostly GI like nausea. Survodutide caused small reductions in many nonalcoholic steatohepatitis (NASH)-related scores [Fib-4 score, APRI, and nonalcoholic fatty liver disease (NAFLD) fibrosis score], Enhanced Liver Fibrosis (ELF) score, and the fibrogenic biomarker Pro-C3. High dose survodutide ≥ 1.2 mg twice weekly led to body weight reduction by ≥ 5% in 50% of the patients and by ≥ 10% in > 25% of the participants.

Major Strengths of the Study

The study was a multicenter, randomized, double-blind, and placebo-controlled study having an additional open-label active comparator semaglutide. This was the first phase 2 dose escalating trial of survodutide. It was a proof-of-concept study to examine the dose–response relationship of survodutide for body weight and HbA1c% reduction and the results can be used to inform the design of further studies. Participants with a wide range of body mass index (BMI) between 25 and 50 kg/m^2 were included.

Limitations of the Study

Being the first trial of survodutide in T2DM, the inclusion/exclusion criteria were quite restrictive thus the results may not be generalizable to all insulin-naive T2DM. Majority of the participants were white, the range of HbA1c was between 7.0 and 10.0%.

Implications of the Findings for the Clinicians

The novel GCGR/GLP-1R dual agonist survodutide has excellent potential for the treatment of NASH, T2DM, and obesity. In spite of rapid dose escalation, apart from GI problems, no other unexpected safety or tolerability concerns were seen.

knowledge Gaps Identified and Scope for Future Research

The findings can guide further larger and longer term trials with survodutide. Slower uptitration with more gradual dose escalations can help mitigate the dose-related GI issues. Discontinuations rates were higher in participants with a baseline bodyweight of <100 kg demanding further studies in more obese individuals.

8. Subcutaneously Administered Tirzepatide vs Semaglutide for Adults with Type 2 Diabetes: A Systematic Review and Network Meta-analysis of Randomised Controlled Trials

Ref: Karagiannis T, Malandris K, Avgerinos I, Stamati A, Kakotrichi P, Liakos A, et al. Subcutaneously administered tirzepatide vs semaglutide for adults with type 2 diabetes: a systematic review and network meta-analysis of randomised controlled trials. Diabetologia. 2024;67(7):1206-22.

ABSTRACT

Objectives and hypotheses: For people of both sexes with type 2 diabetes mellitus, we compared the safety and effectiveness of subcutaneous (SC) administered semaglutide versus SC administered tirzepatide using a network meta-analysis and systematic review.

Techniques: For randomized controlled trials (RCTs) evaluating SC tirzepatide at maintenance doses of 5 mg, 10 mg, or 15 mg once weekly, or SC semaglutide at maintenance doses of 0.5 mg, 1.0 mg, or 2.0 mg once weekly, in adults with type 2 diabetes, regardless of prior glucose-lowering treatment, we searched PubMed and Cochrane until November 11, 2023. Trials that met the eligibility requirements contrasted semaglutide and tirzepatide at any of the recommended dosages with a placebo or other medications that lower blood sugar levels.

Changes from baseline in body weight and hemoglobin A1c (HbA1c) were the main results. Achieving the HbA1c objective of ≤48 mmol/mol (≤6.5%) or <53 mmol/mol (≤7.0%), losing at least 10% of body weight, and avoiding safety complications such severe hypoglycemia and gastrointestinal side events were secondary outcomes. We assessed the risk of bias using version 2 of the Cochrane risk-of-bias tool (ROB 2), performed frequentist random-effects network meta-analyses, and utilized the Confidence In Network Meta-Analysis (CINeMA) framework to evaluate confidence in effect estimates.

Findings: Included were 28 trials with 23,622 participants, 44.2% of whom were female. The most effective treatment for lowering HbA1c was tirzepatide 15 mg [mean difference −21.61 mmol/mol (−1.96%)], followed by tirzepatide 10 mg [−20.19 mmol/mol (−1.84%)], semaglutide 2.0 mg [−17.74 mmol/mol (−1.59%)], tirzepatide 5 mg [−17.60 mmol/mol (−1.60%)], semaglutide 1.0 mg [−15.25 mmol/mol (−1.39%)], and semaglutide 0.5 mg [−12.00 mmol/mol (−1.09%)]. All tirzepatide dosages were better than semaglutide 1.0 mg and 0.5 mg and comparable to semaglutide 2.0 mg in between-drug comparisons. Tirzepatide was more effective than semaglutide at lowering body weight when compared to a placebo; decreases ranged from 9.57 kg (tirzepatide 15 mg) to 5.27 kg (tirzepatide 5 mg).

With decreases ranging from 4.97 kg (semaglutide 2.0 mg) to 2.52 kg (semaglutide 0.5 mg), semaglutide's effect was less noticeable. Tirzepatide 15 mg, 10 mg, and 5 mg were more effective than semaglutide 2.0 mg, 1.0 mg, and 0.5 mg in between-drug comparisons. Neither tirzepatide nor semaglutide raised the risk of severe hypoglycemia or major adverse events, although both medications increased the incidence of gastrointestinal adverse events as compared to a placebo.

Conclusion and interpretation: According to our findings, in individuals with type 2 diabetes, SC tirzepatide had a more noticeable impact on weight loss and HbA1c than SC semaglutide. Both medications increased gastrointestinal side effects, especially greater dosages of tirzepatide.

CRITICAL APPRAISAL

What was Known Prior to this Study?

Semaglutide, both in subcutaneous (SC) and oral forms, has shown superior efficacy compared with most other glucose-lowering agents in reducing hemoglobin A1c (HbA1c) and in facilitating weight loss in individuals with type 2 diabetes mellitus (T2DM). Tirzepatide, a dual agonist of the glucose-dependent insulinotropic peptide (GIP) and glucagon-like peptide-1 receptor agonist (GLP-1 RA) has shown very good efficacy in reducing HbA1c and body weight and has recently received the Food and Drug Administration (FDA) approval for use in people with T2DM and/or obesity. The American Diabetes Association (ADA) Standards of Care recommend semaglutide and tirzepatide as the most efficacious medications for obesity and glycemic benefits in T2DM with obesity. However, there is scarcity of data regarding direct comparison between the subcutaneous formulations of tirzepatide and semaglutide. The current network meta-analysis utilized both direct and indirect comparative data between the two medications in an attempt to compare the glycemic control and weight management as well as adverse effect profile of these two agents.

What this Study Adds?

The authors find all tirzepatide doses to be comparable with semaglutide 2.0 mg but superior to semaglutide 1.0 mg and 0.5 mg in terms of HbA1c% reduction. For body weight reduction, tirzepatide at doses of 15 mg, 10 mg, and 5 mg was more efficacious than semaglutide at doses of 2.0 mg, 1.0 mg, and 0.5 mg, respectively. All doses of both the drugs, particularly tirzepatide 15 mg, was found to increase gastrointestinal adverse effects, but no increase in the risk for serious adverse events or severe hypoglycemia was seen with either tirzepatide or semaglutide.

Major Strengths of the Study

The authors analyzed a large dataset encompassing 28 randomized controlled trials (RCTs), inclusive of trials comparing directly tirzepatide with semaglutide, trials comparing semaglutide with placebo, other GLP-1 RAs, basal insulin, prandial insulin or different doses of semaglutide, as well as trials comparing tirzepatide with placebo, GLP-1 RA (other than semaglutide), basal insulin, prandial insulin, or the multiple doses of tirzepatide. Thus, more accurate comparative estimates between the two treatments could be done.

Limitations of the Study

There was lot of heterogeneity between the comparator molecules used for indirect comparison. The authors acknowledged having low confidence in analysis of the comparisons involving semaglutide 2.0 mg, due to the inclusion of only one RCT assessing this dose of semaglutide. Also, ethnicity could be a confounder since up to five RCTs recruited exclusively Japanese participants. There was a priori exclusion of long-term cardiovascular or mortality outcomes from their analysis, due to the ongoing status of a dedicated ongoing cardiovascular outcomes trial for tirzepatide (SURPASS-CVOT). With regards to the change in HbA1c%, there was variation in the results due to different measurement units used. The trial duration ranged between 26 and 56 weeks for all trials except for two, therefore a subgroup analysis based on duration was unwarranted. A subgroup analyses based on the background glucose-lowering therapy could not be done due to heterogeneity of the treatment arms across trials.

Implications of the Findings for the Clinicians

Using SC tirzepatide can lead to a more pronounced effect on HbA1c% and body weight reduction in T2DM than SC semaglutide. However, both the drugs, especially higher doses of tirzepatide, were associated with a high incidence of gastrointestinal adverse effects.

Knowledge Gaps Identified and Scope for Future Research

Further focused RCTs comparing tirzepatide to subcutaneous as well as oral semaglutide are warranted. Comparison of effect of the two on other parameters such as lipids, blood pressure, and nonalcoholic fatty liver disease (NAFLD)-related outcomes are necessary.

---

9. Ultra-rapid Lispro Improved Postprandial Glucose Control Compared to Insulin Lispro in Predominantly Chinese Patients with Type 1 Diabetes: A Prospective, Randomized, Double-blind Phase 3 Study

Ref: Ma J, Yan X, Feng Q, Liu W, Pérez Manghi F, García-Hernández P, et al. Ultra-rapid lispro improved postprandial glucose control compared to insulin lispro in predominantly Chinese patients with type 1 diabetes: A prospective, randomized, double-blind phase 3 study. Diabetes Obes Metab. 2024;26(1):311-8.

ABSTRACT

Aims: To conduct a prospective, randomized, double-blind, treat-to-target, phase 3 research to compare the safety and effectiveness of insulin lispro and ultra-rapid lispro (URLi) in patients with type 1 diabetes (T1D), who are primarily Chinese.

Materials and methods: Patients were randomized (1:1) to either insulin lispro ($n = 178$) or URLi ($n = 176$), after a lead-in phase where insulin glargine U-100 or insulin degludec U-100 was optimized. The main goal was to determine whether URLi was superior to insulin lispro in terms of 1- and 2-hour postprandial glucose (PPG) excursions during a mixed-meal tolerance test and hemoglobin A1c (HbA1c) change at week 26. The multiplicity-adjusted objectives were to test for noninferiority of URLi to insulin lispro in glycemic control [noninferiority margin = 0.4% for glycated hemoglobin (HbA1c) change from baseline to week 26].

Results: With a least squares mean treatment difference of 0.07% (95% CI −0.11 to 0.24; $p = 0.467$), HbA1c dropped by 0.21% and 0.28% with URLi and insulin lispro, respectively, from baseline to week 26. With least squares mean treatment differences of −1.0 mmol/L (−17.8 mg/dL) and −1.4 mmol/L (−25.5 mg/dL), respectively ($p < 0.005$ for both), URLi showed reduced 1- and 2-hour PPG excursions at week 26 compared to insulin lispro. Insulin lispro and URLi had comparable safety characteristics.

Conclusion: In this trial, URLi given in a basal-bolus regimen showed advantages over insulin lispro in reducing PPG excursions while having no negative effects on HbA1c management in T1D patients who were primarily Chinese.

CRITICAL APPRAISAL

What was Known Prior to this Study?

The current gold standard of care in type 1 diabetes mellitus (T1DM) is basal bolus insulin, of which the prandial insulin, administered at meal-time, takes care of postprandial glucose (PPG) excursions. PPG is a chief contributor to overall glycemic control as measured by and is associated with high risk of cardiovascular disease. The basal-bolus insulin regimen is the most commonly used treatment option. The onset and peak action of the currently available bolus insulins is not fast enough to match carbohydrate absorption. Also, non-adherence to the premeal bolus dosing and administration of postmeal dose is often done. In order to achieve optimal PPG levels, there is need for a prandial insulin with fast-onset and/or fast-offset characteristics. Ultra-rapid lispro (URLi) is a unique formulation of insulin lispro containing two excipients treprostinil, to increase local vasodilatation, and sodium citrate to enhance local vascular permeability thus enhancing absorption of URLi with a faster onset and shorter duration of action than the currently available rapid-acting insulin analogs. In phase 1 study in healthy subjects, URLi has demonstrated faster onset of action and a 2.5-fold increase in early insulin action within the first 30 minutes than insulin lispro. Also, the duration of action was 67.7 minutes shorter compared to insulin lispro.

What this Study Adds?

This phase 3 study was conducted to investigate the efficacy and safety of URLi, if administered as a bolus insulin in combination with basal insulin glargine or degludec, in a population with predominantly Chinese patients with T1DM. When administered in combination with basal insulin, URLi was noninferior to insulin lispro in glycemic control as measured by HbA1c% change from baseline to week 26, and superior to insulin lispro in controlling 1- and 2-hour PPG excursion after a week 26. Notably, the beneficial effects on PPG excursion was also seen 30 and 180 minutes after mixed meal tolerance test (MMTT) and on 10-point self-monitoring of blood glucose (SMBG). Subgroup analyses indicated that there was no difference in results between Chinese patients and the overall population. There was no difference in the incidence of adverse effects including hypoglycemia between the two groups. Injection site reactions were seen but mild.

Major Strengths of the Study

The trial had a treat-to-target design thus keeping HbA1c% within a prespecified target range with insulin titration. This enabled comparison between URLi and insulin lispro with respect to nonglycemic effects and the risk-benefit profile of URLi.

Limitations of the Study

There was no use of continuous glucose monitoring (CGM), which might provide more detailed and more dynamic information through several days. The authors did not evaluate the effects of postmeal administration of URLi. Majority of the population were Chinese.

Implications of the Findings for the Clinicians

When used as a bolus insulin in T1DM patients on basal-bolus regimen, URLi might demonstrated superior results than insulin lispro with respect to postprandial excursions, while maintaining similar effects on HbA1c%.

Knowledge Gaps Identified and Scope for Future Research

Further CGM based studies are needed to understand the effect on intraday and interday glycemic fluctuations. Studies focusing on non-Chinese or multiethnic population are needed.

---

10. Once-daily Oral Small-molecule Glucagon-like Peptide-1 Receptor Agonist Lotiglipron (PF-07081532) for Type 2 Diabetes and Obesity: Two Randomized, Placebo-controlled, Multiple-ascending-dose Phase 1 Studies

Ref: Buckeridge C, Tsamandouras N, Carvajal-Gonzalez S, Brown LS, Hernandez-Illas M, Saxena AR. Once-daily oral small-molecule glucagon-like peptide-1 receptor agonist lotiglipron (PF-07081532) for type 2 diabetes and obesity: Two randomized, placebo-controlled, multiple-ascending-dose Phase 1 studies. Diabetes Obes Metab. 2024;26(8):3155-66.

ABSTRACT

Goals: To find out how people with type 2 diabetes (T2D) and/or obesity respond to lotiglipron (PF-07081532), an oral small molecule glucagon-like peptide-1 receptor agonist taken once daily.

Materials and procedures: The safety, tolerability, pharmacokinetics, and pharmacodynamics of lotiglipron were examined in two Phase 1 randomized, double-blind, placebo-controlled, multiple-ascending-dose investigations.

Results: 74 individuals with T2D received treatment for 28 or 42 days in all investigations, whereas 26 individuals with obesity but no diabetes received treatment for 42 days after being randomly assigned to either a placebo or lotiglipron (target doses ranging from 10 to 180 mg/day, with dose titration to higher target doses).

In both studies, nausea was the most commonly reported adverse event, with the majority of adverse events being moderate (89.6%). Vital signs, electrocardiogram (ECG) parameters, and safety laboratory testing did not show any clinically significant adverse trends. Lotiglipron caused dose-dependent decreases in mean daily glucose in T2D individuals. The 180-mg dose was linked to least squares mean reductions from baseline in body weight [−5.10 kg {90% confidence interval (CI) −6.62, −3.58} vs. −2.06 kg (90% CI −4.47, 0.36) for placebo] and glycated hemoglobin [−1.61% (90% CI −2.08, −1.14) vs. −0.61% (−1.56, 0.34) for placebo] after 42 days; a comparable amount of weight loss was observed in obese participants. Once-daily dosage was supported by the pharmacokinetic profile that was observed.

Conclusion: The safety and tolerability profile of once-daily lotiglipron at doses up to 180 mg, as seen in these two Phase 1 studies, was in line with the mechanism of action. Following multiple doses, there were dose-dependent decreases in body weight and glycemic indices (T2D) in both populations.

CRITICAL APPRAISAL

What was Known Prior to this Study?

Although peptide glucagon-like peptide-1 receptor agonists (GLP-1 RAs) are approved for the treatment of type 2 diabetes mellitus (T2DM) and obesity with high efficacy in lowering glucose and reducing body weight, but they require subcutaneous injections, or the oral formulations have strict fasting requirements before and after administration limiting their patient preference. Oral, non-peptide GLP-1 RAs can be administered without fasting requirements and some of them are in clinical development. Lotiglipron (PF-07081532) is one such a selective and potent oral small-molecule GLP-1 RA that is administered once daily without any fasting requirements.

What this Study Adds?

Lotiglipron caused dose-dependent reductions in mean daily glucose. The 180-mg dose was associated with HbA1c% reduction by 1.6% (vs. 0.6% for placebo) and body weight reduction by 5.10 kg (vs. 2.06 kg for placebo) after 42 days in T2DM and a similar degree of weight loss was also seen in participants with obesity without diabetes mellitus (DM). Pharmacokinetic (PK) profile supported once-daily dosing. Adverse events were mostly mild (89.6%), nausea being the most frequently reported. No clinically meaningful adverse effects were noted in other laboratory tests, vital signs, or electrocardiogram parameters. Treatment emergent adverse events (TEAEs) were reported more with the higher doses of lotiglipron (120 and 180 mg) than placebo. Most were mild in severity, nausea being most common. The dose titration speed was relatively faster than is used clinically for other GLP-1R As in study 1. In study 2, designed to explore tolerability, different starting doses were used and remained at that starting dose for 4 weeks prior to dose escalation and were generally well tolerated.

Major Strengths of the Study

This was the first reported multiple-dose clinical trial with lotiglipron with data gathered during two phase 1, placebo-controlled, multiple-ascending-dose studies that investigated the safety, tolerability, PK, and pharmacodynamic characteristics of lotiglipron in adults with T2DM or obesity without diabetes.

Limitations of the Study

It was a short duration study with rapid dose titration in one of the two studies. There was notable placebo response on glycemic indices in one of the studies, which might be attributed to short run-in period. The studies were conducted at during coronavirus disease 2019 (COVID-19) pandemic, thus indirect effects of the pandemic might have influenced the health and/or background nutritional status of the participants. The response to a liquid meal in the mixed meal tolerance test (MMTT) may not be extrapolatable to the real world where solid meals are eaten. After these phase 1 studies, following elevated transaminases seen in phase 2 and other studies, Pfizer Inc. announced discontinuation of the lotiglipron clinical development program. But there was no clear evidence of elevated transaminases in these phase 1 studies though three participants were noted to have an aspartate aminotransferase (AST) and/or alanine aminotransferase (ALT) >3 upper limit of normal (ULN), after discharge from the clinical research.

Implications of the Findings for the Clinicians

Once-daily administration of multiple oral doses of the GLP-1 RA lotiglipron in these two Phase 1 studies demonstrated a safety and tolerability profile consistent with their mechanism of action. Robust reductions in glycemic indices and body weight were observed in participants with T2DM and obesity without DM. But its clinical development program has been discontinued following reports of elevated transaminases in phase 2 and separate drug–drug interaction studies.

Knowledge Gaps Identified and Scope for Future Research

Similar molecules with slower dose titration intervals need to be studied. The possible mechanism leading to elevated transaminases need research.

11. Effect of Tirzepatide on Body Fat Distribution Pattern in People with Type 2 Diabetes

Ref: Cariou B, Linge J, Neeland IJ, Dahlqvist Leinhard O, Petersson M, Fernández Landó L, et al. Effect of tirzepatide on body fat distribution pattern in people with type 2 diabetes. Diabetes Obes Metab. 2024;26(6):2446-55.

ABSTRACT

Aims: Using sex- and body mass index (BMI)-matched virtual control groups (VCGs) from the UK Biobank imaging study at baseline and week 52, the SURPASS-3 MRI substudy's participants with type 2 diabetes (T2D) were compared to describe their overall fat distribution patterns, independent of body mass index (BMI).

Methods: A VCG of ≥150 persons with the same sex and similar BMI was found from the UK Biobank imaging study ($n = 40,172$) for each study participant at baseline and week 52 ($n = 296$). The paired VCGs were used to compute the average levels of visceral adipose tissue (VAT), abdominal subcutaneous adipose tissue (aSAT), and liver fat (LF), as well as the observed standard deviations (SDs; normalized normal z-scores: z-VAT, z-aSAT, and z-LF).

To characterize possible changes in the fat distribution pattern independent of weight change, differences in z-scores between baseline and week 52 were computed.

Findings: The patterns of baseline fat distribution were comparable in the insulin degludec (IDeg) and pooled tirzepatide (5, 10, and 15 mg) groups. SURPASS-3 individuals showed identical aSAT [z-aSAT −0.13 (1.11); $p = 0.083$] but higher baseline VAT [mean (SD) z-VAT + 0.42 (1.23); $p < 0.001$] and LF [z-LF + 1.24 (0.92); $p < 0.001$] compared to matched VCGs. Participants receiving tirzepatide showed a substantial increase in z-aSAT [+0.11 (0.50); $p = 0.012$] but a significant drop in z-VAT [−0.18 (0.58); $p < 0.001$] and z-LF [−0.54 (0.84); $p < 0.001$]. Only z-LF changed significantly in participants treated with IDeg [−0.46 (0.90); $p = 0.001$], although z-VAT did not alter significantly [+0.13 (0.52); $p = 0.096$] and z-aSAT (+0.09 (0.61); $p = 0.303$].

Conclusion: In this exploratory analysis, tirzepatide treatment in T2D patients led to a significant decrease in z-VAT and z-LF, while z-aSAT increased from a negative initial value. This suggests that treatment may have caused a shift toward a more balanced fat distribution pattern with notable loss of VAT and LF.

CRITICAL APPRAISAL

What was Known Prior to this Study?

Obesity is heterogeneous with different patterns of body fat distribution [visceral fat, subcutaneous fat, and liver fat (LF)] that can impact cardiometabolic risk substantially. Specially, increased visceral rather than subcutaneous fat and increased LF have been established to increase the risk of developing cardiometabolic disease and related complications. The response to weight loss interventions also varies greatly. Though there is concurrent loss of visceral fat, subcutaneous fat, and LF is with successful weight loss, but it is difficult to determine whether the differential compartmental weight loss was in line with the weight change, smaller or greater than expected. It is important to identify a weight-invariant way of describing the body fat distribution phenotype with current weight management options.

In a sub study of the SURPASS-3 trial that compared once-weekly tirzepatide (5, 10, and 15 mg) with once daily basal insulin degludec in patients with type 2 diabetes mellitus (T2DM), participants' visceral fat, subcutaneous fat, and LF were estimated using magnetic resonance imaging (MRI) and it was seen that both treatments reduced LF but there was a mean overall weight loss of 9.6 kg with concurrent visceral and subcutaneous fat reduction with tirzepatide but a mean overall weight gain of +3.2 kg along with visceral and subcutaneous fat increases seen with degludec.

What this Study adds?

The current study was an exploratory analysis to describe the baseline and changes in body fat distribution patterns, independent of body mass index (BMI) and weight change in the SURPASS-3 MRI substudy. It was seen that tirzepatide led to significant decrease in both z-VAT and z-LF, but increased z-aSAT. Thus, with tirzepatide, all fat z-scores moved toward 0 (z-VAT and z-LF decreased from positive values and z-aSAT increased from a negative value) resulting in a change toward a more balanced body fat distribution. Degludec significantly decreased z-LF only, but did not affect z-VAT or z-aSAT. Additionally, this fat redistribution with tirzepatide treatment was accompanied by lowering of triglycerides and very low-density lipoprotein (VLDL) cholesterol concentrations along with a significant increase in high-density lipoprotein (HDL) cholesterol levels.

Major Strengths of the Study

This is the first study to evaluate changes in body fat distribution with weight loss pharmacotherapy independent of weight change. It provides a unique while there is evidence to suggest that a skewed fat distribution pattern between VAT and aSAT (z-aSAT < 0 and z-VAT > 0) is linked to a higher risk of cardiovascular disease (CVD) and T2DM, results of this study show that that both can be modulated by pharmacotherapy. However, the results from this study make fat distribution profiling an interesting end-point for future trials in obesity therapy.

Limitations of the Study

It was an exploratory analysis thus the results need to be interpreted with caution. The SURPASS-3 MRI substudy and UK Biobank imaging study were two separate studies with several differences in baseline demographics. Participants with T2DM in the UK Biobank study were older whereas the skewed fat distribution pattern observed in SURPASS-3 MRI was probably a result of the inclusion criteria for the SURPASS-3 MRI substudy with a fatty liver index of >60. The age difference did not allow for age-matching while calculating the body fat z-scores. Tirzepatide was not compared directly with a Glucagon-like peptide-1 receptor agonist (GLP-1RA) or any other antiobesity agent.

Implications of the Findings for the Clinicians

Tirzepatide, but not insulin degludec, along with weight loss led to a significant reduction of visceral adipose tissue and LF Z scores, irrespective of BMI; making it a very suitable option for obesity in T2DM.

Knowledge Gaps Identified and Scope for Future Research

The study utilized a novel concept to assess fat distribution pattern in terms of z-scores for different fat tissues but more future research is needed in this area. The results can stimulate future research to identify clinically meaningful subphenotypes of obesity.

12. Glucagon-like Peptide-1 Receptor Agonist-based Agents and Weight Loss Composition: Filling the Gaps

Ref: Dubin RL, Heymsfield SB, Ravussin E, Greenway FL. Glucagon-like peptide-1 receptor agonist-based agents and weight loss composition: Filling the gaps. Diabetes Obes Metab. 2024;26(12):5503-18.

ABSTRACT

Type 2 diabetes (T2D) is caused by excessive adiposity. Based on notable weight loss outcomes, glucagon-like peptide-1 receptor agonists (GLP-1RAs) have become the first-line therapies for T2D. Fat-free mass (FFM) loss accounts for <25% of weight loss with most diets, with the remaining portion coming from fat storage. FFM decreases more when weight loss (attained with metabolic bariatric surgery) is larger. Our objective was to evaluate the effects of GLP-1 RA-based therapies on FFM. We examined research that documented alterations in FFM with exenatide, liraglutide, semaglutide, and tirzepatide, a dual incretin receptor agonist. In order to offer a reference for anticipated changes in FFM, we conducted an investigation of different weight loss treatments.

We assessed research that measured FFM (a rough stand-in for skeletal muscle) using dual energy X-ray absorptiometry (DXA). The percentage lost as fat-free mass (%FFML) was equal to ΔFFM/total weight change when assessing the composition of weight loss. Using medicines based on GLP-1 RA, the FFML ranged from 20 to 40%. Although the percentage of FFM loss varied greatly among the 28 clinical trials that were reviewed, most of them reported %FFML >25%. Our review was restricted to DXA, which does not directly assess skeletal muscle mass, and small substudies. The data's heterogeneity may be explained by this indirect measure because FFM has a varied amount of muscle (around 55%). Using magnetic resonance imaging, an advanced imaging technique, to evaluate the amount and quality of skeletal muscle using functional testing will help fill the gaps in our current understanding.

CRITICAL APPRAISAL

What was Known Prior to this Study?

Obesity management is the cornerstone of management of type 2 diabetes mellitus (T2DM). While balanced diet and exercise predominantly lead to loss of fat mass with around 25% loss of fat-free mass (FFM), interventions that lead to more robust weight reduction like bariatric surgery have been associated with some loss of FFM as well. Muscle mass contribute the most significant proportion to FFM and sarcopenic obesity further increases the risk of cardiovascular diseases compared to obesity alone. Glucagon-like peptide-1 receptor agonists (GLP-1 RAs) and dual agonists have emerged as the most efficacious among currently available antiobesity pharmacotherapy agents. Small substudies of semaglutide and liraglutide trials have indeed shown loss of FFM exceeding 40%. Additionally, GLP-1RA by suppressing food intake and appetite may cause a higher than anticipated degree of loss of muscle mass. The authors have written a narrative review summarizing all available data on the impact of GLP-1RA-based treatments on FFM.

What this Study Adds?

The authors have summarized the effects of available GLP-1 RA on FFM. The %FFML using GLP-1 RA-based ranged between 20 and 40% in most of the 28 clinical trials evaluated, majority reporting a %FFML exceeding 25%. The authors also provided a comprehensive review for understanding the importance of skeletal muscle in health, the need to improve measurement of body composition, and the complex interactions between GLP-1RA-based treatments and changes in body composition focusing on loss of FFM including possible mechanisms.

Major Strengths of the Study

First review exploring the possibility, severity, and mechanisms of sarcopenia with GLP-1 RA. They included 28 studies with different GLP-1 RA.

Limitations of the Study

It was a nonsystematic, narrative review and also included several small substudies. Different GLP-1 RAs were studied on different population leading to wide data heterogeneity. The studies used dual energy X-ray absorptiometry (DXA) to measure FFM, a technique that cannot measure skeletal muscle mass directly. Functional indices of sarcopenia were not assessed.

Implications of the Findings for the Clinicians

A significant proportion of weight loss with GLP-1 RA can be attributable to loss of FFM.

Knowledge Gaps Identified and Scope for Future Research

Further research using advanced imaging like MRI to assess quantity and quality of skeletal muscle or functional testing as well as formal tests for sarcopenia in patients using GLP-1 RA must be undertaken for a better understanding of its effects on fat, muscles, and other components of body composition.

13. Oral or Injectable Semaglutide for the Management of Type 2 Diabetes in Routine Care: A Multicentre Observational Study Comparing Matched Cohorts

Ref: Fadini GP, Bonora BM, Ghiani M, Anichini R, Melchionda E, Fattor B, et al.; GLIMPLES study investigators. Oral or injectable semaglutide for the management of type 2 diabetes in routine care: A multicentre observational study comparing matched cohorts. Diabetes Obes Metab. 2024;26(6):2390-400.

ABSTRACT

Aim: The purpose of this study is to better understand the practical ramifications of selecting between injectable and oral semaglutide formulations by examining their real-world use and comparing their clinical outcomes in people with type 2 diabetes (T2D).

Techniques: From a cohort of 14,079 glucagon-like peptide-1 receptor agonist initiators, new users of oral or injectable semaglutide were chosen. To ensure comparability, balanced groups were created using propensity-score matching (PSM). With a follow-up of up to 18 months, the analysis covered dose exposure, drug persistence, and clinical outcomes, such as changes in body weight and glycated hemoglobin A1c (HbA1c).

Results: We examined two matched groups of 107 people each, consisting on average of 63.6% men, 64 years of age, with a body mass index of 29 kg/m^2, a HbA1c level of 7.7–7.8% (61–62 mmol/mol), and a duration of diabetes of about 10 years. The oral and injectable formulations had comparable percentages of low, middle, and high dosages. Both the percentage of those who reached HbA1c < 6.5% (48 mmol/mol) and the reduction in HbA1c (−0.9%/−10 mmol/mol after 18 months) were comparable across groups. At 18 months, the two groups' average weight changes were comparable (3.7 kg with injectable and 3.3 kg with oral), however more new injectable semaglutide users experienced weight loss of at least 5%. With injectables, medication persistence was longer than with oral semaglutide.

Conclusion: Following the start of oral or injectable semaglutide, changes in body weight and HbA1c were comparable in a real-world scenario. With low generalizability across populations with diverse characteristics, these findings might be unique to the characteristics of the matched cohorts being studied.

CRITICAL APPRAISAL

What was Known Prior to this Study?

Glucagon-like peptide-1 receptor agonists (GLP-1 RAs) have emerged as one of the most efficacious agents for the management of obesity with type 2 diabetes mellitus (T2DM). Among the GLP-1 RA, semaglutide has particularly gathered attention, being available in both injectable and, more recently, oral formulations. Oral semaglutide has been formulated utilizing advanced pharmaceutical techniques that ensures efficient gastric absorption, 10 thereby thus offering the benefit of increased patient acceptance. Both weekly subcutaneous injectable semaglutide and oral semaglutide have demonstrated efficacy and safety in a host of clinical situations in the SUSTAIN and PIONEER group of trials respectively and are superior to most other agents for diabetes mellitus (DM) and obesity. In the PIONEER-4 trial, similar degree of hemoglobin A1c (HbA1c)% reduction (1.2% and 1.1%, respectively) but significantly greater weight loss than liraglutide (4.4 vs. 3.1 kg) were seen with oral semaglutide than injectable liraglutide after 26 weeks of treatment. However, more thorough understanding of the comparative efficacy and real-world utilization patterns of the two formulations is necessary. There is lack of direct head-to-head comparisons between the oral and injectable formulations of semaglutide.

What this Study Adds?

The authors conducted a comparative analysis to provide more insights into comparison between the patterns of utilization and clinical outcomes of injectable and oral semaglutide among individuals with T2DM, under real-world circumstances. Among matched cohorts of people with T2DM, oral and injectable semaglutide initiation led to similar degree of glycemic and body weight improvements. Longer persistence with treatment was seen with injectable semaglutide. A significantly greater proportion of new users experienced a ≥5% weight loss with injectable semaglutide which might be due to longer persistence.

Major Strengths of the Study

The current study was the first to address the lack of information about differences between oral and injectable semaglutide in real world settings, building on their differences as noted from the SUSTAIN and PIONEER trial programs and authors explored a wide set of clinical outcomes and metabolic parameters.

Limitations of the Study

There were differences in baseline patient characteristics so a balanced comparison was not possible. While the baseline disparities between the injectable and oral semaglutide groups could be due to diabetes specialists preferentially prescribing oral semaglutide to individuals with a less complex disease. Additionally, there are the inherent limitations of observational research, like unmeasured confounders. Thus, the results may be specifically linked to the phenotype of the matched cohorts, and extrapolations to different populations should be done cautiously. The sample size was small and the study was not powered to reveal subtle differences in change in HbA1c%. The duration of clinical experience with oral semaglutide was shorter, which might affect persistence, clinical outcomes, and dose escalation. Data regarding adverse effects of the two formulations was not compared. Due to its retrospective design, the study could not assess patient-reported outcomes, patient-centered perspectives, and patient preferences.

Implications of the Findings for the Clinicians

Both the oral and injectable formulations of semaglutide can be equally effective for glycemic control and weight management in T2DM in real-life settings. While injectable semaglutide potential scored better in terms of persistence, it needs to be mentioned that there was lesser clinical experience with oral semaglutide prior to this trial.

Knowledge Gaps Identified and Scope for Future Research

Further research to comprehensively compare the oral and injectable formulations of semaglutide in randomized head-to-head trials is necessary.

---

14. Effectiveness of Switching from Dipeptidyl Peptidase-4 Inhibitor to Oral Glucagon-like Peptide-1 Receptor Agonist in Japanese Participants with Type 2 Diabetes Mellitus: Prospective Observational Study Using Propensity Score Matching

Ref: Iwamoto H, Kimura T, Fushimi Y, Iwamoto M, Tatsumi F, Sanada J, et al. Effectiveness of switching from dipeptidyl peptidase-4 inhibitor to oral glucagon-like peptide-1 receptor agonist in Japanese participants with type 2 diabetes mellitus: Prospective observational study using propensity score matching. Diabetes Obes Metab. 2024;26(10):4366-74.

ABSTRACT

Goal: The development of semaglutide, an oral glucagon-like peptide-1 receptor agonist, has garnered a lot of attention lately. The purpose of this study was to evaluate the effects of dipeptidyl peptidase-4 (DPP-4) inhibitors and oral glucagon-like peptide-1 receptor agonist semaglutide on glycemic management and a number of metabolic parameters in patients with type 2 diabetes mellitus over a 6-month period.

Methods: We recruited 59 people and, in "study 1" (prepost comparison), we evaluated a number of clinical parameters before and after switching from DPP-4 inhibitors to oral semaglutide. In "study 2", we established the control group using the propensity score matching approach.

Results: In "study 1", the body mass index dropped from 29.7 to 28.8 kg/m^2, and the glycated hemoglobin value dropped dramatically from 7.5 to 7.0% six months after the changeover. Participants with poor glycemic control showed these effects more obviously. 51 participants from each group were matched in "study 2" with 1:1 propensity score matching. During the 6-month observation period, the switching group's glycemic control and body weight management were better than those of the DPP-4 inhibitor continuing group.

Conclusion: Regardless of age, body weight, or length of diabetes, moving from DPP-4 inhibitors to oral semaglutide had greater positive benefits on weight and glycemic control in this trial, which included obese people with poor glycemic control. Thus, it would be preferable to begin utilizing oral semaglutide in clinical practice, especially in obese participants who have poor glycemic control when using DPP-4 inhibitors.

CRITICAL APPRAISAL

What was Known Prior to this Study?
Over the past few years, glucagon-like peptide-1 receptor agonists (GLP-1 RAs) have shown massive benefits with regards to glucose control, weight reduction, reduction in cardiorenal outcomes, and mortality benefits. Recently, oral GLP-1 RA semaglutide has drawn a great deal of attention. Additionally, basic research has reported that early introduction of GLP-1 RA is important for β-cell preservation if given early in the disease, an effect which was not observed at an advanced stage. A retrospective study has shown that switching from dipeptidyl peptidase-4 (DPP-4) inhibitors to the GLP-1 RA dulaglutide led to improved glycemic control. DPP-4 inhibitors are known to be neutral with respect to atherosclerotic cardiovascular events, heart failure, and renal function and do not seem to have any benefits beyond glycemic control. The PIONEER 3 compared semaglutide to sitagliptin and its subanalysis targeting only Japanese participants reported slightly stronger hypoglycemic events with oral semaglutide than sitagliptin. Oral semaglutide can offer the additional benefits of GLP-1 RA with the convenience of oral administration, unlike the other GLP-1 RA.

What this Study Adds?
The authors examined the effectiveness of switching to oral semaglutide from DPP-4 inhibitors on hemoglobin A1c (HbA1c)%, body weight, lipid profile, liver enzymes, and renal function in T2DM (study 1). In a subsequent study 2, patients who continued to receive DPP-4 inhibitors in study 1 were matched at a ratio of 1:1 using the propensity score (PS) matching method and used as controls. It was seen that switching from DPP-4 inhibitors to semaglutide significantly improved glycemic and lipid control and reduced body weight in participants with type 2 diabetes mellitus (T2DM) in both the studies. Results were seen even at the lowest dose 3 mg of semaglutide. Notably however, no significant difference was observed in HbA1c or body mass index (BMI) was seen between the lowest and higher doses of semaglutide.

Major Strengths of the Study
The study showed the effectiveness of switching from DPP-4 inhibitors to oral GLP-1 RAs. Instead of the dosage of medicine being determined beforehand, the attending physician in this trial adjusted the dosage of semaglutide depending on efficacy and side effects, making the data close to real-life settings. Indeed, no differences in efficacy or safety were seen between the lower and higher doses of semaglutide.

Limitations of the Study
The study was performed only on Japanese participants. The effects of the switching to oral GLP-1 RA semaglutide on residual pancreatic β-cell function were not seen.

Implications of the Findings for the Clinicians
Switching from DPP-4 inhibitor to oral GLP-1 RA leads to greater degree of glycemic control and weight reduction. No additional benefits were seen with higher doses of semaglutide which might mean that continuing the drug without increasing the dose may be useful, especially if using higher dose is difficult due to side effects or drug costs.

Knowledge Gaps Identified and Scope for Future Research
Further research is required to understand the effect of the switch on cardiorenal outcomes, glycemic durability, and also important adverse effects such as pancreatitis. Cost-effective analysis of this switch should also be considered given the high cost of oral semaglutide.

15. Inclisiran in Individuals with Diabetes or Obesity: Post Hoc Pooled Analyses of the ORION-9, ORION-10 and ORION-11 Phase 3 Randomized Trials

Ref: Leiter LA, Raal FJ, Schwartz GG, Koenig W, Ray KK, Landmesser U, et al. Inclisiran in individuals with diabetes or obesity: Post hoc pooled analyses of the ORION-9, ORION-10 and ORION-11 Phase 3 randomized trials. Diabetes Obes Metab. 2024;26(8):3223-37.

ABSTRACT

Goals: To do a pooled analysis of Phase 3 trials examining inclisiran's safety and effectiveness across body mass index (BMI) and glycemic strata.

Materials and procedures: With background oral lipid-lowering treatment, participants were randomized 1:1 to receive 300 mg inclisiran sodium or a placebo twice a year following initial and 3-month doses up to 18 months. Glycemic status (normoglycemia, prediabetes, and diabetes) or BMI (<25, ≥25 to <30, ≥30 to <35, and ≥35 kg/m^2) were used to stratify the analyses. The percentage and time-adjusted percentage change in low-density lipoprotein (LDL) cholesterol from baseline were the co-primary objectives. Safety was evaluated as well.

Findings: Baseline characteristics were uniform across strata and between treatment arms. Across glycemic/BMI strata, the percentage change in LDL cholesterol (placebo-corrected) with inclisiran from baseline to day 510 varied from −47.6 to −51.9% and from −48.8 to −54.4%, respectively. Similarly, across glycemic/BMI strata, time-adjusted percentage changes varied from −46.8% to −52.0% after day 90 and from −48.6% to −53.3% up to day 540. Across the glycemic/BMI strata, inclisiran significantly decreased proprotein convertase subtilisin/kexin type 9 as well as other atherogenic lipids and lipoproteins when compared to a placebo.

As glycemic and BMI strata increased, so did the percentages of people who achieved LDL cholesterol criteria of <1.8 mmol/L and <1.4 mmol/L with inclisiran. More people experienced mild/moderate treatment emergent adverse events (TEAEs) at the injection site with inclisiran (2.8–7.7%) than with a placebo (0.2–2.1%) across all glycemic/BMI strata.

Conclusion: Despite a slight overabundance of temporary mild-to-moderate TEAEs at the injection site, inclisiran significantly and continuously reduced LDL cholesterol across glycemic/BMI strata.

CRITICAL APPRAISAL

What was Known Prior to this Study?

Recent guidelines on dyslipidemia from the American College of Cardiology Expert Consensus Decision Pathway 2022 and the 2023 American Heart Association advisory for management of cardiovascular (CV)-kidney-metabolic syndrome provide practical recommendations regarding the use of novel nonstatin therapies for lowering low-density lipoprotein (LDL) cholesterol for atherosclerotic cardiovascular disease (ASCVD) risk management. Important barriers to LDL cholesterol goal attainment include the underutilization of combination therapies and also poor long-term adherence to lipid-lowering medication, leading to prolonged, and cumulative LDL cholesterol exposure.

Use of statins along with novel nonstatin therapies in combination can lead to consistent reduction in LDL cholesterol and useful for long-term treatment compliance and LDL cholesterol goal attainment. Inclisiran is one novel lipid-lowering agent which is a small interfering ribonucleic acid (RNA) targeting the PCSK9 messenger RNA (mRNA). By binding to the RNA-induced silencing complex, and directing it to degrade the PCSK9 mRNA, it leads to inhibition of its translation into the PCSK9 protein.

What this Study Adds?

The currents study presents findings from three phase 3 trials—ORION-9, ORION-10, and ORION-11 of inclisiran and demonstrated that twice-yearly inclisiran, when added to other maximally tolerated background oral lipid-lowering therapies (LLTs), can facilitate the attainment of LDL cholesterol targets, with >61% and >48% achieving LDL cholesterol <1.8 mmol/L and <1.4 mmol/L, respectively after 18 months, regardless of glycemic status and body mass index (BMI) category. A greater proportion of individuals treated with inclisiran achieved ≥50% LDL cholesterol reduction from baseline across all BMI and glycemic strata. Baseline factors such as diabetes mellitus (DM) medication, the triglyceride levels, BMI, waist circumference or background lipid-lowering medication did not influence LDL cholesterol. Additionally, significant reductions in PCSK9 levels (>80%), along with reductions in other atherogenic lipid components were also achieved with inclisiran across different glycemic and BMI strata.

Notably, slightly greater percentage reductions in most atherogenic lipid components with inclisiran were observed in those with DM versus those with normoglycemia or prediabetes, and in those with a higher BMI compared to lower BMI. Since in these populations, LDL cholesterol levels often remain in the normal range, necessitating the measurement of non-high-density lipoprotein (HDL) cholesterol and ApoB measurements as better surrogate markers for cardiovascular disease (CV) risk.

With inclisiran use, >76% and >60% of individuals achieved ApoB levels within the targets of <1,454.5 nmol/L (<80 mg/dL) and <1,181.8 nmol/L (<65 mg/dL), respectively, whereas >68% and >57% achieved non-HDL cholesterol levels of <2.6 mmol/L and <2.2 mmol/L, respectively. Inclisiran was generally well tolerated irrespective of the glycemic or BMI category. Mild-moderate injection site TEAEs were more common with inclisiran than with placebo.

Major Strengths of the Study

It provides a pooled analysis of three trials with a novel molecule inclisiran and demonstrates its efficacy in LDL cholesterol lowering across all categorized of BMI and glycemic status. It also highlights its effects on other atherogenic components like ApoB and non-HDL cholesterol.

Limitations of the Study

The current analysis was not powered to identify a relationship between Lp(a) lowering by inclisiran and changes in glycemic status. Since BMI and glycemic status are closely related, it was not possible to determine whether glycemic and BMI categories were independently associated with the effects of inclisiran treatment.

Implications of the Findings for the Clinicians

Inclisiran is an effective novel lipid-lowering agent that can lead to attainment of LDL cholesterol, ApoB, and non-HDL cholesterol goals in high-risk individuals with metabolic disorders when added as when added as twice yearly injections to maximally tolerated statins with or without other oral lipid lowering agents. The effects are seen irrespective of the glycemic and BMI status with the mean reductions in atherogenic lipoproteins being as high as or higher in individuals with DM compared to those without DM. Inclisiran is well tolerated in each of these population subgroups without an increase in adverse effects.

Knowledge Gaps Identified and Scope for Future Research

The effect of inclisiran on CV outcomes remains to be explored and is currently being investigated in the ongoing ORION-4 and VICTORION-2 prevent trials.

16. Pioglitazone Reduces Serum Ketone Bodies in Sodium-glucose Cotransporter-2 Inhibitor-treated Non-obese Type 2 Diabetes: A Single-centre, Randomized, Crossover Trial

Ref: Yang M, Yue H, Xu Q, Shao S, Chen Y. Pioglitazone reduces serum ketone bodies in sodium-glucose cotransporter-2 inhibitor-treated non-obese type 2 diabetes: A single-centre, randomized, crossover trial. Diabetes Obes Metab. 2024;26(8):3137-46.

ABSTRACT

Goal: To investigate how the sodium-glucose cotransporter-2 (SGLT-2) inhibitor canagliflozin affects the reduction of ketone bodies in nonobese patients with type 2 diabetes treated with thiazolidinedione (TZD) pioglitazone.

Methods: Two-period crossover studies were carried out, with a 4-week washout interval in between each treatment period. Participants were randomized in a 1:1 ratio to receive either canagliflozin monotherapy (CANA group) or pioglitazone plus canagliflozin (PIOG + CANA group). Change (Δ) in β-hydroxybutyric acid (β-HBA) before and after the CANA or PIOG + CANA treatments was the main result.

Δchanges in serum acetoacetate and acetone, the rate of conversion into urine ketones, and Δchanges in SGLT-2 inhibitor-induced ketone body production-related factors, such as glucagon, noradrenaline (NA), glucagon to insulin ratio, and nonesterified fatty acids (NEFAs), were the secondary outcomes. In accordance with the intention-to-treat concept, analyses were conducted.

Results: There were 25 patients with a body mass index of 25.35 ± 2.22 kg/m^2 and a mean age of 49 ± 7.97 years. During the washout phase, one patient stopped participating in the trial. Following both interventions, analyses showed a significant increase in the rate of conversion into urine ketones and in the amounts of serum ketone bodies.

With the exception of acetoacetate, however, the PIOG + CANA group's differences in ketone body levels were substantially less than those of the CANA group (219.84 ± 80.21 μmol/L vs. 317.69 ± 83.07 μmol/L, $p < 0.001$ in β-HBA; 8.98 ± 4.17 μmol/L vs. 12.29 ± 5.27 μmol/L, $p = 0.018$ in acetone). Following both CANA and PIOG + CANA treatments, there was a considerable increase in NEFA, glucagon, the glucagon to insulin ratio, and NA; however, only NEFAs showed a meaningful difference between the two groups. The differences in Δchanges in Δketone levels of β-HBA and acetoacetate were shown to be significantly correlated with the differences in Δchanges in serum NEFA levels, according to correlation analyses.

Conclusion: Canagliflozin-induced ketone bodies may be lessened by pioglitazone supplementation. This advantage might be more directly linked to lower substrate NEFAs than to other elements such as glucagon, fasting insulin, and NA.

CRITICAL APPRAISAL

What was Known Prior to this Study?

Although sodium-glucose cotransporter-2 (SGLT-2) inhibitors have shown multiple pleiotropic benefits in type 2 diabetes mellitus (T2DM) patients including weight loss, good effect on blood pressure (BP), cardiorenal outcomes, etc., in addition to their glycemic control, a concern with their use is the predisposition to ketosis with/without ketoacidosis, often in euglycemic state. This may be related to their lipolytic effects with nonesterified fatty acid (NEFA) elevation, decrease in circulating insulin levels and the increase of noradrenaline (NA) and glucagon have also been proposed to contribute to lipolysis and ketosis. The risk is believed to be higher in the nonobese and insulinopenic individuals. Though low levels of ketosis are considered beneficial in metabolism of a failing myocardium, but excess ketone bodies may be harmful for their predisposition to ketoacidosis as well as blunting of the hypoglycemic action of sodium-glucose cotransporter-2 inhibitors (SGLT-2is). It is necessary to explore strategies that can offset SGLT-2i-associated ketosis.

What this Study Adds?

This cross-over randomized controlled trial (RCT) studied the effect of pioglitazone on SGLT-2i-induced elevation of ketone bodies in nonobese T2DM. Participants who received the combination of pioglitazone and canagliflozin demonstrated significantly lower elevation in serum and urinary ketones than patients receiving canagliflozin monotherapy. There was also a trend toward better insulin sensitivity and better glycemic control in those receiving the combination.

Additionally in this study, it was identified that NEFAs were remarkably elevated after canagliflozin monotherapy, along with altering trends of insulin, glucagon to insulin ratio, and NA after 4-weeks of canagliflozin use, which are consistent with previous findings regarding the mechanism of ketosis with SGLT-2i. Addition of pioglitazone efficiently lowered NEFA concentrations in the present study. The correlation analysis also found a significant association of decreased NEFAs with reduction in ketone bodies, including β-hydroxybutyric acid (β-HBA), and acetoacetate.

While pioglitazone reduced NEFA levels, its supplementation did not significantly affect the levels of glucagon, glucagon to insulin ratio and NA, hinting at the possibility that NEFA reduction with pioglitazone might explain the reduced ketosis in this group. There was a nonsignificant decreasing trend in body weight after canagliflozin monotherapy, which was possibly related to the nonobese participants or short treatment time. Interestingly, patient weight in the pioglitazone + canagliflozin group also presented a downward trend. Pioglitazone as an add-on treatment did not significantly alter changes in body weight, blood pressure or plasma lipids occurring with canagliflozin.

Major Strengths of the Study

The current study was the first to investigate the effect of pioglitazone treatment on SGLT-2i-induced ketosis in nonobese T2DM. The randomized crossover trial allowed for removal of many confounders and study multiple parameters as well as possible mechanisms. While the exact mechanism and risk factors for SGLT-2i-induced ketosis remain unknown, NEFA elevation seems to be a reasonable predictor and also target for treatment to prevent ketosis as evidenced from this study.

Limitations of the Study

It was an open-label and single-center study, thus limiting the generalizability of its results. It is not clear whether the findings would be consistent among obese participants or those with long-course or poor β-cell function. The short intervention period of only 4 weeks did not allow testing for significant alteration in metabolic indicators such as BMI, blood pressure, and blood lipids. While serum and urinary ketone bodies were assessed, the short observation period was insufficient to observe for events of diabetic ketoacidosis (DKA). Additionally, to confirm the exclusion of potential carryover effects of pioglitazone on lipogenesis, a longer washout period would be appropriate.

Implications of the Findings for the Clinicians

Add-on treatment of pioglitazone to nonobese patients with T2DM receiving SGLT-2is lowered serum ketone bodies. This might be possibly due to reduction in levels of the substrate NEFAs.

Knowledge Gaps Identified and Scope for Future Research

Longer duration clinical trials are necessary to explore if addition of pioglitazone could actually reduce the risk of DKA with SGLT-2i and also their influence on cardiovascular outcomes. Basic science research on fat metabolism pathways is necessary to undersstand the actual mechanisms driving this benefit.

---

17. Are the Cardiovascular Properties of GLP-1 Receptor Agonists Differentially Modulated by Sulfonylureas? Insights from Post-hoc Analysis of EXSCEL

Ref: Gooding KM, Stevens S, Lokhnygina Y, Giczewska A, Shore AC, Holman RR. Are the cardiovascular properties of GLP-1 receptor agonists differentially modulated by sulfonylureas? Insights from post-hoc analysis of EXSCEL. Diabetes Res Clin Pract. 2024;212:111685.

ABSTRACT

Goals: In a post hoc analysis of the Exenatide Study of Cardiovascular Event Lowering (EXSCEL), investigate whether concurrent sulfonylurea (SU) medication mitigates the cardiovascular effects of glucagon-like peptide-1 (GLP-1) receptor agonists.

Techniques: In intent-to-treat analyses of all trial participants classified as SU users or nonusers, we examined whether SUs, either as a class or by kind, modified the effects of once-weekly exenatide (EQW) on EXSCEL cardiovascular outcomes. To determine whether EQW effects varied by SU category on major adverse cardiovascular events (MACEs) based on the length of SU consumption (6, 12, and 18 months), marginal structural models were employed. Hazard ratios [95% confidence intervals (CIs)] and EQW-by-SU type interaction p-values for EQW versus placebo for each baseline SU type (glibenclamide, gliclazide, glimepiride, and other SUs) were calculated.

Findings: Individual SU types, such as glibenclamide (a systemically wide-acting SU), did not alter the effect of EQW on time to MACE, nor did SU use or baseline SU type ($P_{interaction}$ = 0.88 and 0.78, respectively).

Conclusion: SUs did not modify the impact of EQW on cardiovascular outcomes, indicating that individuals with type 2 diabetes do not require a change in SU treatment options to maximize the cardiovascular benefits of GLP-1 receptor agonists.

CRITICAL APPRAISAL

What was Known Prior to this Study?

Several cardiovascular outcome trials with glucagon-like peptide-1 receptor agonists (GLP-1 RAs) have highlighted their cardiovascular benefits. Multiple mechanisms have been reported, one of which is the possibility of direct GLP-1 RA effect on the vasculature. GLP-1 receptors have been found to be expressed in the human vasculature. It has been postulated that opening of KATP channels may mediate the improvement of endothelial function induced by exenatide and by GLP-1.

It has been seen in healthy individuals that pretreatment with the sulfonylurea (SU) glibenclamide is associated with the abolishment of the incretin-based improvements in endothelial function. Notably however, the vascular actions of GLP-1 were not modified by another

SU glimepiride. This might be due to the fact that different SUs act on different KATP channel subtypes.

While the KATP channels consist of two subunits, the Kir channel (Kir 6.1/6.2) and the SU receptor subunit (SUR1, SUR2A, and SUR2B), the distribution of these subtypes vary in different organ like the Kir 6.2/SUR1 on the pancreas and the Kir 6.2/SUR2B on the cardiovascular system.

Since SUs are still prescribed widely across the globe, it becomes important to determine if their use might actually attenuate the beneficial cardio-vascular effects of the GLP-1 RAs. The authors analyzed data from the Exenatide Study of Cardiovascular Event Lowering (EXSCEL) trial to examine whether the use of SU as a class or any particular type of SU, especially glibenclamide and glimepiride, impacts the effects of once-weekly exenatide (EQW) on time to occurrence of the primary cardiovascular outcome and some other secondary outcomes.

What this Study Adds?

This post hoc analysis of the EXSCEL trial showed that treatment with SUs, as a class, had no modulating effect on the impact of EQW on time-to-event of the 3-point MACE outcome or any of the prespecified secondary cardiovascular outcomes. Additionally, impact of the glibenclamide did not differ from that of the more pancreatic-specific SU gliclazide or SU nonuse on the effects of EQW on cardiovascular events.

Major Strengths of the Study

The EXSCEL was a large trial enrolling 14,752 patients with T2DM, of whom a large proportion (73.1%) had pre-existing cardiovascular disease. All EXSCEL participants were included by post hoc intent-to-treat analysis strategy. A number of predefined EXSCEL time-to-event cardiovascular outcomes were noted including 3-P MACE (composite of cardiovascular death, nonfatal myocardial infarction, or nonfatal stroke), cardiovascular mortality, occurrence of fatal or nonfatal myocardial infarction, occurrence of fatal or nonfatal stroke, hospitalization for heart failure (hHF); and hospitalization for acute coronary syndrome (hACS).

Limitations of the Study

Limitations of the study included the fact that SU use was not randomly assigned, and it was not possible to fully rule out the presence of some unobserved confounders. Also, among SU users, continuous use of SU was assumed unless there was no documented SU use for a period ≥2 years.

Implications of the Findings for the Clinicians

Use of SUs, including glibenclamide, do not have modulating effect on the cardiovascular effects of the GLP-1 RA EQW.

Knowledge Gaps Identified and Scope for Future Research

Focused clinical trials of long duration with prespecified study design and outcomes are necessary for a meaningful comparison between SU users and nonusers among those on GLP-1 RA. Basic science research to elucidate the effects of SU on the K+ ATP channels of endothelial vascular cells exposed to GLP-1 is necessary.

18. Tirzepatide 5, 10 and 15 mg versus Injectable Semaglutide 0.5 mg for the Treatment of Type 2 Diabetes: An Adjusted Indirect Treatment Comparison

Ref: Osumili B, Fan L, Paik JS, Pantalone KM, Ranta K, Sapin H, et al. Tirzepatide 5, 10 and 15 mg versus injectable semaglutide 0.5 mg for the treatment of type 2 diabetes: An adjusted indirect treatment comparison. Diabetes Res Clin Pract. 2024;212:111717.

ABSTRACT

Goals: Using adjusted indirect treatment comparisons (aITCs), compare the safety and effectiveness of tirzepatide 5, 10, and 15 mg with subcutaneous semaglutide 0.5 mg as a second-line treatment for people with type 2 diabetes mellitus following metformin monotherapy.

Methods: Based on trial data from SURPASS-2 (NCT03987919) and SUSTAIN 7 (NCT02648204), the Bucher technique was used to examine the relative safety and efficacy of tirzepatide 5, 10, and 15 mg with semaglutide 0.5 mg using a common comparator (subcutaneous semaglutide 1.0 mg) in the aITCs.

Findings: From baseline to week 40, all tirzepatide dosages demonstrated statistically significant increases in glycated hemoglobin, body weight, and body mass index decreases. The adverse event (AE) profile was similar, and there were no statistically significant variations in the likelihood of gastrointestinal AEs in contrast to 0.5 mg of semaglutide. Additionally, compared to semaglutide 0.5 mg, all tirzepatide doses demonstrated higher probabilities of patients reaching weight reduction targets of ≥5% and ≥10% and hemoglobin A1c (HbA1c) targets of ≤6.5% (≤48 mmol/mol) and <7.0% (<53 mmol/mol).

Conclusion: Compared to semaglutide 0.5 mg with a similar AE profile, glycated hemoglobin, and weight reductions were considerably higher for all tirzepatide doses in these aITCs. In the absence of a head-to-head clinical trial, these results offer insights on comparative effectiveness.

CRITICAL APPRAISAL

What was Known Prior to this Study?

While guidelines recommend that in all patients with type 2 diabetes mellitus (T2DM) who are overweight or obese, in addition to diet and lifestyle interventions, treatment must include a medication that is highly efficacious for both glycemic control and body weight reduction. The best agents with these effects include glucagon-like peptide-1 receptor agonists (GLP-1 RAs) like semaglutide and more recently, dual GIP-GLP-1 RA agonist like tirzepatide. Semaglutide provides the most appropriate comparator for tirzepatide as a first line monotherapy or as the best second or third line pharmacotherapy, in combination with other agents in the treatment of T2DM. In the SURPASS-2 trial, tirzepatide in 5, 10, and 15 mg doses showed superior glycemic reduction and weight loss compared to subcutaneous semaglutide 1.0 mg injections.

Additionally, head-to-head comparison data collected from the SURPASS group of trials have shown the efficacy and safety of tirzepatide versus comparators like subcutaneous semaglutide 1.0 mg injection. However, there is no data on direct or indirect comparison between tirzepatide and 0.5 mg dose of subcutaneous semaglutide, which is the initial maintenance dose that is often used in clinical practice. While the SURPASS-2 (NCT03987919) compared different doses of tirzepatide to semaglutide 1.0 mg, the SUSTAIN

7 (NCT02648204) compared semaglutide 0.5 mg and semaglutide 1.0 mg in patients with T2D receiving background metformin monotherapy. In the current study, aggregated data from two randomized controlled trials (RCTs), SURPASS-2, and SUSTAIN 7 were used to compare the adjusted indirect treatment comparisons (aITCs) of the efficacy and safety of tirzepatide 5, 10, and 15 mg doses to semaglutide 0.5 mg using the Bucher method.

What this Study Adds?

Upon comparison with subcutaneous semaglutide 0.5 mg, all doses of tirzepatide showed significantly greater reductions in hemoglobin A1c (HbA1c), body weight, and body mass index (BMI) from baseline after 40 weeks. In prior trials and meta-analysis though tirzepatide was compared to 1 mg semaglutide, there was no direct or indirect comparison with 0.5 mg semaglutide, which is a commonly used maintenance dose in many patients. All tirzepatide doses were found to demonstrate significantly greater reductions in HbA1c, weight, and BMI and also greater odd of patients achieving the HbA1c targets of ≤6.5% and <7.0%, and weight loss targets of ≥5% and ≥10%, in comparison to semaglutide 0.5 mg.

Major Strengths of the study

The Bucher method for aITCs were conducted using a statistical methodology has been supported by widespread published literature and multidisciplinary workshop discussions. Both the SURPASS-2 and SUSTAIN 7 trials were open-label, active-controlled, multinational trials including patients from Asia, Europe, and the United States. Choosing SUSTAIN 7 as the comparator study allowed similarity in baseline characteristics (age, HbA1c, and BMI) between the two study population as well as sample size of the tirzepatide and semaglutide treatment arms, thus supporting the appropriateness of the Bucher approach.

Limitations of the Study

The results were derived from indirect evidence, and there were residual confounding factors that could not be adjusted. Two endpoints were identified as inconsistent across the common comparator arms of the two trials—the proportion of patients with treatment discontinuation due to side effects, and the proportion who experienced at least one episode of hypoglycemia. Due to fewer patients with treatment discontinuations in the semaglutide 1.0 mg arm of SURPASS-2 than in SUSTAIN 7 trial, the results are likely to be statistically biased in favor of semaglutide 0.5 mg. However, there were very low number of hypoglycemia events across all treatment arms.

Implications of the Findings for the Clinicians

All three doses of tirzepatide demonstrated significantly greater reductions in HbA1c%, body weight, and BMI, with comparable safety profile in terms of adverse effects, compared to semaglutide 0.5 mg.

These may be relevant for choice of second line pharmacotherapy for patients with T2DM and inadequate glycemic control on metformin monotherapy.

Knowledge Gaps Identified and Scope for Future Research

There is need for cost-effectiveness analyses for an effective comparison between semaglutide 0.5 mg and all doses of tirzepatide.

19. Continuous Glucose Monitoring-based Metrics and the Duration of Hypoglycaemia Events with Once-weekly Insulin Icodec versus Once-daily Insulin Glargine U100 in Insulin-naive Type 2 Diabetes: An Exploratory Analysis of ONWARDS 1

Ref: Bergenstal RM, Ásbjörnsdóttir B, Watt SK, Lingvay I, Mader JK, Nishida T, et al. Continuous glucose monitoring-based metrics and the duration of hypoglycaemia events with once-weekly insulin icodec versus once-daily insulin glargine U100 in insulin-naive type 2 diabetes: an exploratory analysis of ONWARDS 1. Lancet Diabetes Endocrinol. 2024;12(11):799–810.

ABSTRACT

Background: Glycemic control can be thoroughly evaluated by continuous glucose monitoring (CGM). In this exploratory analysis of the ONWARDS 1 study, insulin-naive people with type 2 diabetes treated with subcutaneous once-weekly insulin icodec (icodec) versus once-daily insulin glargine U100 (glargine U100) were evaluated for CGM-based metrics and CGM-derived hypoglycemia duration.

Techniques: ONWARDS 1 was a 78-week, randomized, open-label, treat-to-target, and phase 3a trial conducted at 143 locations (hospital departments and outpatient clinics) in 12 countries. It consisted of a 52-week main treatment phase, a 26-week treatment extension phase, and a 5-week follow-up. An interactive web-response system was used to randomly assign (1:1) adults (≥18 years old) with type 2 diabetes (HbA1c: 7.0–11.0%) who had never received insulin to once-daily glargine U100 or once-weekly icodec.

Treatment beginning (weeks 0–4), midtrial (weeks 22–26), end of main phase (weeks 48–52), end of extension phase (weeks 74–78), and follow-up (weeks 78–83) all involved the collection of double-masked CGM data. CGM-based metrics, such as the mean percentages of time in glycemic range [TIR; sensor glucose 3.9–10.0 mmol/L (70–180 mg/dL)], time in tight range [TITR; 3.9–7.8 mmol/L (70–140 mg/dL)], time above range [TAR; >10.0 mmol/L (>180 mg/dL)], and time below range [TBR; <3.9 mmol/L (<70 mg/dL) and <3.0 mmol/L (<54 mg/dL)], as well as CGM-derived hypoglycemic episode durations [episodes defined by sensor glucose <3.9 mmol/L (<70 mg/dL for ≥15 consecutive minutes)]. The whole analytic set, which included all randomly assigned participants, was used for the analyses. The ONWARDS 1 trial is finished and filed with ClinicalTrials.gov with the number NCT04460885.

Results: Between November 25, 2020 and December 1, 2022, participants ($n = 492$ in each treatment group) were recruited and allocated at random to ONWARDS 1. We found no statistically significant differences between the mean percentages of TIR, TITR, TAR, and TBR with icodec and glargine U100 at the start of treatment. The mean percentages of TIR and TITR were statistically considerably higher and the mean percentages of TAR were statistically significantly lower with icodec compared to glargine U100 at the midtrial, end of main phase, and end of extension phase periods. During the three periods, the mean percentages of TIR with icodec but not with glargine U100 reached the globally advised CGM target (>70%). Throughout all study periods, both treatment groups' TBRs [<3.9 mmol/L (<70 mg/dL) and <3.0 mmol/L (<54 mg/dL)] were low and below suggested targets (<4% and <1%, respectively). For the lower threshold [<3.0 mmol/L (<54 mg/dL)], there were no statistically significant differences between treatment groups. The mean percentages of TIR, TITR, TAR, and TBR did not differ statistically significantly between icodec and glargine U100 during the course of the follow-up period. Throughout the experiment, the median duration of total hypoglycemic episodes (≤35 minutes) was comparable among treatment groups.

Interpretation: These CGM results showed no increase in the length of individual hypoglycemic episodes with icodec compared to glargine U100 in insulin-naive type 2 diabetics, and they corroborated the long-term safety and effectiveness of icodec over glargine U100 throughout therapy.

CRITICAL APPRAISAL

What was Known Prior to this Study?
Continuous glucose monitoring (CGM) use is incorporated in all guidelines for the management of patients with diabetes on insulin therapy and the assessment of CGM-metrics including the time spent in, above, or below the target glycemic range, as also the duration of hypoglycemic episodes provide a more comprehensive assessment of glycemic control than self-monitored blood glucose or hemoglobin A1c (HbA1c%) measurements, with greater sensitivity in detecting hypoglycemia. The ONWARDS (ONWARDS 1–5) group of clinical trials evaluated the safety and efficacy of once-weekly insulin icodec (icodec) against different comparators in type 2 diabetes mellitus (T2DM). It was seen that compared to once-daily basal insulin comparators (insulin degludec, insulin glargine U100, and insulin glargine U300), icodec was noninferior in achieving glycemic control (ONWARDS 4; basal-bolus regimen) or statistically superior glycemic control (ONWARDS 1–3 and 5) with a low combined rate of clinically significant or severe hypoglycemia, which remained below one event per person-year of exposure in all trials except ONWARDS 4. ONWARDS 1 evaluated the efficacy and long-term safety of icodec versus glargine U100 in insulin-naïve individuals with inadequately controlled T2DM. During the end of main phase (weeks 48–52) and end of extension phase (weeks 74–78) CGM periods, the percentages of time in glycemic range [TIR; sensor glucose 3.9–10.0 mmol/L (70–180 mg/dL)] were statistically significantly greater with icodec versus glargine U100, whereas percentages of time above range [TAR; sensor glucose >10 mmol/L (>180 mg/dL)] were statistically significantly lower in favor of icodec.

What this Study Adds?
This analysis builds on the data from ONWARDS 1 regarding the long-term efficacy and safety of icodec versus glargine U100 including effects on CGM-based metrics in insulin-naïve patients with T2DM. Although CGM-based metrics have previously been reported for the end of main phase and extension phase, authors in the current analysis also included CGM data collected during treatment initiation (weeks 0–4), midtrial (weeks 22–26), and follow-up (weeks 78–83) and included CGM-derived hypoglycemia duration.

During all the phases, time-in-range (TIR) and time-in-tight-range (TITR) were significantly greater with icodec than with glargine U100, whereas TAR was statistically significantly lower. Proportion of participants achieving the recommended TIR target or >70% was also higher with icodec. Time below range (TBR) was below the recommended targets in both treatment groups and hypoglycemia duration, prolonged hypoglycemia (≥1.20 minutes duration) or nocturnal hypoglycemia was not increased with the use of icodec during the phase of initiation, ongoing treatment, or discontinuation.

Major Strengths of the Study
Data from a large, randomized trial in insulin-naive people with T2DM was used. Notably, ONWARDS 1 was the longest trial of the ONWARDS group of trials, including a 78-week treatment period, thus allowing for the assessment of long-term icodec treatment across multiple CGM periods. Also, the CGM data was masked and not used for insulin dose titration, minimizing potential bias.

Limitations of the Study
Limitations included an open-label trial design, making it susceptible to bias, and exploratory analyses. The ONWARDS 1 only enrolled patients who were insulin-naive, this result cannot be extrapolates to individuals willing to switch to icodec from another basal insulin. However, analysis of data from ONWARDS 2 and 4, including insulin-experienced participants initiating icodec treatment, give idea regarding these. ONWARDS 1 was not statistically powered to assess significant differences between the treatment arms for the evaluated CGM-based metrics. CGM data collection was only collected during specified periods rather than throughout the entire trial or at baseline.

Implications of the Findings for the Clinicians

This exploratory analysis highlights the efficacy and safety of icodec in different phases—during treatment initiation as well as for long-term use as the first insulin to be used in patients of T2DM. The study also reiterates the fact that CGM-based metrics including time spent in hypoglycemia duration are complementary to widely accepted measures of glycemic control such as HbA1c, as also self-reported hypoglycemia. The mean TIR could meet the recommended target of >70% with icodec but not U-100 glargine insulin during different phases, with similar TBR and hypoglycemia duration in both groups.

Knowledge Gaps Identified and Scope for Future Research

Studies for comparison of icodec to ultra-long-acting insulin like U-300 glargine and degludec should be undertake.

20. Efficacy and Safety of SGLT2 Inhibitors with and without Glucagon-like Peptide 1 Receptor Agonists: A SMART-C Collaborative Meta-analysis of Randomised Controlled Trials

Ref: Apperloo EM, Neuen BL, Fletcher RA, Jongs N, Anker SD, Bhatt DL, et al. Efficacy and safety of SGLT2 inhibitors with and without glucagon-like peptide 1 receptor agonists: a SMART-C collaborative meta-analysis of randomised controlled trials. Lancet Diabetes Endocrinol. 2024;12(8):545-57.

ABSTRACT

Background: In individuals with type 2 diabetes, sodium-glucose cotransporter-2 (SGLT-2) inhibitors and glucagon-like peptide-1 (GLP-1) receptor agonists both enhance renal and cardiovascular outcomes. Our goal was to determine if individuals receiving GLP-1 receptor agonists and those not getting them would consistently benefit from SGLT-2 inhibitors.

Techniques: As part of the SGLT-2 inhibitor Meta-Analysis Cardio-Renal Trialists' Consortium, we conducted a collaborative meta-analysis of trials that were limited to individuals with diabetes. Inverse variance weighted meta-analysis was used to aggregate treatment effects from individual trials, which were derived from Cox regression models. Hospitalization for heart failure or cardiovascular death, as well as significant adverse cardiovascular events (nonfatal myocardial infarction, nonfatal stroke, or cardiovascular death), were the two primary cardiovascular outcomes evaluated.

Chronic kidney disease progression [≥40% drop in estimated glomerular filtration rate (eGFR), kidney failure (eGFR <15 mL/min/1.73 m^2), chronic dialysis, or kidney transplantation], or death from kidney failure were the primary kidney outcomes evaluated, as was the pace at which eGFR changed over time. Safety results were evaluated as well.

Results: GLP-1 receptor agonists were used at baseline by 3,065 (4.2%) of 73,238 diabetic patients in 12 randomized, double-blind, and placebo-controlled trials. In participants receiving and not receiving GLP-1 receptor agonists, SGLT-2 inhibitors decreased the incidence of major adverse cardiovascular events [hazard ratio (HR) 0.81; 95% CI 0.63–1.03 vs. 0.90, 0.86–0.94; p-heterogeneity = 0.31]. GLP-1 receptor agonist use did not affect the chronic rate of change in eGFR over time (heterogeneity = 0.92), hospitalization for heart failure or cardiovascular death (0.76, 0.57–1.01 vs. 0.78, 0.74–0.82; p-heterogeneity = 0.90), or the progression of chronic kidney disease (0.65, 0.46–0.94 vs. 0.67, 0.62–0.72; p-heterogeneity = 0.81). Regardless of the usage of GLP-1 receptor agonists, SGLT-2 inhibitors were associated with fewer major adverse events than placebo (relative risk 0.87; 95% CI 0.79–0.96 vs. 0.91, 0.89–0.93; p-heterogeneity = 0.41).

> **Interpretation:** Regardless of prior use of GLP-1 receptor agonists, SGLT-2 inhibitors consistently affect kidney and cardiovascular outcomes. These results support clinical practice guidelines that urge using these drugs in combination to benefit cardiovascular and kidney metabolic outcomes, and they also demonstrate independent effects of these evidence-based therapies.

CRITICAL APPRAISAL

What was Known Prior to this Study?

Several large randomized controlled trial (RCT) have shown that both sodium-glucose cotransporter-2 inhibitor (SGLT-2i) and glucagon-like peptide-1 receptor agonists (GLP-1 RAs) lead to the reduction in the rates of cardiovascular events and improve renal outcomes in type 2 diabetes mellitus (T2DM). The mechanisms by which the pleiotropic effects of both these agents occur on the heart and kidney are totally different, raising further interest in usage of this combination leading to synergistic beneficial effects on cardiorenal outcomes. Some small, randomized trials of relatively short duration have studied the combination of SGLT-2i and GLP-1 RAs and found that together they improve cardiometabolic risk factors to a larger degree than either alone, but there is limited data on clinical events from these trials.

Also, since the event-driven trials with each of these agents were conducted prior to the demonstration of benefits with these agents, therefore the proportion of patients on GLP-1 RA at baseline was too less in any individual trial for a meaningful subgroup analysis to be conducted based on the presence or absence of background use of GLP-1 RA. The current meta-analysis was conducted to study the effects of SGLT-2i on cardiovascular, kidney, along with their safety outcomes in patients with T2DM based on whether or not they received GLP-1 RAs at baseline.

What this Study Adds?

Twelve large RCTs involving 73,238 participants with T2DM were included in this collaborative meta-analysis, in which 3,065 were receiving GLP-1 RAs at baseline. In comparison to placebo, SGLT-2i were found to reduce the occurrence of major adverse cardiovascular events (a composite of myocardial infarction, stroke, or cardiovascular death) by 11% and the composite of hospitalization for heart failure/cardiovascular death by 23%, and these beneficial effects were consistently seen, irrespective of baseline use of GLP-1 RAs. Similarly, the beneficial effects of SGLT-2i on the kidney including reduction in the risk of chronic kidney disease progression [a composite of ≥40% decline in estimated glomerular filtration rate (eGFR), renal failure, or renal deaths] by 33% and attenuation in the rate of annual eGFR decline were seen irrespective of baseline use of GLP-1 RA. Neither did the rates of serious adverse events, hypoglycemia or volume depletion differs based on baseline use of GLP-1 RA.

Major Strengths of the Study

This was the largest and most comprehensive assessment of the impact of GLP-1 RA use on the cardiorenal benefits and safety of SGLT-2i in T2DM and found that the cardiorenal benefits with SGLT-2i were independent of baseline GLP-1 RA use.

Limitations of the Study

The number of outcomes among the patients who were using GLP-1 RA was much lower than among those not using GLP-1 RA. Therefore, the number of composite renal endpoints in participants receiving GLP-1 RAs was low. However, the authors also looked at eGFR decline as an additional endpoint.

The treatment effects were not estimated from one-stage meta-analysis. Also, they did not assess whether the effects of GLP-1 RAs on clinical outcomes were similar with and without SGLT-2 inhibitors but only the reverse.

Implications of the Findings for the Clinicians

The benefits of SGLT-2i on cardiorenal outcomes in T2DM can be seen irrespective of baseline GLP-1 RA use. This provides promise for a synergistic beneficial effect on cardiac and renal events in T2DM if both SGLT-2i and GLP-1 RA are used together, without any additional safety concerns.

Knowledge Gaps Identified and Scope for Future Research

This study provides indirect evidence toward the independent beneficial effects of SGLT-2i and GLP-1 RA in T2DM, but direct support toward their use and impact on cardiorenal outcomes if used together is necessary. With increasing evidence of the role of both these agents for cardiorenal benefits in people without diabetes, that is another interesting area to explore. Economic evaluation of this combination using cost-effective analysis in different countries across different healthcare should also be assessed to address potential barriers to their widespread implementation.

21. Once-weekly Insulin Icodec as Compared to Once-daily Basal Insulins: A Meta-analysis

Ref: Mukhopadhyay P, Chatterjee P, Pandit K, Sanyal D, Ghosh S. Once-weekly Insulin Icodec as Compared to Once-daily Basal Insulins: A Meta-analysis. Endocr Pract. 2024;30(2):128-34.

ABSTRACT

Background: In various clinical contexts for type 2 diabetes, once-weekly basal insulin icodec has been evaluated in clinical studies for safety and effectiveness in comparison to currently available glargine-100 and degludec. Using all known randomized controlled trials, we conducted this meta-analysis to assess its overall safety and effectiveness in comparison to glargine-100 and degludec (nonicodec).

Techniques: Included were seven trials that contrasted once-weekly basal insulin icodec with once-daily basal insulin analogs. Results in terms of hemoglobin A1c (HbA1c), reduction in fasting plasma glucose, and increase in time in range (TIR) were compared based on the information that was available. The consequences of weight growth, severe hypoglycemia, and general hypoglycemia were compared. A decrease in "estimated differences in mean (with 95% CI)" was used to calculate the pooled effect size for continuously distributed data.

The Mantel–Haenszel risk ratio [with 95% confidence interval (CI)] was used to calculate the pooled effect size for categorical data.

Findings: The "estimated mean changes" in HbA1c and fasting plasma glucose favoring icodec, when compared to the nonicodec comparators combined, were −0.22% (−0.35, −0.10) and −1.59 mg% (−9.26, 6.08), respectively. Icodec's weight "estimated mean increment" was 0.64 kg (0.61, 0.67). Icodec's TIR increased by 4.24%, or the "estimated mean percentage" (2.99, 5.49). Indicating a 24% higher incidence of all hypoglycemia with icodec, the Mantel–Haenszel risk ratios for severe hypoglycemia and all hypoglycemic episodes were 0.81 (0.31, 2.08) (P is not significant) and 1.24 (1.02, 1.50) ($p = 0.03$), respectively.

Conclusion: Compared to once-daily basal insulin analogs, once-weekly basal insulin icodec had a somewhat higher risk of weight gain and general hypoglycemia, but no difference in severe hypoglycemia and comparable glycemic control (measured by fasting plasma glucose, HbA1c, and TIR).

CRITICAL APPRAISAL

What was Known Prior to this Study?
Multiple subcutaneous insulin injections using once daily basal insulin treatment followed by the addition of single or multiple bolus doses is the cornerstone to achieving and maintaining adequate glycemic control. Icodec is a novel basal insulin which has a very long half-life, allowing it to be used potentially as a once-weekly insulin dose regimen. Several observational and randomized clinical trials (phase 2 and phase 3a) have compared icodec either with degludec or U-100 glargine-100 in terms of glycemic control and side effect profile. These studies have mostly included subjects naive to insulin therapy, for whom the currently used basal insulin has been swapped to icodec.

What this Study Adds?
The current meta-analyses focusing on once weekly insulin icodec, and comparing it to currently used basal insulins U-100 glargine and degludec found that icodec led to similar glycemic control with a slightly increased risk for hypoglycemia a weight gain.

The HbA1c% change was 0.22% lower with insulin icodec compared to once-daily basal insulin analogs, and the fasting plasma glucose (FPG) reduction for icodec versus the nonicodec comparator insulins was −1.59, though there was a slight increase in FPG. The TIR was also 4.88% greater in those receiving insulin icodec. But there was an additional 0.64 kg weight gain and up to 16% increased risk for overall hypoglycemia. However, severe hypoglycemia rates were similar in both groups.

Major Strengths of the Study
The current is one of the first and largest meta-analysis including only studies that focused on comparing icodec to other long- or ultra-long-acting basal insulins.

Limitations of the Study
A limitation of this study was the lack of comparison of other parameters like differences in dose requirement of insulin and bolus insulin, in nocturnal hypoglycemia, recurrent hypoglycemia due to lack of this data in all the studies included. The meta-analysis was conducted using the results of published trials, not by using individual patient data. Also, long-term data in relation to icodec are not currently available.

Implications of the Findings for the Clinicians
Once weekly icodec, a once-weekly insulin, is noninferior to U-100 glargine or glycemic control (HbA1c%, FPG, and TIR) with slightly higher risk of hypoglycemia, albeit similar rates of serious hypoglycemia.

Knowledge Gaps Identified and Scope for Future Research
Additional studies regarding long-term safety of icodec insulin and its effects in diabetes other than T2DM need to be studied.

---

22. Insulin Efsitora versus Degludec in Type 2 Diabetes without Previous Insulin Treatment

Ref: Wysham C, Bajaj HS, Del Prato S, Franco DR, Kiyosue A, Dahl D, et al; QWINT-2 Investigators. Insulin Efsitora versus Degludec in Type 2 Diabetes without Previous Insulin Treatment. N Engl J Med. 2024;391(23):2201-11.

ABSTRACT

Overview: Insulin efsitora alfa, often known as efsitora, is a novel basal insulin that is intended to be administered once every 7 days. Only modest, phase 1 or phase 2 trials have provided data on safety and efficacy.

Methods: We randomized persons with type 2 diabetes who had never used insulin before to a 52-week, phase 3, parallel-design, open-label, treat-to-target trial. Efsitora or degludec were given to participants at random in a 1:1 ratio. Glycated hemoglobin level change from baseline to week 52 was the main outcome, and we predicted that efsitora would be noninferior to degludec (noninferiority margin, 0.4 percentage points).

The percentage of time that the glucose level was in the target range of 70–180 mg per deciliter in weeks 48 through 52, the change in the glycated hemoglobin level in subgroups of participants using and not using glucagon-like peptide-1 (GLP-1) receptor agonists, and hypoglycemic episodes were secondary and safety endpoints.

Outcomes: Randomization was used to 928 participants, 466 of whom were assigned to the efsitora group and 462 to the degludec group. With efsitora, the mean glycated hemoglobin level dropped from 8.21% at baseline to 6.97% at week 52 (least-squares mean change, −1.26 percentage points), and with degludec, it dropped from 8.24 to 7.05% (least-squares mean change, −1.17 percentage points) [estimated treatment difference −0.09 percentage points; 95% confidence interval (CI) −0.22 to 0.04], results that demonstrated noninferiority. Regarding the change in the glycated hemoglobin level between persons using and not taking GLP-1 receptor agonists, efsitora was not inferior to degludec. 64.3% of the time with efsitora and 61.2% of the time with degludec, respectively, had the glucose level within the desired range (estimated treatment difference 3.1% points; 95% CI 0.1 to 6.1). There were 0.58 and 0.45 instances of combined clinically significant or severe hypoglycemia for every participant year of efsitora and degludec exposure, respectively (estimated rate ratio 1.30; 95% CI 0.94 to 1.78). Efsitora did not cause any severe hypoglycemia; nevertheless, degludec caused six episodes. The two groups had adverse events at comparable rates.

Conclusion: Once-weekly efsitora was not less effective than once-daily degludec in lowering glycated hemoglobin levels in persons with type 2 diabetes who had never taken insulin before. (Promoted by Eli Lilly; NCT05362058 is the QWINT-2 ClinicalTrials.gov number.)

CRITICAL APPRAISAL

What was Known Prior to this Study?

Although a significant proportion of patients with type 2 diabetes mellitus (T2DM) require insulin after some years of diagnosis due to loss of β cell secretory function. The first insulin to be used is usually a long-acting basal insulin followed by bolus doses, if required. However, multiple barriers at the level of the physician and patient exist to insulin therapy, one important one being the burden of multiple daily injections, along with fear of hypoglycemia and weight gain. Some patients are unable to take daily injections of insulin in a timely way, themselves or through caregivers. Efsitora is a novel basal insulin made of insulin chains which are linked to an Fc fragment of a human antibody. Since it is not readily cleared from the circulation by the usual insulin-degrading mechanisms, it has a long duration of action enabling once weekly injection making it a promising agent for several patients.

What this Study Adds?

The QWINT-2 trial provides evidence of non-inferiority once-weekly insulin efsitora alfa (efsitora) to once-daily ultra-long-acting insulin degludec for glycemic control at

52 weeks. Similar reduction in HbA1c% were seen with efsitora and degludec in patients with T2DM, without any reported excess in clinically significant hypoglycemia episodes.

Major Strengths of the Study

First phase 3 trial on insulin efsitora alpha which confirmed its efficacy and safety echoing the findings of phase 2 trials.

Limitations of the Study

It was an open-label study with treat-to-target design, leaving room for bias. Treatment-related differences in adverse events like hypoglycemia were not prespecified as a primary end point. The participants wore a blinded continuous glucose monitoring (CGM) intermittently during the study thereby not allowing dose adjustments based on CGM findings.

Implications of the Findings for the Clinicians

Efsitora alpha is noninferior to degludec insulin in terms of glycemic efficacy in adults with T2DM.

Knowledge Gaps Identified and Scope for Future Research

Though the current trial showed the noninferiority of weekly efsitora to daily degludec insulin, the ONWARDS-6 trial in patients with T1DM showed disproportionate rise in hypoglycemia with efsitora-alpha which led the Food and Drug Administration (FDA) advisory panel to publish an advisory that its benefits do not outweigh the risk. Thus, further trials are necessary to establish the long-term safety of weekly efsitora and also its efficacy and safety in different types of insulin dependent diabetes.

Section 8: NEWER TECHNOLOGIES

Section Editor: Anirban Sinha

1. Efficacy and Safety of Continuous Glucose Monitoring and Intermittently Scanned Continuous Glucose Monitoring in Patients with Type 2 Diabetes: A Systematic Review and Meta-analysis of Interventional Evidence

Ref: Seidu S, Kunutsor SK, Ajjan RA, Choudhary P. Efficacy and Safety of Continuous Glucose Monitoring and Intermittently Scanned Continuous Glucose Monitoring in Patients With Type 2 Diabetes: A Systematic Review and Meta-analysis of Interventional Evidence. Diabetes Care. 2024;47(1):169-79.

ABSTRACT

Background: Inconvenient finger pricks are a part of traditional diabetes self-monitoring of blood glucose (SMBG). Type 2 diabetes (T2D) management is improved by continuous glucose monitoring (CGM) and intermittently scanned CGM (isCGM) devices, which provide easy access to thorough data.

Purpose: To evaluate the possible advantages and disadvantages of CGM and compare it to standard care or SMBG in patients with type 2 diabetes.

Data sources: Up until August 2023, we thoroughly searched bibliographies, Web of Science, the Cochrane Library, MEDLINE, and Embase.

Study selection: We examined research that satisfied the following criteria: Randomized controlled trials (RCTs) that compared at least two therapies for 8 weeks in patients with type 2 diabetes, including SMBG, short- and long-term CGM, isCGM, and real-time/retrospective CGM, and that reported glycemic and pertinent data.

Data extraction: We extracted information such as author, year, study design, baseline characteristics, intervention, and results using a standardized data collecting form.

Synthesis of data: 26 RCTs with 2,783 T2D patients were included (17 CGM and 9 isCGM) (CGM 632 vs. usual care/SMBG 514 and isCGM 871 vs. usual care/SMBG 766). CGM decreased the risk of adverse events [relative risk (RR) 1.22 (95% confidence interval (CI) 1.01, 1.47)], decreased user satisfaction [20.54 (20.98, 20.11)], and decreased hemoglobin A1c (HbA1c) [mean difference 20.19% (95% CI 20.34, 20.04)] and glycemic medication effect score [20.67 (21.20 to 20.13)]. CGM improved CGM measures, raised the risk of adverse events [RR 1.30 (0.05, 1.62)], decreased HbA1c by 20.31% (20.46, 20.17), and enhanced user satisfaction [0.44 (0.29, 0.59)]. Neither CGM nor isCGM significantly affected lipid levels, blood pressure, or body composition.

Limitations: Small sample sizes, results from a single study, population differences, and uncertainty for younger adults are among the limitations. Additionally, thorough analysis was limited by the inclusion of <10 studies for the majority of endpoints, and technical developments over time must be taken into account.

Conclusion: In people with type 2 diabetes, both CGM and isCGM showed a decrease in HbA1c levels; however, the use of isCGM was linked to higher user satisfaction than CGM. While the effects of these devices on blood pressure, cholesterol levels, and body composition are still unknown, both CGM and its use were linked to a higher risk of adverse outcomes.

CRITICAL APPRAISAL

What was Known Prior to this Study?
This is a study which compares continuous glucose monitoring (CGM) versus intermittently scanned CGM (isCGM) and this is a meta-analysis. Prior to this publication there have been several small studies with variable results in terms of both of the safety and the benefits of CGM versus isCGM.

What this Study Adds?
This study demonstrated that, when it comes to improvement of hemoglobin A1c (HbA1c) both CGM and isCGM were equally efficacious and additionally isCGM data demonstrated that it causes greater patient satisfaction. So, these are the two main positives points in terms of the benefits. What this study fails to show is that other benefits, e.g., improvement in other metabolic parameters, body composition, and lipid profile; there was no additional benefit. And when it comes to harm, it suggests that there is no difference in reduction in hypoglycemia risk between two groups. And the local side effects and adverse effects in terms of site infection and other things there is no difference or there is no reduction in favor of either.

Implications of the Findings for the Clinicians
So, from a clinician's point of view, what this study adds is that both CGM and isCGM are useful tools for better glycemic control to be achieved. But remember it does not reduce hypoglycemia risk and local side effects of the both the systems are almost the same. Probably isCGM could score slightly over the continuous CGM in the sense that it has better patience satisfaction and we maybe need further studies in future.

The importance of these findings warrants reconsideration of the integration of CGM and isCGM into clinical practice guidelines to perfectly manage type 2 diabetes (T2D) while being aware of their safety profiles.

2. Estimating Glycemia from HbA1c and CGM: Analysis of Accuracy and Sources of Discrepancy

Ref: Tozzo V, Genco M, Omololu SO, Mow C, Patel HR, Patel CH, et al. Estimating Glycemia From HbA1c and CGM: Analysis of Accuracy and Sources of Discrepancy. Diabetes Care. 2024;47(3):460-6.

ABSTRACT

Objective: To assess the precision of hemoglobin A1c (HbA1c), various continuous glucose monitoring (CGM) intervals, and their combination in determining mean glycemia over ninety days (AG90).

Design and methods of research: We examined 985 90-day CGM periods with <10% missing data from 315 persons with paired HbA1c values, 86% of whom had type 1 diabetes. In order to evaluate the influence of mean red blood cell age as a stand-in for nonglycemic effects on HbA1c, published theoretical models were compared with actual data. Since there is no gold standard measurement for AG90, we created a reference (eAG90) using correction techniques, which we then utilized to evaluate the accuracy of HbA1c and CGM.

Results: When comparing 14 days of CGM with eAG90 at the conclusion of the 90-day period, the mean absolute error (95th percentile) was 14 (34) mg/dL. The average glucose derived from HbA1c had a mean absolute error of 12 (29) mg/dL due to nonglycemic influences on HbA1c. The inaccuracy was decreased to 10 (26) mg/dL when 14 days of CGM and HbA1c were combined. More than 5% of the time, there were discrepancies between CGM and HbA1c >40 mg/dL.

> **Conclusion:** By extending the monitoring duration beyond ~26 days or averaging with a HbA1c-based estimate, the accuracy of eAG90 estimates from brief CGM periods can be increased. Significant discrepancies between HbA1c and eAG90 calculated by CGM are common and could last because of steady nonglycemic factors.

CRITICAL APPRAISAL

What was Known Prior to this Study?

Normally we look at hemoglobin A1c (HbA1c) as a marker of glucose control over a 3 months period. And when initially the continuous glucose monitoring (CGM) data came or even the HbA1c came on earlier, we tried to extrapolate the estimated average glucose from the HbA1c. Even some of the laboratories still talk about HbA1c is so-and-so and the estimated average glucose is so-and-so. And that was first established in a study called the ADAG study (*A1c-Derived Average Glucose* study). There we tried to figure out a relationship between average estimated glucose over 3 months period with the HbA1c. Now this study tried for a similar estimation with 14 days CGM data. This tries to give us an idea about what would be the HbA1c or the average glucose estimate from that report. So we are all trying to give an estimate either from the HbA1c report or from the CGM report.

What this Study Adds?

In this study essentially, we are trying to get an idea of the glycemic excursions over a set 3 months period. This study actually compares the analysis and the prediction of estimated glucose from each of these two methods and tries to compare how good they are in terms of prediction and also tries to highlight what are the causes of discrepancies and how we can probably improve our prediction by doing certain things. So if we observe, this study first of all identifies that there are some sources of error for this estimation whether it is from CGM or from HbA1c. For HbA1c, there are factors such as the lifespan of the red blood cell (RBC), the differences in essay and the essay error methods. For the CGM, it talks about the sensor bias depending on what sensor you are using, where you are placing it and the accuracy of each of the sensors; because of a parameter called mean absolute relative difference (MARD) which assesses the common sources of errors in CGMs. Also we know that the CGM is done only for a 2 week period. Therefore, from 2 weeks data you are trying to extrapolate what it could have been be in 3 months. This study demonstrates that, whichever of the two methods you are looking at—it is always going to be an estimation and it is never ever going to be perfectly predictive of what the real glycemic story is, because there are too many variables involved. The study tells us that one of the changes that we can do is if we extend the monitoring period from 2 to 4 weeks. Then the CGM data might be giving better predictions, as suggested by the study in terms of prediction in the way forward of research. The biases or the inaccuracies of HbA1c cannot be changed by any other newer intervention in the prediction model.

Limitations of the Study

Several limitations warrant consideration in current study. The absence of a definitive gold standard for mean glycemia over ninety days (AG90) requires the utilization of correction methods, while limited data on CGM sensor bias further confound the accuracy of the findings. The study's findings primarily utilize individuals with diabetes who shows extensive CGM use (>90 days with <10% missing data), with the chance of generating biases in the generalizability of results to the common diabetic population.

3. Relationship between Sensor-detected Hypoglycemia and Patient-reported Hypoglycemia in People with Type 1 and Insulin-treated Type 2 Diabetes: The Hypo-METRICS Study

Ref: Divilly P, Martine-Edith G, Zaremba N, Søholm U, Mahmoudi Z, Cigler M, et al.; Hypo-RESOLVE Consortium. Relationship Between Sensor-Detected Hypoglycemia and Patient-Reported Hypoglycemia in People With Type 1 and Insulin-Treated Type 2 Diabetes: The Hypo-METRICS Study. Diabetes Care. 2024;47(10):1769-77.

ABSTRACT

Objective: The clinical significance of the increased detection of hypoglycemia due to the use of continuous glucose monitoring (CGM) is still unclear. In order to better understand the prevalence and duration of sensor-detected hypoglycemia (SDH) and its correlation with person-reported hypoglycemia (PRH) in individuals with type 1 diabetes (T1D) and insulin-treated type 2 diabetes (T2D) who have previously experienced hypoglycemia, the Hypo-METRICS (Hypoglycemia -Measurement, Thresholds and Impacts) study was created.

Design and methods of research: We enrolled 276 T1D and 321 T2D participants who wore blinded CGMs and used the Hypo-METRICS app to monitor PRH over a 10-week period. SDH < 70 mg/dL, SDH < 54 mg/dL, and PRH rates were reported as weekly median episodes. SDH episodes were correlated with PRH episodes that occurred within 1 hour.

The median (interquartile range) rates of hypoglycemia were considerably greater in T1D compared to T2D; this was true for PRH [3.9 (2.4–5.9) vs. 1.1 (0.5–2.0)], SDH < 70 mg/dL [6.5 (3.8–10.4) vs. 2.1 (0.8–4.0)], and SDH < 54 mg/dL [1.2 (0.4–2.5) vs. 0.2 (0.0–0.5)]. PRH was not linked to SDH in 43% of cases, while SDH <70 mg/dL was not linked to PRH in 65% of cases overall. Compared to T2D, the median percentage of SDH linked to PRH in T1D was greater for SDH < 70 mg/dL (40% vs. 22%) and SDH < 54 mg/dL (47% vs. 25%).

Conclusion: According to the new research, many documented symptomatic hypoglycemia events occur above 70 mg/dL, whereas at least half of CGM hypoglycemia is silent, even below 54 mg/dL. These episodes cannot be used in therapeutic or research settings.

CRITICAL APPRAISAL

What was Known Prior to this Study?

While historical data regarding hypoglycemic rates are available, they primarily are from the generation before widespread continuous glucose monitoring (CGM) implementation. Thus, the results of Hypo-METRICS (Hypoglycemia-Measurement, Thresholds and Impacts) study may detect a novel context, specifically correlating with the transition from conventional capillary glucose monitoring methods to more advanced CGM, likely influencing the detected rates of both sensor-detected hypoglycemia (SDH) and person-reported hypoglycemia (PRH) together.

What this Study Adds?

The Hypo-METRICS study, part of the European Union Innovative Medicines Initiative Hypoglycaemia—Redefining Solutions for Better Lives (Hypo-RESOLVE) program, represents a multicenter observational investigation aimed at elucidating the clinical, psychological, and economic consequences of both symptomatic and asymptomatic hypoglycemic episodes, while also striving to offer an evidence-based definition of SDH through the prospective assessment of PRH alongside blinded CGM data. This gives a novel opportunity to give graded importance to patient-reported hypoglycemia, which was previously ignored.

Further elaboration of the data predicts that PRH reported by participants is associated with a psychosocial impact regardless of the presence of independent SDH, suggesting the complex relationship between subjective symptoms and objective measures of glucose levels in the population. Knowing the prevalence of asymptomatic hypoglycemia available, it is likely that experiencing such hypoglycemia could be a normal aspect of living with diabetes as detected by CGM data analysis. The presence of these asymptomatic episodes does not inherently suggest diminished awareness of hypoglycemia, as similar situation have been observed in nondiabetic populations as well.

It is noteworthy that the elevated SDH rates observed in the T2D study population may be attributable to the inclusion criteria focusing on individuals with a recent hypoglycemic history and an increased interest in the subject matter from the patient's perspective.

Limitations of the Study

These findings, however, are derived from only a predominantly White European cohort, suggesting that the applicability of results may be difficult when generalized to another demographic zone, especially for Indians. Future research is needed to further find the implications of these findings across different populations and clinical settings.

Implications of the Findings for the Clinicians

The findings from the study help us to conclude that we need to individually assess the CGM hypoglycemia and patient reported hypoglycemia in our clinical settings. This orientation could be more important in research settings.

4. Does Fully Closed-loop Automated Insulin Delivery Improve Glycemic Control in Patients with Type 2 Diabetes? A Meta-analysis of Randomized Controlled Trials

Ref: Amer BE, Yaqout YE, Abozaid AM, Afifi E, Aboelkhier MM. Does fully closed-loop automated insulin delivery improve glycaemic control in patients with type 2 diabetes? A meta-analysis of randomized controlled trials. Diabet Med. 2024;41(1):e15196.

ABSTRACT

Objectives: The effectiveness and safety of fully closed-loop automated insulin delivery (AID) in individuals with type 2 diabetes were examined in this meta-analysis.

Materials and procedures: From the beginning until April 26, 2023, we conducted a systematic search of PubMed, Scopus, Web of Science, and Cochrane Central. Randomized controlled trials (RCTs) that contrasted fully closed-loop AID with traditional insulin therapy were included. In the random effect model, the results were combined as the risk ratio and mean difference (MD) with 95% confidence interval (CI). The percentage of time spent in the target glucose range (5.6–10 mmol/L, 3.9–10 mmol/L, or 3.9–8 mmol/L, depending on the study) was our main result. The percentage of time spent in hyperglycemia or hypoglycemia was one of the important secondary outcomes.

Results: We compromised 390 individuals in seven RCTs, three of which were crossover and four of which were parallel design. According to our analysis, fully closed-loop AID increased the amount of time spent within the target glucose range by 337 minutes per 24 hours [MD = 23.39%, 95% CI (16.64%, 30.14%), $p < 0.01$], 108 minutes overnight [MD = 22.40%, 95% CI (12.88%, 31.91%), $p < 0.01$], and 258 minutes during the day [MD = 26.85%, 95% CI (21.06%, 32.63%), $p < 0.01$] in comparison to the control group. The total duration of hyperglycemia was reduced by 326 minutes per 24 hours in comparison to the control group [MD = −22.67%, 95% CI (−30.87%, −14.46%), $p < 0.01$]. Overall, nighttime, and daytime durations spent in each group did not significantly differ from one another.

Conclusion: According to our meta-analysis, people with type 2 diabetes who receive fully closed-loop AID may have better glycemic control, especially if their diabetes management is more difficult. To determine whether putting these systems into clinical practice is feasible, more investigation is needed. [Addition made on August 26, 2023, following initial online publication: The first sentence under Results, "We included seven RCTs (three crossover and one parallel designs)," has been modified to "We included seven RCTs (three crossover and four parallel designs)"]

CRITICAL APPRAISAL

What was Known Prior to this study?

Closed-loop insulin delivery systems have been of extensive importance in the management of type 1 diabetes; however, their efficacies in type 2 diabetes were less investigated. Automated insulin delivery (AID) systems have evolved as a promising therapeutic option, particularly for patients having challenging diabetes management with fluctuation. These systems function almost as an automated artificial pancreas, where insulin administration is monitored and regulated in a physiological system, utilizing real-time glucose sensor data tailored by software. The likely benefits of AID systems include improved glycemic control, less risk of hypoglycemia, improved quality of life for patients, and less healthcare provider workload in clinic. Since the start of the first closed-loop AID system in the early 1960s, various generations of these systems have been used, encompassing single-hormone, dual-hormone, hybrid, and fully closed-loop configurations in different models.

What this Study Adds?

The present meta-analysis encompassed seven RCTs (four parallel and three crossover design), involving a total sample of 390 patients. The analysis revealed no statistically significant differences between the fully closed-loop group and the control group concerning the overall, overnight, and daytime duration spent below the target glycemic range. Conversely, participants assigned to the fully closed-loop cohort demonstrated a significant reduction in total time spent in hyperglycemia compared to the control intervention (overall time in hyperglycemia was reduced by nearly 5.5 hours in 24 hours). It is important to note that incidences of device deficiencies were markedly higher in the closed-loop group, with a relative risk (RR) of 3.77 (95% CI). While comparing the time spent in hyperglycemia across the two groups yielded significant results, the proportion of time with glucose concentrations below the target range remained consistent between the groups. Furthermore, the fully closed-loop AID systems significantly decreased glucose variability, as evidenced by a reduction in the standard deviation (SD) of glucose measurements.

Limitations of the Study

Unfortunately, all studies were conducted within Switzerland and the United Kingdom. Of these, four studies utilized a parallel-group design, and the remaining three employed a crossover design. Also, four studies were single-centric, contrasting with three that used across multiple centers. So, there is patient selection bias and may not be represented globally, especially Indian population.

Implications of the Findings for the Clinicians

Fully closed-loop AID systems are a safe and likely more effective alternative for achieving enhanced glycemic control as compared to traditional methods in patients with type 2 diabetes. The utilizations of the results may be limited to complex cases of type 2 diabetes, particularly those patients who are more to use insulin therapy.

Knowledge Gaps Identified and Scope for Future Research

Further investigations are warranted to assess the practical feasibility of implementing such systems in routine clinical practice and to generalize these findings across different populations and settings.

---

5. Real Time Continuous Glucose Monitoring in High-risk People with Insulin-requiring Type 2 Diabetes: A Randomised Controlled Trial

Ref: Lever CS, Williman JA, Boucsein A, Watson A, Sampson RS, Sergel-Stringer OT, et al. Real time continuous glucose monitoring in high-risk people with insulin-requiring type 2 diabetes: A randomised controlled trial. Diabet Med. 2024;41(8):e15348.

ABSTRACT

Goal: The purpose of this study is to examine how real-time continuous glucose monitoring (rtCGM) affects glycemia in a group of persons with insulin-requiring type 2 diabetes (T2D) in New Zealand who are primarily indigenous (Māori).

Methods: A multicenter, 12-week randomized controlled trial (RCT) of persons with type 2 diabetes who received insulin at a rate of 0.2 units/kg/day and had elevated glycated hemoglobin A1c (HbA1c) of 6.4 mmol/mol (8.0%). Participants were randomized to either rtCGM or control [self-monitoring blood glucose (SMBG)] after a 2-week blinded CGM run-in period. Time in the target glucose range [3.9–10 mmol/L; time in range (TIR)] during weeks 10–12 was the main endpoint, and blinded rtCGM was used to collect data for the control group.

Findings: The RCT phase involved 67 people (54% Māori, 57% female), with a median age of 53 (range 16–70 years), a body mass index of 36.7 ± 7.7 kg/m^2, and a HbA1c of 85 (IQR 74, 94) mmol/mol (9.9 [IQR 8.9, 10.8]%). The mean (±SD) TIR did not change in the SMBG group [45 (21)% to 45 (25)%, Δ 2.5%, 95% confidence interval (CI) −6.1 to 11, $p = 0.84$], but it did increase in the rtCGM group from 37 (24)% to 53 (24)% [Δ 13%; 95% CI 4.2 to 22; $p = 0.007$]. The TIR difference between groups, corrected for baseline, was 10.4% (95% CI −0.9 to 21.7; $p = 0.070$).

Between the rtCGM arm and the SMBG arm, the mean HbA1c (±SD) dropped from 85 (18) mmol/mol (10.0 [1.7]%) to 64 (16) mmol/mol (8.0 [1.4]%) and from 81 (12) mmol/mol (9.6 [1.1]%) to 65 (13) mmol/mol (8.1 [1.2]%), respectively ($p < 0.001$ for both groups). Neither group experienced any severe episodes of ketoacidosis or hypoglycemia.

Conclusion: Under a population with insulin-treated type 2 diabetes and increased HbA1c, real-time CGM use under a supportive treat-to-target care approach probably improves glycemia.

CRITICAL APPRAISAL

What was Known Prior to this Study?

Real-time continuous glucose monitoring (rtCGM) assesses interstitial glucose concentrations and wirelessly transmits glucose readings via Bluetooth to a connected device (such as a smartphone or insulin pump). This device also displays glucose trends and the rate of change, allowing users to customize alerts. Nonetheless, consistent utilization of contemporary rtCGM systems has been shown to enhance time in the target glucose range [time in range (TIR); 3.9–10.0 mmol/L and lower hemoglobin A1c (HbA1c) levels in recent large randomized controlled trials (RCTs) involving individuals with insulin-requiring type 2 diabetes (T2D). However, there is currently no RCT data examining the application of rtCGM in T2D patients who self-titrate insulin.

What this Study Adds?

Evidence of benefit of the use of rtCGM in patients with T2D who are on insulin therapy is not well documented. In this current study, in an indigenous Māori population who were having T2D and requiring insulin; first underwent a CGM and on the basis of the data of that CGM the entire population was randomized into two groups. One who would continue to be on rtCGM and the other group that would be on self-monitoring blood glucose (SMBG) testing so that is the control group. And adjustments were made by the patients according to the readings in the treatment arm according to the real-time CGM and in the control arm in terms of the SMBG readings. After 10–12 weeks another CGM was put on the control group but the patients were blinded to it so that you could document what was happening in terms of the TIR and the time below range (TBR) in both the groups. What this study demonstrates is that real-time CGM users benefited in terms of improvement in time in range because it probably helped them in better titration of their insulin dosage. Therefore, this study particularly underscores the effectiveness of the use of rtCGM when improving glucose control in type two diabetes.

Limitations of the Study

There was wider variability in participant glycemia and a lower starting TIR than expected. Due to this variability and the difficulties of recruitment during the coronavirus disease 2019 (COVID-19) pandemic, the study had inadequate power. Also, the care model employed in this investigation is not broadly available in primary care, which limits the generalizability of the findings. No validated instruments were used to measure participant self-efficacy or self-management practices, which could have shed light on the reasons behind improved glycemia for participants, considering that the mean daily insulin dosage and dietary habits appeared mostly unchanged during the study. Finally, the data presented is from a relatively brief follow-up period of 12 weeks.

---

6. Continuous Glucose Monitoring with Structured Education in Adults with Type 2 Diabetes Managed by Multiple Daily Insulin Injections: A Multicentre Randomised Controlled Trial

Ref: Kim JY, Jin SM, Sim KH, Kim BY, Cho JH, Moon JS, et al. Continuous glucose monitoring with structured education in adults with type 2 diabetes managed by multiple daily insulin injections: a multicentre randomised controlled trial. Diabetologia. 2024;67(7):1223-34.

ABSTRACT

Objectives and hypotheses: The purpose of this study was to evaluate the efficacy of blood glucose monitoring (BGM) and stand-alone intermittently scanned continuous glucose monitoring (isCGM) in persons with type 2 diabetes receiving multiple daily insulin injections (MDI) with or without a structured education program.

Techniques: Adults with type 2 diabetes receiving intensive insulin therapy and having hemoglobin A1c (HbA1c) levels between 58 and 108 mmol/mol (7.5% and 12.0%) were randomly assigned in a 1:1:1 ratio to one of three groups: isCGM with conventional education (control group 1), BGM with conventional education (control group 2), or isCGM with a structured education program on adjusting insulin dose and timing according to graphical patterns in CGM (intervention group). An independent statistician performed the block randomization.

Participants and researchers could not be blinded because of the nature of the intervention. Using ANCOVA and the baseline value as a covariate, the main outcome was the change in HbA1c from baseline at 24 weeks. The whole analysis set had 148 individuals, of whom 52 were in the intervention group, 49 were in control group 1, and 47 were in control group 2. A total of 159 participants were randomly assigned ($n = 53$ for each group). At baseline, the HbA1c level was 68.19 ± 10.94 mmol/mol ($8.39 \pm 1.00\%$) on average ($\pm$ SD).

At 24 weeks, the intervention group's least squares mean change ($\pm$ SEM) from baseline HbA1c was -10.96 ± 1.35 mmol/mol ($-1.00 \pm 0.12\%$), control group 1's was -6.87 ± 1.39 mmol/mol ($-0.63 \pm 0.13\%$; $p = 0.0367$ vs. intervention group), and control group 2's was -6.32 ± 1.42 mmol/mol ($-0.58 \pm 0.13\%$; $p = 0.0193$ vs. intervention group). Of those in the intervention group, 28.85% (15/52) experienced adverse events, compared to 26.42% (14/53) in control group 1 and 48.08% (25/52) in control group 2.

Conclusion and interpretation: In people with type 2 diabetes on MDI, stand-alone CGM provides a higher reduction in HbA1c when instruction is given on how to interpret the graphical patterns in CGM.

CRITICAL APPRAISAL

What was Known Prior to this Study?

Continuous glucose monitoring (CGM) helps us to get valuable insights into the fluctuation of glucose levels, trends, and variability that traditional hemoglobin A1c (HbA1c) or intermittent daily blood glucose checks cannot find out. Research has found out the importance of a systematic educational program specifically structured to help patients in adjusting their insulin doses based on CGM data trends. This approach is essential for achieving the long-term benefits of real-time CGM for individuals with type 1 diabetes who rely on multiple daily injections (MDI). The necessity for educational support in optimizing the use of CGM may vary significantly; it can be influenced by factors such as the patient's endogenous insulin production and the specific insulin treatment protocols employed.

What this Study Adds?

There is still a degree of uncertainty of whether individuals with type 2 diabetes who are on MDI can derive additional advantage from a structured education program in association with what is typically offered in standard care. This consideration is particularly relevant given that these patients may retain some residual insulin secretion, which could help to offset minor errors in insulin dosing. Notably, this study marks the first multicenter randomized controlled trial (RCT) to successfully demonstrate a reduction in HbA1c levels through the use of standalone intermittently scanned CGM (isCGM) in type 2 diabetes patients using MDI. We know prior studies reported improvements in glycemic control with CGM usage among type 2 diabetes patients on MDI.

Limitations of the Study

The trial was performed in tertiary centers where patient education was conducted by specialist doctors and generalization of these findings to primary care settings on periphery where expertise may vary. The participants exclusively from South Korea may make it difficult the applicability of the results to other populations like India, and it is worth noting the absence of sex-based analyses within the study.

Implications of the Findings for the Clinicians

This RCT shows that the combination of stand-alone isCGM and a structured educational program helps in significant reduction in HbA1c levels among adults with type 2 diabetes on MDI as compared to isCGM when it is accompanied by conventional education or blood glucose monitoring along with standard educational practices. This knowledge may help us in specific cases or situations whenever feasible.

---

7. Comparison between a Tubeless, On-body Automated Insulin Delivery System and a Tubeless, On-body Sensor-augmented Pump in Type 1 Diabetes: A Multicentre Randomised Controlled Trial

Ref: Kim JY, Jin SM, Kang ES, Kwak SH, Yang Y, Yoo JH, et al. Comparison between a tubeless, on-body automated insulin delivery system and a tubeless, on-body sensor-augmented pump in type 1 diabetes: a multicentre randomised controlled trial. Diabetologia. 2024;67(7):1235-44.

ABSTRACT

Aim: The purpose of this study is to compare the safety and effectiveness of an automated insulin delivery (AID) system that uses a tubeless on-body system with that of a on-body sensor-augmented pump (SAP).

Techniques: Thirteen tertiary medical facilities in South Korea participated in this multicenter, parallel-group randomized controlled trial (RCT). Eligible participants were adults with type 1 diabetes aged 19–69 with hemoglobin A1c (HbA1c) levels <85.8 mmol/mol (<10.0%). For 12 weeks, the subjects were randomized 1:1 to either receive a tubeless, on-body SAP (control group) or an AID system (intervention group). An independent statistician performed stratified block randomization. Because of the nature of the technique, blinding was not possible.

The proportion of time in range (TIR) or blood glucose between 3.9 and 10.0 mmol/L, as determined by continuous glucose monitoring, was the main result. Study centers and baseline data were included as covariates for ANCOVA.

Findings: A total of 104 individuals were randomly assigned to one of two groups: 53 were placed in the intervention group and 51 in the control group. The participants' average age (±SD) was 40 ± 11 years. Over the course of the 12-week trial, the intervention group's mean (±SD) TIR rose from 62.1 ± 17.1% at baseline to 71.5 ± 10.7%, whereas the control group's grew from 64.7 ± 17.0% to 66.9 ± 15.0% {difference between the adjusted means: 6.5% [95% confidence interval (CI) 3.6%, 9.4%], $p < 0.001$}. Additionally, the intervention group's compared with the control group, time below range, time above range, CV, and mean glucose levels were significantly better. With a difference between the adjusted means of −0.7 mmol/mol (95% CI −2.0, 0.8 mmol/mol) [−0.1% (95% CI −0.2%, 0.1%)], $p = 0.366$, HbA1c dropped from 50.9 ± 9.9 mmol/mol (6.8 ± 0.9%) at baseline to 45.9 ± 7.4 mmol/mol (6.4 ± 0.7%) after 12 weeks in the intervention group and from 48.7 ± 9.1 mmol/mol (6.6 ± 0.8%) to 45.7 ± 7.5 mmol/mol (6.3 ± 0.7%) in the control group. Neither group experienced severe hypoglycemia or diabetic ketoacidosis.

Conclusion/Interpretation: Compared to using a tubeless, on-body SAP, using an AID system was safer and linked to better glycemic profiles, such as TIR, time below range, time above range, and CV.

CRITICAL APPRAISAL

What was Known Prior to this Study?
Automated insulin delivery (AID) systems, which employ continuous glucose monitoring (CGM) to automatically adjust insulin delivery rates, have demonstrated notable benefits in both glycemic control and psychosocial well-being. Current guidelines from leading organizations recommend their use for all eligible patients with type 1 diabetes, based on a robust evidence base. A previous single arm study with tubeless on-body AID system has shown improved glycemic control compared to standard care in type 1 diabetes mellitus (T1DM) patients.

What this Study Adds?
This multicenter randomized controlled trial (RCT) compared a tubeless, on-body AID system with a tubeless, on-body sensor-augmented pump (SAP) to compare the glycemic management in adults with type 1 diabetic populations. As conducted in South Korea, the study included individuals with type 1 diabetes who were insulin users along with specific criteria, such as low fasting C-peptide levels and positive autoantibody tests. The study looked for the percentage of time in range (TIR) time above range (TAR), and time below range (TBR). During our 12 week multicenter RCT, the use of the tubeless on-body AID system was associated with greater improvement in glycemic profiles than the use of the tubeless, on-body SAP. The AID system increased TIR more than the SAP without serious adverse events. TAR, TBR, mean glucose, and CV were also improved more with the AID system than the SAP. No cases of diabetic ketoacidosis or severe hypoglycemia were documented and device-related skin changes seen in 15.1% of the intervention group versus 11.8% of the control group. Patient unwillingness to use pumps often arises from discomfort caused by insulin infusion sets and devices, which end up in kinking or leakage. While the AID system shows improved CGM data during night time, there were no significant changes in hemoglobin A1c (HbA1c) levels, as there are low baseline measurements.

Limitations of the Study
The study was conducted only in South Korea, which could limit the generalizability of the results. Moreover, the study cohort had excellent mean glucose control at baseline; thus, they may not be representative of the broader population of people with T1DM.

Implications of the Findings for the Clinicians
Automated insulin delivery systems, which use CGM to adjust insulin delivery rates automatically, have shown important benefits in both glycemic control along mental well-being. The use of a tubeless, on-body AID system was found to be safe and associated with superior glycemic outcomes, including TIR, TBR, TAR, and CV, compared to a tubeless, on-body SAP.

Knowledge Gaps Identified and Scope for Future Research
Studies are required that include various age groups and pregnant individuals as well. Analysis of sex was not conducted here.

8. Performance of the MiniMed 780G System on Mitigating Menstrual Cycle-dependent Glycaemic Variability

Ref: Elhenawy YI, Abdel Kader MS, Thabet RA. Performance of the MiniMed 780G system on mitigating menstrual cycle-dependent glycaemic variability. Diabetes Obes Metab. 2024;26(11):4916-23.

ABSTRACT

Aim: The purpose of this study is to map the insulin requirements and glycemic variabilities over the various menstrual cycle phases and evaluate the effectiveness of the MiniMed 780G system in reducing glycemic variabilities during these periods.

Materials and procedures: 15 female adolescents and young adults with type 1 diabetes were recruited for a pilot research. In this study, only women who experienced regular and spontaneous menstruation were included. The follicular and luteal phases of each menstrual cycle were identified. The open loop period (OLP) and the advanced hybrid closed-loop (AHCL) periods, each lasting 3 consecutive months, were the two study periods during which continuous glucose monitoring parameters were analyzed.

Findings: The mean time in range (TIR) during the OLP was substantially lower during the luteal phase than during the follicular phase (65.13% ± 3.07% vs. 70.73% ± 2.05%) ($p < 0.01$, respectively). From 21.07% ± 2.58% in the follicular phase to 24.87% ± 2.97% in the luteal phase, the mean time above range increased significantly ($p < 0.01$). TIR was similar in both menstrual cycle phases after the AHCL period began ($p = 0.72$), but the amount of time spent below 70 mg/dL did not increase ($p > 0.05$). The percentage of Auto basal and Auto correction supplied by the algorithm during the luteal phase rose by 13.55% and 30.6%, respectively ($p < 0.01$), in relation to insulin administration during the AHCL period.

Conclusion: The MiniMed 780G system's completely automated adaptive algorithm successfully achieved the targeted glycemic results with a TIR >70% during the whole menstrual cycle, reducing menstrual cycle-dependent glycemic variability.

CRITICAL APPRAISAL

What was Known Prior to this Study?

The pathophysiological mechanisms for glycemic variability during different phases of the menstrual cycle are very important topics of ongoing debate. There is increasing evidence indicating the effect of sex hormones on insulin requirements in women, both with type 1 diabetes (T1D) as well as normal populations; however, this association is not thoroughly studied.

What this Study Adds?

The current use of insulin delivery and the effort of automated insulin delivery (AID) systems on glycemic control throughout the various phases of the menstrual cycle is less studied. It is important to evaluate the efficacy of AID systems in premenopausal women who detect fluctuations in blood glucose levels and changes in insulin needs throughout their menstrual cycles. Such a study is essential to find out that whether these systems can meet specific requirements and provide structured insulin delivery during this complex duration.

The present study aimed to detect glycemic variability and insulin needs during different times of the menstrual cycle along with assessing the efficacy and performance of the MiniMed 780G system. This study had only women with a history of regular, spontaneous menstruation for at least 2 years, and cycles occurring every 25–30 days. Findings from this study detects an increased risk of hyperglycemia during the luteal phase of the menstrual cycle, along with a significant reduction in the time spent within the target glycemic range. Moreover, the overall glycemic risk, as measured by the glycemic risk index (GRI), significantly increased during the luteal phase, with this increase primarily attributable to hyperglycemic episodes. This study gives us an insight into targeting glycemic control in a more natural way during menstruation and avoiding hypoglycemia and hyperglycemia.

Section 9: OTHERS

Section Editor: Nisha Batra

1. Optimal Dose and Type of Physical Activity to Improve Glycemic Control in People Diagnosed With Type 2 Diabetes: A Systematic Review and Meta-analysis

Ref: Gallardo-Gómez D, Salazar-Martínez E, Alfonso-Rosa RM, Ramos-Munell J, Del Pozo-Cruz J, Del Pozo Cruz B, et al. Optimal Dose and Type of Physical Activity to Improve Glycemic Control in People Diagnosed With Type 2 Diabetes: A Systematic Review and Meta-analysis. Diabetes Care. 2024;47(2):295-303.

ABSTRACT

History: It is yet unknown what kind of physical activity is best for controlling glycated hemoglobin (HbA1c) in diabetics. Baseline HbA1c is not taken into account when prescribing activities according to current guidelines.

Purpose: To investigate the dose-response association between type 2 diabetics' HbA1c (%) and physical activity.

Sources of data: Embase, MEDLINE, Scopus, CINAHL, SPORTDiscus, and Web of Science were all thoroughly searched.

Selection of study: Trials that used physical activity of any kind as an intervention for individuals with type 2 diabetes were included in our analysis.

Extraction of data: Change scores for each trial arm were computed using pre- and postintervention HbA1c data, demographic and intervention characteristics, and descriptive statistics.

Synthesis of data: We compiled high-quality data from 126 research (6,718 participants) using Bayesian random-effects meta-analyses. HbA1c decreased from 21.02 to 20.66% in severe uncontrolled diabetes, from 20.64 to 20.49% in uncontrolled diabetes, from 20.47 to 20.40% in controlled diabetes, and from 20.38 to 20.24% in prediabetes when the ideal physical activity dose was 1,100 MET min/week.

Restrictions: Because of the variety in the duration and protocols of therapies as well as the interpersonal variability of this result, it was not possible to estimate the time needed to achieve these HbA1c decreases.

Results: The findings of this meta-analysis offer important insights into the best weekly physical activity levels for diabetics, taking into account their baseline HbA1c level, as well as the efficacy of various active intervention methods. Clinicians can now recommend specialized physical activity programs for this population because to these findings.

CRITICAL APPRAISAL

Type 2 diabetes is a prevalent and growing global health issue, significantly impacting mortality and healthcare costs. Lifestyle interventions, particularly physical activity, play a key role in managing the condition. Existing guidelines from the American Diabetes Association (ADA), World Health Organization (WHO), and the American College of Sports Medicine have recommended a certain amount of aerobic physical activity along with muscle-strengthening activities for diabetic patients. However, the precise recommendations for the amount and type of activity necessary to ensure the most effective reduction in glycated hemoglobin (HbA1c) levels have not been studied and remain unclear.

Hence, this systematic review and meta-analysis were conducted to explore the relationship between physical activity and glycemic control in individuals with type 2 diabetes. To achieve this, the researchers conducted a comprehensive search across multiple databases, including Embase, MEDLINE, Scopus, CINAHL, SPORTDiscus, and Web of Science. Eligible studies were randomized controlled trials that focused on participants with type 2 diabetes and used physical activity as the sole intervention. Eligible studies examined any type of physical activity as the intervention, included a control group (usual care or alternate activity), and reported HbA1c as the outcome. Trials combining multiple treatments (e.g., diet or supplements), involving participants with severe comorbidities, or focusing on acute effects (<4 weeks duration) were excluded. Final analysis included 126 studies involving 6,718 participants.

Physical activity was quantified using MET minutes per week, a measure of energy expenditure. The data were analyzed using Bayesian random-effects dose-response models to estimate the relationship between physical activity and HbA1c changes.

The analysis found a nonlinear J-shaped dose-response relationship between physical activity dose and HbA1c reduction across all ADA categories. The optimal dose of physical activity to achieve meaningful reductions in HbA1c was 1,100 MET minutes per week, which corresponds to approximately 244 minutes of moderate-intensity aerobic activity per week or 36 minutes of brisk walking per day. This dose was found to be effective across all categories of diabetes severity.

For individuals with severe uncontrolled diabetes (HbA1c > 8%), the HbA1c reduction ranged from 1.02 to 0.66%, for uncontrolled diabetics (HbA1c 7-8%), the reduction in HbA1c was between 0.64 and 0.49% and for controlled diabetics (HbA1c 6.5-7%), the reduction ranged from 0.47 to 0.40%, while those with prediabetes (HbA1c <6.5%) saw a reduction from 0.38 to 0.24%. These findings indicate that physical activity was particularly effective for those with higher baseline HbA1c levels, with greater reductions in individuals with more severe forms of the condition.

Additionally, the study identified the minimal effective doses of physical activity required to shift individuals between different glycemic categories. For instance, moving someone from severe uncontrolled to uncontrolled diabetes required as little as 150-810 MET minutes per week, while transitioning from uncontrolled to controlled diabetes required 330-990 MET minutes per week. Similarly, to move from controlled diabetes to prediabetes, the required dose ranged from 570 to 900 MET minutes per week.

The study's strengths include its rigorous methodology, using Bayesian random-effects dose-response meta-analysis, which provided precise insights into the optimal dose of physical activity for reducing HbA1c. With data from 126 studies and 6,718 participants, the study is robust and generalizable. It also included a range of physical activity types and controlled for bias using tools like Cochrane Risk of Bias 2.

However, the study has limitations due to heterogeneity in the intervention protocols, such as varying types, durations, and intensities of physical activity, which complicates the generalizability of the results. Additionally, despite efforts to assess and account for bias, a significant portion of the studies had high or unclear risks of bias, often due to the use of per-protocol analyses, which can distort the results. These factors may affect the certainty of the results and suggest that further research with more standardized protocols and longer follow-up periods is needed.

The study got significant clinical implications, providing clear guidance on the optimal dose of physical activity (1,100 MET minutes per week) to improve glycemic control in people with type 2 diabetes. Healthcare providers can use these findings to tailor physical activity prescriptions based on patients' baseline HbA1c levels, particularly recommending multicomponent exercises for better outcomes.

As for future prospects, the study paves the way for further research into how different types of physical activities can be optimized for long-term health outcomes in diabetes care. This includes exploring the longitudinal effects of activity doses, their impact on cardiovascular health and cognitive function, and assessing feasibility and adherence in diverse populations. Further studies are also needed to understand the sustainability of the optimal dose and its effects on other comorbid conditions associated with type 2 diabetes.

2. Suicidal Ideation, Suicide Attempts, and Suicide Deaths in Adolescents and Young Adults with Type 1 Diabetes: A Systematic Review and Meta-analysis

Ref: Renaud-Charest O, Stoljar Gold A, Mok E, Kichler J, Nakhla M, Li P. Suicidal ideation, suicide attempts, and suicide deaths in adolescents and young adults with type 1 diabetes: A systematic review and meta-analysis. Diabetes Care. 2024;47(7):1227-37.

ABSTRACT

Background: There is insufficient data regarding the risk of suicide-related behaviors in young people with type 1 diabetes (T1D), including suicidal thought, suicide attempt, and suicide death.

Goal: Our objectives were to (1) compare the prevalence of suicide-related behavior in youth with and without T1D; (2) ascertain the factors linked to suicide-related behaviors; and (3) ascertain the prevalence of suicidal ideation, suicide attempts, and suicide deaths among adolescents and young adults (AYA) with T1D, aged 10–24.

Sources of data: Up until September 3, 2023, MEDLINE, Embase, and PsycInfo were thoroughly searched.

Selection of studies: We included observational studies in which researchers documented the prevalence of behaviors associated to suicide among AYA with T1D aged 10–24.

Extraction of data: We gathered information on study characteristics, the prevalence of behaviors related to suicide, and related factors.

Synthesis of data: 31 studies were included. Suicidal ideation was 15.4% (95% CI 10.0–21.7; $n = 18$ studies) versus 11.5% (0.4–33.3; $n = 4$), and suicide attempts were 3.5% (1.3–6.7; $n = 8$) versus 2.0% (0.0–6.4; $n = 5$) in AYA with and without T1D. Among young people with T1D, the prevalence of suicide fatalities varied from 0.04 to 4.4%. Higher incidence of behaviors related to suicide have often been linked to challenges with T1D self-management. However, there was conflicting evidence regarding the relationship between glycemic levels and behaviors related to suicide.

Restrictions: The meta-analysis of suicide attempts and suicidal ideation revealed a significant degree of heterogeneity.

Results: Among AYA with T1D, suicidal thoughts and attempts are common. These rates are not greater among AYA with T1D than among those without, according to the available data.

CRITICAL APPRAISAL

Depression, suicidal ideation, and suicide attempts are common in adolescents with chronic conditions such as type 1 diabetes (T1D), negatively affecting self-management and health outcomes. In adolescents and young adults (AYA) with T1D, physiological and psychological changes, such as deteriorating glycemic control, decreased adherence to self-care, and increased psychiatric risks, often occur simultaneously. While previous reviews have examined suicide risk in T1D, no systematic review or meta-analysis has estimated the prevalence of suicide-related behaviors in AYA with T1D.

The aim of this study was to synthesize the existing evidence on the prevalence of these behaviors and the factors associated with them in this population.

A systematic search was conducted in MEDLINE, Embase, and PsycInfo for studies published up to September 3, 2023. The inclusion criteria focused on participants aged 10–24 years with a diagnosis of T1D and studies reporting the prevalence of suicide-related behaviors (suicidal ideation, suicide attempts, or suicide deaths), assessed with any tool. Case reports and studies, where most participants had type 2 diabetes or were followed for a depressive episode, were excluded. Eligible study designs included cross-sectional, case-control, and cohort studies. The prevalence of suicidal ideation and suicide attempts was calculated for all timeframes, with a subgroup analysis for the timeframe (past 12 months vs. lifetime).

Meta-regression and subgroup analysis were used to explore heterogeneity, focusing on categorical variables such as timeframe and sex. A total of 31 studies were included, with 20 studies contributing to the quantitative analysis. Among these, 18 were cross-sectional studies, 8 were retrospective cohort studies, 2 were prospective cohort studies, and 1 was a case-control study.

In the 18 studies reporting the prevalence of suicidal ideation, the pooled estimate from the random-effects meta-analysis was 15.4% in AYA with T1D versus 11.5% in those without T1D. The prevalence of suicide attempts was found to be 3.5% in T1D versus 2.0% in those without T1D. However, data was reported in a handful of studies only. The study did not find consistent evidence that the rates of suicidal ideation or attempts were higher in AYA with T1D compared to their peers without T1D. Suicide deaths were infrequently reported, with limited data to estimate prevalence accurately. Stigma and the potential reluctance of youth with T1D to disclose suicide-related behaviors may have contributed to underreporting.

Challenges in T1D self-management were identified as key contributors to suicide-related behaviors. Daily tasks such as blood glucose monitoring and insulin management often result in diabetes distress, characterized by negative emotions associated with managing the condition. High rates of depression and anxiety further compounded the psychological burden in AYA with T1D. Feelings of loneliness, burdensomeness, and social stigma—exacerbated by the visibility of medical equipment and hypoglycemic symptoms—were also highlighted as factors increasing the risk of suicidal ideation and attempts. The availability of insulin, a potentially lethal medication, was frequently noted in methods used for suicide attempts, emphasizing the need for targeted prevention strategies.

Sex differences were noted in the data. While females exhibited a higher prevalence of suicidal ideation (17.6%) than males (7.0%), the difference was not statistically significant. Suicide attempts were more common in females, whereas suicide deaths were more frequent in males, consistent with patterns observed in general youth populations. Interestingly, the study found no consistent association between glycemic levels [glycated hemoglobin (HbA1c)] and suicide-related behaviors, suggesting that glycemic control should not be relied upon as a marker for suicide risk.

The review acknowledged several limitations, including significant heterogeneity in study methodologies, variations in tools used to assess suicide-related behaviors, and the lack of control groups in most studies. Although some studies included control groups, the overall number was limited, and comparisons between AYA with and without T1D were restricted. Furthermore, subgroup analyses were constrained by the availability of data on variables such as sex and developmental stages. Differences between AYAs were potentially overlooked by combining these groups in the analysis.

This review underscores the need for tailored mental health support for AYA with T1D, incorporating validated tools for assessing suicide-related behaviors and addressing both psychological and social challenges associated with the condition. Longitudinal studies are required to explore the evolution of suicide-related behaviors over time, particularly from the point of T1D diagnosis through young adulthood. These studies should account for factors such as sex, glycemic control, and structural and social determinants of health to inform more effective prevention strategies. While the findings suggest no clear difference in the prevalence of suicide-related behaviors between AYA with and without T1D, the prevalence remains significant, warranting increased attention to the mental health needs of this vulnerable population.

3. Individualizing Treatment of Type 2 Diabetes after Metformin: More Insights from GRADE

Ref: Riddle MC. Individualizing Treatment of Type 2 Diabetes After Metformin: More Insights From GRADE. Diabetes Care. 2024;47(4):556-61.

ABSTRACT

Objective: The GRADE (Glycemia Reduction Approaches in Diabetes) study sought to evaluate the efficacy of four common second-line treatments—(1) glargine, (2) liraglutide, (3) glimepiride, and (4) sitagliptin—for managing type 2 diabetes (T2D) not adequately controlled by metformin alone. The study focused on glycemic durability and patient outcomes.

Methodology: This extensive, randomized trial involved 5,047 T2D patients [average disease duration: 4.2 years, glycated hemoglobin (HbA1c): 7.5%, body mass index (BMI): 34.3]. Participants continued metformin use and were randomly assigned to one of the four treatments. The main outcome measure was glycemic control durability, defined as maintaining HbA1c below 7%. Additional measures included safety, adverse events, and patient-reported outcomes. Insulin rescue therapy was introduced when HbA1c surpassed 7.5%.

Findings: Liraglutide and glargine showed superior glycemic control durability, lowering the risk of HbA1c exceeding 7% by 16% and 13%, respectively, compared to glimepiride and sitagliptin. Liraglutide led to weight reduction and initial quality-of-life improvements, but 44% of patients experienced gastrointestinal side effects. Glargine and glimepiride caused more hypoglycemic events, though severe cases were infrequent. Sitagliptin, while safe, proved least effective, particularly in insulin-resistant patients. Cardiovascular events and mortality rates were low, with no significant intertreatment differences. By the study's conclusion, 71% of participants had HbA1c ≥ 7%.

Conclusion: The research emphasizes the need for personalized treatment approaches, as no single therapy emerged as universally superior. Liraglutide may be beneficial for patients with obesity or cardiovascular risk, while glargine is effective for fasting hyperglycemia. The findings underscore T2D's progressive nature and the necessity for tailored therapeutic strategies to optimize patient outcomes.

CRITICAL APPRAISAL

The GRADE (Glycemia Reduction Approaches in Diabetes) study was conducted to identify the most effective second-line therapy for managing type 2 diabetes (T2D) when metformin alone fails to achieve glycemic control. Its goal was to provide guidance in selecting second line therapy for individuals in this important group, which has not previously been evaluated in a large, long-term comparative effectiveness study.

The trial included 5,047 participants with a mean diabetes duration of 4.2 years, an average glycated hemoglobin (HbA1c) of 7.5%, and a body mass index (BMI) of 34.3. The study compared four treatments—glargine (long-acting insulin), liraglutide [glucagon-like peptide 1 (GLP-1) receptor agonist)], glimepiride (sulfonylurea), and sitagliptin [dipeptidyl peptidase 4 (DPP-4) inhibitor]. Participants were randomized to one of these treatments while continuing metformin. The primary endpoint was the durability of glycemic control, defined as maintaining HbA1c levels below 7.0%. Secondary outcomes included safety, adverse effects, quality of life, and cardiovascular and microvascular complications.

The study found that liraglutide and glargine were slightly more effective in maintaining glycemic control compared to glimepiride and sitagliptin. Liraglutide reduced the risk of HbA1c rising above 7.0% by 16%, while glargine reduced it by 13%. However, glycemic control declined steadily in all groups, and by the end of the study, 71% of participants had HbA1c levels above the target. Liraglutide also led to significant weight loss and early improvements in quality of life, although these effects were not sustained. It was associated with gastrointestinal side effects in 44% of participants. Glargine and glimepiride were linked to a higher risk of hypoglycemia, though severe events were rare. Sitagliptin had the fewest side effects but was the least effective at maintaining glycemic control, especially in patients with insulin resistance.

The study observed low rates of cardiovascular events and mortality, with no significant differences between treatments. However, liraglutide showed a nonsignificant trend toward lower cardiovascular risks and mortality. Emotional distress and quality of life measures improved slightly with liraglutide and glargine, and none of the treatments worsened these outcomes.

The findings highlight the need for individualized therapy in T2D management. Liraglutide may be preferable for patients with obesity or cardiovascular risk factors, while glargine is effective for fasting hyperglycemia. Glimepiride may suit those with higher baseline HbA1c, but its risk of hypoglycemia requires caution. Sitagliptin, despite its lower efficacy, may be an option for older patients or those concerned about side effects. It is noteworthy that this class of drugs has been reported to provide better glycemic control for Asian populations than for other populations.

While the GRADE Study provides valuable guidance, its exclusion of newer therapies, such as SGLT-2 inhibitors, limits its applicability to current clinical practice. The study underscores the importance of tailoring therapy to individual patient needs, focusing on safety, lifestyle considerations, and the progressive nature of T2D.

4. Diabetes Management in Detention Facilities: A Statement of the American Diabetes Association

Ref: Lorber DL, ElSayed NA, Bannuru RR, Shah V, Puisis M, Crandall J, et al. Diabetes Management in Detention Facilities: A Statement of the American Diabetes Association. Diabetes Care. 2024;47:544-55.

ABSTRACT

Guidelines for diabetes care in correctional facilities are provided in this statement. Key points are included at the conclusion of each section, which focuses on areas where the procedures for providing treatment to diabetics in correctional facilities may differ from those in the community. (1) Timely identification or diagnosis of diabetes treatment needs and continuity of care (at reception/intake, during transfers, and upon discharge); (2) physical activity and nutrition; (3) timely access to diabetes management tools (insulin, blood glucose monitoring, tracking data, current diabetes management technologies, etc.); and (4) treatment of the individuals with diabetes as a whole (self-management education, mental health support, monitoring and addressing long-term complications, specialty care, etc.) are areas of emphasis that inform multiple aspects discussed in this statement.

CRITICAL APPRAISAL

An estimated 9% of the incarcerated population has been diagnosed with diabetes. As the incarcerated population ages and the incidence of diabetes among young people rises, the prevalence of diabetes and its related comorbidities and complications is expected to increase further within this group. Additionally, the detained population includes a disproportionately high number of individuals from minoritized or marginalized ethnic groups, who also have a higher likelihood of being diagnosed with diabetes.

Considering all these aspects, American Diabetes Association (ADA), in this statement, provided a comprehensive guide for managing diabetes in detention facilities. The document emphasizes early diagnosis, uninterrupted access to treatment, and holistic care to meet national diabetes care standards.

One of the key recommendations is timely identification of diabetes at intake. Detention facilities are urged to perform thorough health screenings on arrival, termed as Reception Screening to detect diabetes and assess immediate treatment needs. These include blood glucose monitoring, ensuring access to insulin or other diabetes medications, and checking for signs of complications like diabetic ketoacidosis (DKA). Early diagnosis and intervention can prevent serious, sometimes life-threatening complications. Intake procedures should also consider behavioral health issues, substance use, and any existing diabetes-related complications.

Nutrition plays a vital role in managing diabetes, and the statement calls for balanced meals with consistent carbohydrate levels. Facilities are encouraged to offer meals that meet the nutritional needs of people with diabetes and to provide snacks for those on insulin or glucose-lowering medications to prevent low blood sugar (hypoglycemia). However, implementing these recommendations may be difficult in facilities with limited budgets or strict meal plans that do not allow much flexibility.

Another focus is on access to diabetes technologies, such as continuous glucose monitors (CGMs) and insulin pumps. These tools are effective for managing blood sugar levels, especially in individuals with type 1 diabetes. The ADA advises that detainees already using these devices before incarceration should continue to have access unless specific safety concerns arise. However, logistical challenges, such as replacing supplies or ensuring proper use, can limit their implementation in detention facilities.

The document also highlights the importance of mental health support. People with diabetes often experience higher rates of depression, stress, and other mental health challenges, which can make managing their condition harder. Regular mental health assessments and counseling are recommended, along with diabetes self-management education. Through structured education programs, detainees can learn essential skills such as blood sugar monitoring, medication management, and how to handle emergencies such as low blood sugar.

Continuity of care during transfers and upon release is a critical part of the ADA's recommendations. When detainees are moved between facilities or released into the community, delays in medication or treatment can have serious consequences. The ADA advises facilities to prepare detailed medical summaries, including the individual's current treatment plan, recent blood sugar levels, and any special care needs. Detainees should also receive enough medication and supplies to last until their first medical appointment postrelease. Such measures help ensure that treatment is not interrupted during these transitions.

In addition to managing diabetes itself, the statement addresses the prevention and treatment of diabetes-related complications, such as heart disease, kidney damage, and eye problems. Routine screenings for these complications, along with timely referrals to specialists, are crucial for maintaining the health of detainees with diabetes.

The statement also highlights the need for foot care, as people with diabetes are at risk for ulcers and amputations. Regular foot examinations and protective footwear are recommended to prevent complications.

Staff training is another significant focus. The ADA calls for both medical and security staff to be educated about diabetes management. This includes recognizing and responding to emergencies, such as severe low or high blood sugar levels, and understanding how medications and technologies like CGMs work. Such training ensures that staff are prepared to support detainees' health needs effectively.

The statement also outlines challenges in detention settings. Resource limitations, overcrowding, and variability in staff training can make it difficult to implement these recommendations consistently. Some facilities may lack access to diabetes specialists or the infrastructure needed to provide advanced care. Additionally, while the document emphasizes the need to address racial and socioeconomic disparities—since diabetes disproportionately affects marginalized groups—it provides limited actionable strategies for tackling these systemic issues.

Despite these challenges, the ADA's recommendations represent a significant step forward in improving diabetes care for incarcerated individuals. By addressing all aspects of care—nutrition, mental health, emergency preparedness, and continuity of treatment—the statement aims to create a framework that supports better health outcomes.

In conclusion, this guidance offers a clear and thorough plan to improve diabetes care in detention facilities, recognizing the unique needs and challenges of this population. While some recommendations may be difficult to implement due to systemic and resource-related barriers, the document provides a strong foundation for advancing equitable and effective care for people with diabetes in custody.

5. Dapagliflozin Improves Erectile Dysfunction in Patients with Type 2 Diabetes Mellitus: An Open-label, Non-randomized Pilot Study

Ref: Cannarella R, Condorelli RA, Leanza C, Garofalo V, Aversa A, Papa G, et al. Dapagliflozin improves erectile dysfunction in patients with type 2 diabetes mellitus: An open-label, non-randomized pilot study. Diabet Med. 2024;41(1):e15217.

ABSTRACT

Aim: The study's objective was to assess how dapagliflozin, either by itself or in conjunction with tadalafil, affected erectile dysfunction (ED) in patients with type 2 diabetes.

Techniques: 30 white male patients with type 2 diabetes and severe ED participated in this open-label, nonrandomized pilot trial. Group 1 received tadalafil 5 mg/day, Group 2 received tadalafil 5 mg/day with dapagliflozin 10 mg/day, and Group 3 received dapagliflozin 10 mg/day for 3 months. They were equally split into three groups. The International Index of Erectile Function 5-item (IIEF-5) questionnaire and the dynamic penile echo color Doppler ultrasound (PCDU) examination were used to assess the presence and severity of ED at enrollment and following treatment.

Results: The three groups' IIEF-5 scores significantly improved at the end of treatment, increasing by 294%, 375%, and 197% for Groups 1, 2, and 3, respectively. Peak systolic velocity increased significantly by 178.9%, 339%, and 153%, according to PCDU evaluation; acceleration time was significantly reduced in Group 2 (−26.2%) compared to Groups 1 and 3 (−7.2% and −6.6%), but end-diastolic velocity did not significantly change after treatment. For every end goal, Group 2 showed the highest rates of progress.

Conclusion: Dapagliflozin increases the effectiveness of tadalafil and improves ED in people with type 2 diabetes. Additional research is required to validate our findings and clarify the mechanism or mechanisms by which dapagliflozin affects ED.

CRITICAL APPRAISAL

An estimated 150 million men globally experience erectile dysfunction (ED), most frequently present in patients with DM. A recent meta-analysis of 145 studies showed that the overall prevalence of ED among diabetic patients is 52.5%. Factors contributing to this connection include microvascular disease, diabetic neuropathy, hypogonadism, medication side effects, and psychogenic conditions. Hyperglycemia increases oxidative stress, lowering nitric oxide (NO) levels and fostering conditions leading to ED. ED is linked to cardiovascular diseases (CVDs) and can predict coronary artery disease (CAD) onset by 2–5 years, emphasizing the need for early diagnosis in diabetic patients.

First-line treatments for ED typically involve phosphodiesterase type 5 inhibitors (PDE5i) like sildenafil and tadalafil. Some antidiabetic medications, such as metformin and pioglitazone, may also help manage ED. While empagliflozin has shown promise in improving erectile function in diabetic rats, the effects of dapagliflozin remain uncertain. Given dapagliflozin's cardiovascular and renal benefits, this study aimed to evaluate its effects on ED in patients with type 2 diabetes mellitus (T2DM) when used alone or with tadalafil.

This was an open-label, nonrandomized pilot study wherein male patients of Caucasian origin with T2DM, severe ED [International Index of Erectile Function 5-item (IIEF-5) score < 7] and mild lower urinary tract symptoms (LUTS) [International Prostate Symptom Score (IPSS) score ≤ 7] aged 58–60 year were taken.

In this open-label, nonrandomized pilot study, 30 Caucasian male patients aged 58–60 with T2DM and severe ED (IIEF-5 score < 7) were included. Only those taking metformin at 3 g/day were selected, while patients with significant comorbidities were excluded. Participants were divided into three groups (10 in each group): Group 1 received tadalafil 5 mg/day, Group 2 received tadalafil plus dapagliflozin 10 mg/day, and Group 3 received dapagliflozin alone, all for 3 months, alongside a 20% caloric reduction and minimal exercise.

Primary endpoints included IIEF-5 scores and penile echo color Doppler ultrasound parameters—peak systolic velocity (PSV), acceleration time (AT), and end-diastolic velocity (EDV)—measured at baseline and after 3 months. Glycated hemoglobin (HbA1c) levels were also assessed at the beginning and end of treatment period, while age, body mass index (BMI), and waist circumference (WC) were recorded at enrollment.

The mean age of the participants was 59.6 ± 5.9 years, with most being overweight or mildly obese. After 3 months, HbA1c values showed significant improvements in all groups: Group 1 from 7.8 to 7.3%, Group 2 from 8.0 to 6.5%, and Group 3 from 8.1 to 7.3%.

By the end of the study, all groups demonstrated significant increases in IIEF-5 scores by 294%, 375% and 197%, in Groups 1, 2 and 3, respectively with Group 2 showing the greatest improvement in PSV (+339%) compared to Groups 1 (+178%) and 3 (+153%). Group 2 also had a greater reduction in AT (−26.2%) than the other groups, highlighting dapagliflozin's potential benefits for managing ED in patients with T2DM.

The study suggests that dapagliflozin improves ED in patients with T2DM by reducing penile microvascular damage and endothelial dysfunction, contributing to enhanced erectile function. While glycemic control plays a role in improving ED, dapagliflozin's effects may also be due to its ability to restore NO levels in the penile arteries. This could explain why combination therapy with tadalafil showed the greatest improvements, as dapagliflozin may enhance tadalafil's efficacy by increasing NO-mediated vasodilation. The other mechanism that is postulated is Dapagliflozin might act by reducing low-grade systemic inflammation, a key contributor to ED. Increased levels of inflammatory markers such as interleukin 6 (IL-6), tumor necrosis factor α (TNF-α), and C-reactive protein are often found in patients with ED, while lower levels of IL-10 suggest disturbed inflammation. Dapagliflozin is known for its anti-inflammatory properties, as demonstrated in other studies, such as those on rats with lung injury and in arrhythmogenic cardiomyopathy.

Although there was an inverse correlation between HbA1c levels and erectile function (IIEF-5 score and PSV), adjustments for confounding factors reduced statistical significance, suggesting that improvements in erectile function might not solely rely on HbA1c reduction.

However, the study has notable limitations. As a pilot study, it involved a small sample size, and the use of the IIEF-5 questionnaire introduces subjectivity, while PCDU was performed in a nonblinded manner, increasing the risk of bias. Furthermore, the nonrandomized design prevents establishing causal effects. Despite these limitations, the findings suggest that dapagliflozin could be a promising treatment for ED in T2DM patients, particularly when combined with PDE5 inhibitors (like tadalafil), offering potential benefits for both sexual function and cardiovascular risk.

The study provides a foundation for future, more robust research to better understand how dapagliflozin affects erectile function and to confirm these initial positive results. The potential dual benefits of dapagliflozin—improving ED and mitigating cardiovascular risk—could make it an important addition to clinical practice for patients with T2DM and ED.

6. Footwear Fit as a Causal Factor in Diabetes-related Foot Ulceration: A Systematic Review

Ref: Jones PJ, Armstrong DG, Frykberg R, Davies M, Rowlands AV. Footwear fit as a causal factor in diabetes-related foot ulceration: A systematic review. Diabet Med. 2024;41(10):e15407.

ABSTRACT

Goals: Diabetes-related at-risk feet are at risk for harm from incorrectly fitting footwear (IFF). This systematic review's objective was to evaluate and summarize the data supporting the claim that IFF is a statistically significant cause of ulcers.

Methods: We looked for English-language peer-reviewed research that included a physical inspection of the footwear worn and reported the number or proportion of individuals with diabetes-related foot ulceration (DFU) attributable to wearing IFF. We searched PubMed, Scopus, Web of Science, and Google Scholar. The Newcastle–Ottawa scale was used by two independent reviewers to evaluate the possibility of bias.

Findings: 45 studies were picked from 4,318 findings that were obtained after duplicates were removed. The inclusion criteria were met by 10 studies, the majority of which were evaluated as good ($n = 3$) or fair ($n = 6$). There is some evidence that DFU and IFF are strongly related, but it is restricted because only 3 out of 10 included studies indicated that a statistically significant percentage of DFU patients wore improper footwear, including footwear that was not adequate in terms of fit, type, fastening, or material (15.0–93.3%). In these three investigations, the risk of bias varied from "fair" to "poor". IFF definitions were inconsistent or sometimes unreported. Only one investigation identified ulcer locations linked to IFF, with 10% occurring at the plantar metatarsal heads and 70% occurring at the plantar hallux/toes.

Conclusion: There is some indication that IFF contributes to DFU, but more study is required to define IFF and systematically document physical activity, ulcer location, and footwear assessment. Researchers must determine whether the use of IFF is influenced by economic considerations, the need for footwear education, or other factors.

CRITICAL APPRAISAL

Diabetes-related foot ulceration (DFU) is a significant complication affecting an estimated 9–26 million people worldwide, with a lifetime incidence of 19–34%. Mortality rates can reach 30–50% within 5 years. Incorrectly fitting footwear (IFF) may contribute to foot ulcers. Tight shoes can cause blisters and increase pressure, while loose shoes can heighten friction and exposure to heat. A lack of protective sensation may also lead to the use of ill-fitting footwear, although this remains unconfirmed.

The International Working Group on Diabetic Foot (IWGDF) guidelines state that inadequate footwear can cause ulceration. Still, no systematic review has specifically examined the extent to which poorly fitting shoes are linked to ulcers. Most reviews have focused on whether therapeutic footwear reduces diabetes-related foot ulcers, with limited discussion on footwear fit. Research on the impact of nontherapeutic footwear on ulcer risk is lacking, and a systematic review by Monteiro-Soares predominantly addressed adherence to therapeutic footwear.

Hence, this study was planned to explore the percentage of diabetes-related foot ulcers associated with IFF, the strength of the evidence for this relationship, and the quantification of improperly fitting footwear. It also tried to investigate the locations of ulcers correlated with ill-fitting shoes.

This systematic review examined articles from the PubMed, Scopus, Google Scholar, and Web of Science databases up until August 2023. Initially, 45 papers were shortlisted, and after full-text reviews, 10 studies were selected. Two reviewers (PJ and AR) independently assessed the risk of bias using the Newcastle–Ottawa Scale.

Most studies were cohort, observational, or cross-sectional ($n = 8$), with one case series and one case-control study. 60% of the studies originated from developed countries. The primary focus of most of the studies was to identify broadly the causes and risk factors for DFUs, including footwear, with only two studies specifically addressed poorly fitting footwear.

Study durations varied from 2–6 months ($n = 4$) to over 2 years ($n = 5$), with participant ages ranging from 50.6 ± 6.3 years to 67.2 ± 12.5 years.

Three of the ten included studies found a statistically significant percentage (15.0–93.3%) of those with DFU were wearing IFF that included IFF and unsuitable footwear type, fastening, or material (57.0%). The risk of bias in these three studies ranged from "fair" or "poor". In one of these studies, the focus was primarily related to outcomes concerning factors such as foot surgery, debridement, Wagner grade of ulcer at inclusion, and independent living, rather than footwear.

Definitions of IFF were inconsistent in all studies, and risky types included flip-flops, unsuitable materials, or footwear that was one size too small. Footwear depth was not discussed, and methods for measuring foot dimensions varied.

Only one study reported the location on feet where the ulcers associated with IFF or socks occurred–the most common being plantar hallux (37.5%) or toes (34.2%).

Similarly, the severity of ulcers caused by IFF or socks was only reported in this study where two-thirds are superficial and deep ulcers (69.1%), with 10.6% classified as abscess/osteomyelitis and 20.3% as minor and major gangrene. Ulcer healing outcomes were not stratified by location on feet. Where IFF or socks were a precipitating factor, 70% of ulcers healed, 25% of ulcers led to amputations and 5%, died before healing but severity and healing outcomes were not stratified by location.

Most studies did not record physical activity levels, such as the number of daily steps or hours wearing IFF or economic factors that could influence the purchase of properly fitting footwear.

This systematic review was the first of its kind and ensured the quality of chosen criteria, explored in various databases; however, articles were restricted due to the chosen language being English only.

To conclude, there was evidence that IFF is a cause of DFU, however, it was found to be weaker than anticipated. Often it is not possible to determine causality and studies assessing relationships with inappropriate or IFF are adversely affected when either standards or methodologies are unreported or ambiguous. Admittedly, ascribing inappropriate or IFF as a principal cause of ulceration can also be challenging due to its multifactorial nature. Only 1 study described the severity, but considering high rates of amputation and mortality underlines the seriousness of the problem and further research in this area. Even the trained medical experts have limited education regarding foot self-care rather than specific knowledge about footwear.

Robust research is needed to make a clear definition of IFF and devise a methodology for assessing footwear fit. Ulcer location, physical activity, severity, and healing outcomes of these ulcers are some other relevant points that need to be further explored to reach a conclusion and devise further strategies to prevent the onset of DFU and its complications as well.

7. Effectiveness and Safety of Empagliflozin: Final Results from the EMPRISE Study

Ref: Htoo PT, Tesfaye H, Schneeweiss S, Wexler DJ, Everett BM, Glynn RJ, et al. Effectiveness and safety of empagliflozin: final results from the EMPRISE study. Diabetologia. 2024;67:1328-42.

ABSTRACT

Objectives and hypotheses: There is little data on how safe and effective empagliflozin is in comparison to other glucose-lowering drugs in people with type 2 diabetes who have a wide range of cardiovascular risks. Using data gathered from electronic health databases, the EMPagliflozin Comparative Effectiveness and Safety (EMPRISE) cohort study was created to periodically assess the safety and efficacy of empagliflozin over a 5-year period.

Techniques: Using US Medicare and commercial claims databases, we found people with type 2 diabetes who were at least 18 years old and started taking empagliflozin or dipeptidyl peptidase 4 inhibitors (DPP-4i) between 2014 and 2019.

Four a priori-defined effectiveness outcomes were identified following 1:1 propensity score matching using 143 baseline characteristics—(1) myocardial infarction (MI) or stroke; (2) hospitalization for heart failure (HHF); (3) major adverse cardiovascular events (MACE); and (4) cardiovascular mortality or HHF. Lower limb amputations, nonvertebral fractures, acute kidney injury (AKI), diabetic ketoacidosis (DKA), severe hypoglycemia, the advancement of retinopathy, and short-term kidney and bladder malignancies were among the safety results. Overall and stratified by age, sex, baseline atherosclerotic cardiovascular disease (ASCVD), and heart failure, we calculated HRs and rate differences (RDs) per 1,000 person-years.

Findings: 115,116 matching pairings were found. Empagliflozin was linked to lower risks of heart failure [HR 0.50 (0.44, 0.56); RD −5.35 (−6.22, −4.49)], MI/stroke [HR 0.88 (95% CI 0.81, 0.96); RD −2.08, 95% CI (−3.26, −0.90)], MACE [HR 0.73 (0.62, 0.86); RD −6.37 (−8.98, −3.77)], and cardiovascular mortality/HHF [HR 0.57 (0.47, 0.69); RD −10.36 (−12.63, −8.12)] when compared to DPP-4i. Older people and those with ASCVD/heart failure benefited more in absolute terms. Empagliflozin was linked to reduced risks of AKI [HR 0.62 (0.54, 0.72); RD −2.39 (−3.08, −1.71)], hypoglycemia [HR 0.75 (0.67, 0.84); RD −2.46 (−3.32, −1.60)], retinopathy progression [HR 0.78 (0.63, 0.96); RD −9.49 (−16.97, −2.10)], and comparable risks of other safety events.

Conclusions and interpretations: Empagliflozin was linked to lower risks of MI or stroke, HHF, MACE, and the composite of cardiovascular mortality or HHF when compared to DPP-4i. Older people and those with a history of heart failure or ASCVD showed greater absolute risk decreases. There was no difference in the short-term risks of lower-extremity amputation, non-vertebral fractures, kidney and renal pelvis cancer, and bladder cancer; however, empagliflozin was linked to a higher risk of DKA and a lower risk of AKI, hypoglycemia, and progression to proliferative retinopathy.

CRITICAL APPRAISAL

Atherosclerotic cardiovascular disease (ASCVD) and heart failure (HF) are the leading causes of illness and death among individuals with type 2 diabetes. Placebo-controlled trials have shown that empagliflozin, a sodium-glucose cotransporter-2 inhibitor (SGLT-2i), offers cardiovascular benefits for those with established ASCVD or HF. However, there are still questions about how its benefits and safety compare to other glucose-lowering medications in individuals with type 2 diabetes, especially considering the diversity of patient characteristics that differ from those in the randomized controlled trials (RCTs) conducted so far. To date, no RCTs have directly compared the effectiveness and safety of empagliflozin with alternative glucose-lowering medications. Previous studies highlighting the benefits of SGLT-2i in routine care have included only a small number of empagliflozin users, provided limited data on safety events, or focused on individuals with specific conditions. Therefore, gathering comparative evidence on the safety and effectiveness of empagliflozin versus alternative medications could help weigh their benefits against potential adverse effects.

The EMPagliflozin Comparative Effectiveness and Safety (EMPRISE) study is a sequential cohort study designed to monitor the safety and effectiveness of empagliflozin over a period of five years (2014–2019) using three U.S. electronic healthcare databases.

The study included individuals with type 2 diabetes initiated on empagliflozin or dipeptidyl peptidase 4 inhibitors (DPP-4i) between August 1, 2014, and September 30, 2019. Participants were over 65 years old for those in Medicare and over 18 for others. They entered the study after a 12-month period without SGLT-2i or DPP-4i prescriptions and needed continuous insurance coverage. Individuals with type 1 diabetes, malignancies, end-stage kidney disease (ESKD), or those prescribed both drug classes were excluded.

Follow-up continued until participants discontinued their medication or reached a study outcome. Primary outcomes included composite events of myocardial infarction (MI) or stroke, hospitalization for heart failure (HHF), major adverse cardiovascular events (MACE), and composite outcomes of cardiovascular death or HHF. Secondary outcomes considered broader definitions of HHF and various MACE components, while safety outcomes included lower-limb amputation, acute kidney injury (AKI), diabetic ketoacidosis (DKA), severe hypoglycemia, and cancer diagnoses.

After matching on propensity scores, the study analyzed 115,116 individuals in each treatment group, with about 33% having a history of ASCVD or HF. The median follow-up was approximately 5 months.

The rates for composite MI or stroke events were 13.2 per 1,000 person-years (PY) for empagliflozin and 15.3 for DPP-4i, resulting in a hazard ratio (HR) of 0.88. HHF rates were 5.0 per 1,000 PY for empagliflozin compared to 10.3 for DPP-4i (HR 0.50). In Medicare beneficiaries, MACE rates were lower for empagliflozin (22.4 vs. 28.7 events/1,000 PY; HR 0.73). While safety outcomes showed similar rates of lower-limb amputation, empagliflozin was associated with a higher risk of DKA (HR 1.78) but lower risks for AKI (HR 0.62) and severe hypoglycemia (HR 0.75).

Overall, absolute risk reductions were greater in patients with baseline ASCVD or HF. Stratified analyses indicated slightly larger relative risk reductions in older individuals for the composite outcome of MI or stroke.

The study enhances the evidence regarding the cardiovascular effectiveness and safety of empagliflozin, building on findings from other RCTs. The EMPA-REG OUTCOME trial indicated a 13% risk reduction in MI, similar to the 12% reduction found in this study. A greater absolute risk reduction for MI or stroke was observed in participants with a history of ASCVD or HF, supporting the current recommendation of SGLT-2 inhibitors for these individuals.

Regarding HHF outcomes, the study confirms that empagliflozin consistently reduces risk across various subgroups, including those without prior HF. However, prior trials lacked sufficient power to assess safety events, the large sample size in this study allowed for precise estimates of relative risk for most safety events.

Increased risk of hospitalization for DKA among individuals starting empagliflozin was seen as compared to those on DPP-4i, consistent with the known class effect. Nevertheless, the number needed to treat for one additional case of DKA was high ($n = 693$).

This study got some limitations as well, including the potential for residual confounding. Efforts were made to achieve balance in laboratory results, the possibility of bias still cannot be ruled out. Evolving treatment indications over time were accounted for, matching participants within each time block and cardiovascular disease subgroup to strengthen the study findings.

The definition of cardiovascular death was accurate, but death data were limited to Medicare enrollees aged over 65. The follow-up period might be insufficient to detect long-term outcomes for MI or stroke, only 20% of the participants remained on medication after 1 year.

In conclusion, the study showed that empagliflozin significantly reduced the risks of HHF, cardiovascular mortality, and MACE compared to DPP-4i, particularly in patients with previous heart issues or older age.

However, it was associated with a higher risk of DKA, while also lowering risks of AKI, severe hypoglycemia, and retinopathy progression.

---

8. Impact of the Timing of Metformin Administration on Glycaemic and Glucagon-like Peptide-1 Responses to Intraduodenal Glucose Infusion in Type 2 Diabetes: A Double-blind, Randomised, Placebo-controlled, Crossover Study

Ref: Xie C, Iroga P, Bound MJ, Grivell J, Huang W, Jones KL, et al. Impact of the timing of metformin administration on glycaemic and glucagon-like peptide-1 responses to intraduodenal glucose infusion in type 2 diabetes: a double-blind, randomised, placebo-controlled, crossover study. Diabetologia. 2024;67:1260-70.

ABSTRACT

Objectives and hypotheses: In people with type 2 diabetes, metformin reduces postprandial glycemic excursions by gastrointestinal function modulation, including glucagon-like peptide 1 (GLP-1) activation. It is unclear how changing the time at which metformin is administered affects postprandial glucose metabolism. We assessed how metformin, given at various times before to an intraduodenal glucose infusion, affected the glycemic, insulinemic, and GLP-1 responses that followed in patients with type 2 diabetes treated with metformin.

Techniques: In a crossover approach, 16 individuals with type 2 diabetes who were comparatively well-controlled with metformin monotherapy were examined over 4 different days. Participants were randomly assigned to receive either saline at all timepoints (control) or a bolus infusion of metformin (1,000 mg in 50 mL 0.9% saline) via a nasoduodenal catheter at $t = 0$–60 minutes, then an intraduodenal glucose infusion of 12.56 kJ/min (3 kcal/min) at $t = 0$–60 minutes. Participants and researchers involved in the study procedures were blinded to the treatments. Measurements of total GLP-1, insulin, and plasma glucose were made every 30 minutes from $t = -60$ to 120.

Findings: Metformin decreased plasma glucose levels and raised plasma GLP-1 and insulin levels in a treatment-by-time interaction ($p < 0.05$ for each). When metformin was given at $t = -60$ or -30 minutes as opposed to $t = 0$ minutes, there was a higher decrease in plasma glucose levels ($p < 0.05$ for each), and only when metformin was given at $t = -60$ or -30 minutes ($p < 0.05$ for each) were there rises in plasma GLP-1 levels. Metformin increased glucose-induced insulin production ($p < 0.05$) but had no effect on insulin sensitivity. The increases in plasma insulin levels during the 3 days when metformin was administered were similar.

Conclusions and interpretations: When metformin is administered before enteral glucose instead of with it, it lowers blood sugar levels more effectively in type 2 diabetes that is well-controlled and is linked to a higher GLP-1 response. These findings imply that taking metformin prior to meals may maximize its impact on enhancing postprandial glycemic management.

CRITICAL APPRAISAL

Metformin is the primary treatment for type 2 diabetes and is often recommended as the first-line medication. Its glucose-lowering effects are mainly attributed to reducing liver glucose production. However, recent studies have uncovered several other mechanisms including stimulation of the incretin hormone glucagon-like peptide 1 (GLP-1), slowing of gastric emptying, suppression of intestinal glucose absorption, inhibition of bile acid resorption and modulation of the gut microbiota. GLP-1, an incretin hormone that enhances insulin secretion, suppresses glucagon release, slows gastric emptying, and reduces appetite. This is particularly important for managing postprandial (after meal) hyperglycemia, a key factor in overall glycemic control.

Strategies to improve postprandial glycemia often focus on optimizing the timing of therapeutic interventions relative to nutrient ingestion. While guidelines recommend taking metformin with meals to minimize gastrointestinal side effects, this practice may limit its effectiveness in lowering postprandial glucose. Preliminary studies indicate that taking metformin before meals could improve its efficacy. However, the impact of timing on glucose control and GLP-1 responses is not well understood, and existing studies often have limitations such as small sample sizes and inadequate control over meal factors.

Addressing this knowledge gap has the potential to refine clinical guidelines, improve postprandial glycemic control, and reduce long-term complications in individuals with type 2 diabetes. Hence, this study was designed to evaluate the effects of varying the timing of metformin administration relative to an intraduodenal glucose infusion on glycemic, insulinemic, and GLP-1 responses in patients with well-controlled type 2 diabetes.

16 adults with well-controlled type 2 diabetes on stable metformin therapy participated in a double-blind, randomized, placebo-controlled crossover trial. Participants underwent four sessions where metformin or a placebo was administered intraduodenally at different intervals (−60, −30, or 0 minutes before glucose infusion) or received a saline control. A nasoduodenal catheter ensured precise delivery, eliminating variability due to gastric emptying rates. The glucose infusion occurred at a rate of 12.56 kJ/min (3 kcal/min) for 60 minutes. Blood samples were collected from baseline (−60 minutes) to 120 minutes after the glucose infusion to measure plasma glucose, GLP-1, and insulin levels.

The results demonstrated that metformin effectively lowered postprandial plasma glucose levels when compared to the saline control. The glucose-lowering effect was significantly greater when metformin was administered 30 or 60 minutes before the glucose infusion, compared to administration at the start of the infusion. Metformin given 60 minutes prior showed the most pronounced effect at the end of the glucose infusion. This reduction in glycemia was accompanied by an increase in GLP-1 secretion, which was only observed when metformin was administered before glucose infusion, specifically at −30 and −60 minutes. GLP-1 levels peaked at 60 minutes postinfusion and gradually declined thereafter.

Metformin also enhanced glucose-induced insulin secretion across all administration times, but there were no significant differences in insulin levels between the three timing intervals. Notably, metformin did not improve whole-body insulin sensitivity, as measured by the Matsuda index. Additionally, the study found that metformin administration did not lead to significant gastrointestinal symptoms such as nausea, nor did it affect appetite.

The findings suggest that administering metformin 30–60 minutes before meals could enhance its efficacy in lowering postprandial glucose levels. This benefit is likely mediated through a stronger GLP-1 response and increased glucose-induced insulin secretion. Current recommendations to take metformin with meals may, therefore, limit its potential benefits in controlling postprandial glycemia.

Despite its strengths, the study has limitations. The use of intraduodenal metformin infusion bypasses the normal gastric phase, limiting the direct application of findings to routine oral administration. The small sample size, predominantly male participants, and the acute nature of the study further constrain its generalizability. Future research should assess the long-term effects of premeal metformin administration in diverse populations and its impact on overall glycemic control, particularly in real-world settings.

In conclusion, this study provides compelling evidence that altering the timing of metformin administration can optimize its glucose-lowering effects. Administering metformin 30-60 minutes before meals could be a simple and effective strategy to improve postprandial glycemia in patients with type 2 diabetes.

9. Efficacy and Safety of Oral Semaglutide Monotherapy versus Placebo in a Predominantly Chinese Population with Type 2 Diabetes (PIONEER 11): A Double-blind, Phase IIIa, Randomised Trial

Ref: Wang W, Bain SC, Bian F, Chen R, Gabery S, Huang S, et al. Efficacy and safety of oral semaglutide monotherapy vs placebo in a predominantly Chinese population with type 2 diabetes (PIONEER 11): a double-blind, Phase IIIa, randomised trial. Diabetologia (2024) 67:1783-99.

ABSTRACT

Objectives and hypotheses: In a primarily Chinese population with type 2 diabetes that was not adequately managed with diet and exercise alone, the study's objective was to compare the safety and effectiveness of oral semaglutide monotherapy versus a placebo.

Techniques: 52 sites in the China region (mainland China and Taiwan), Hungary, Serbia, and Ukraine participated in the double-blind, randomized, Phase IIIa Peptide Innovation for Early Diabetes Treatment (PIONEER) 11 trial. Participants who were ≥18 years old (≥20 years old in Taiwan), diagnosed with type 2 diabetes with a HbA1c of 53–86 mmol/mol (7.0–10.0%), and not on any glucose-lowering medications were eligible.

Participants who met the randomization criteria were randomly assigned (1:1:1:1) using a web-based randomization system to receive once-daily oral semaglutide 3 mg, 7 mg, or 14 mg or a placebo for 26 weeks (using a 4-week dose-escalation regimen for the higher doses) following a 4-week run-in period during which they were treated with diet and exercise alone. Depending on whether participants were from the China region or not, the randomization process was tiered. Changes in body weight (kg) and glycated hemoglobin (HbA1c) from baseline to week 26 were the primary and confirmatory secondary objectives, respectively. Every participant who received at least one dose of the study product had their safety evaluated.

Findings: The majority of participants (92.5%, n = 482) finished the trial, while 39 participants stopped treatment too soon. A total of 774 participants were screened between October 2019 and October 2021, and 521 participants were randomly assigned to oral semaglutide 3 mg (n = 130), 7 mg (n = 130), 14 mg (n = 130), or placebo (n = 131). The total number of participants who were randomly assigned at the start of the trial served as the basis for the number of participants who contributed to the trial analysis. The mean age of participants was 52 years, and the majority were male (63.7%). The mean body weight was 79.6 kg and the mean HbA1c was 63 mmol/mol (8.0%) at baseline. At week 26, oral semaglutide significantly reduced HbA1c compared to placebo ($p < 0.001$ for all dosages).

When comparing oral semaglutide 3 mg, 7 mg, and 14 mg to a placebo, the estimated treatment differences [ETDs (95% Cis)] were −11 (−13, −9) mmol/mol, −16 (−18, −13) mmol/mol, and −17 (−19, −15) mmol/mol, respectively. In percentage points (95% CI), the equivalent ETDs versus placebo were −1.0 (−1.2, −0.8), −1.4 (−1.6, −1.2), and −1.5 (−1.8, −1.3). At week 26, oral semaglutide 7 mg and 14 mg also showed significantly higher reductions in body weight than placebo [ETD (95% CI) −1.2 kg (−2.0 kg, −0.4 kg; $p < 0.01$) and −2.0 kg (−2.8 kg, −1.2 kg; $p < 0.001$), respectively], but not oral semaglutide 3 mg [ETD (95% CI) −0.0 kg (−0.9 kg, 0.8 kg; not significant)].

The Chinese subgroup, which accounted for 74.9% of participants in the total population, showed comparable decreases in body weight and HbA1c. Participants who received oral semaglutide (at all doses) experienced adverse events (AEs) in 65.4–72.3% of cases, compared to 57.3% of those who received a placebo. Few serious AEs were observed, and the majority of AEs were mild to moderate in intensity. Gastrointestinal AEs were the most frequently reported AEs, and they were more common with semaglutide (at all dosages) than with a placebo. The Chinese group had a marginally greater percentage of AEs.

Conclusions/Interpretation: In primarily Chinese participants with type 2 diabetes that was not adequately controlled by diet and exercise alone, oral semaglutide led to significantly higher reductions in HbA1c at all doses and in significant body weight reductions for the 7 mg and 14 mg doses when compared with placebo. The safety profile of oral semaglutide was in line with the worldwide PIONEER trials, and it was generally well tolerated.

CRITICAL APPRAISAL

In China, the prevalence of diabetes is rising, with around 140 million cases of diabetes in 2021. Achieving and maintaining glycemic targets and weight loss are essential for individuals with type 2 diabetes to reduce the risk of complications. Both international guidelines [American Diabetes Association–European Association for the Study of Diabetes (ADA/EASD)] and the Chinese Diabetes Society (CDS) recommend glucagon-like peptide 1 receptor agonists (GLP-1 RAs) or sodium-glucose cotransporter-2 inhibitors as adjuncts to metformin, especially for those with established cardiovascular disease or high risk. However, the use of subcutaneous GLP-1 RAs is less common in China than other glucose-lowering medications.

The efficacy and safety of once-daily oral semaglutide have been well-studied in the global PIONEER Phase IIIa trial program. Although it included Asian populations, there is limited evidence specifically for predominantly Chinese populations. Distinct differences in the clinical characteristics of type 2 diabetes between East Asian and Western populations may affect treatment responses, highlighting the need for tailored strategies.

The PIONEER 11 Phase IIIa trial evaluated the efficacy and safety of oral semaglutide compared to placebo in in a predominantly Chinese cohort with type 2 diabetes inadequately managed by diet and exercise. Conducted across 52 sites in China, Hungary, Serbia, and Ukraine, the 26-week randomized, double-blind study included 521 participants who were randomized to receive oral semaglutide (3 mg, 7 mg, or 14 mg) or placebo. Participants were aged 18 or older with an glycated hemoglobin (HbA1c) level between 53 and 86 mmol/mol (7.0–10.0%) with specific exclusion criteria related to prior glucose-lowering treatments, renal impairment, pancreatitis, malignancies, and certain histories of endocrine disorders or diabetic retinopathy. Eligible participants were randomized in a 1:1:1:1 ratio using a web-based system to receive once-daily oral semaglutide (3 mg, 7 mg, or 14 mg) or a placebo for 26 weeks, with a follow-up visit at week 31.

The primary endpoint was the change in HbA1c from baseline to week 26, with the confirmatory secondary endpoint being the change in body weight. Additional secondary endpoints included achieving HbA1c targets, weight loss of ≥5% or ≥10%, and various metabolic measures. Safety was monitored through adverse events (AEs) and vital signs.

Between October 2019 and October 2021, 774 participants were screened, and 521 were randomized to receive oral semaglutide at 3 mg ($n = 130$), 7 mg ($n = 130$), 14 mg ($n = 130$), or placebo ($n = 131$). The results showed significant reductions in HbA1c for all semaglutide doses compared to placebo: −12 mmol/mol for 3 mg, −16 mmol/mol for 7 mg, and −17 mmol/mol for 14 mg (all $p < 0.001$). Weight loss was also observed, with significant reductions for the 7 mg and 14 mg doses (1.2 kg and 2.0 kg, respectively). The study demonstrated that oral semaglutide was effective in improving both glycemic control and body weight in patients with type 2 diabetes. The trial had a 92.5% completion rate, with 7.5% discontinuing early. Most participants were from China (74.9%), and the majority were male (63.7%), with a mean age of 52 years.

Oral semaglutide 14 mg resulted in significant reductions in total cholesterol, low-density lipoprotein (LDL) cholesterol, and triglycerides compared to placebo ($p < 0.05$). AEs occurred more frequently with oral semaglutide (3 mg: 16.2%, 7 mg: 32.3%, and 14 mg: 31.8%) than placebo (9.2%), mainly gastrointestinal disorders. Most AEs were mild to moderate, and the rate of serious AEs was low. Mean estimated glomerular filtration rate (eGFR), calcitonin, creatine kinase levels, and the bilirubin ratio were similar between treatment groups. Overall, the Chinese subpopulation experienced a higher proportion of AEs (73.2–80.6% with oral semaglutide) compared to 65.3% with placebo.

This double-blind, randomized trial found that once-daily oral semaglutide significantly reduced HbA1c levels in a predominantly Chinese population with type 2 diabetes, showing results similar to those in the global PIONEER 1 trial. Body weight reductions from baseline to week 26 were greater with 7 mg and 14 mg doses of oral semaglutide compared to placebo, though the reductions were smaller in the Chinese subpopulation.

Previous studies, such as the PIONEER 9 trial (in a predominantly Japanese population) and SUSTAIN China (in a Chinese population), have suggested that body weight reductions with semaglutide are generally less pronounced in Asian populations compared to global trials. While cross-trial comparisons should be cautious due to differences in study designs, these trends highlight a need for further investigation. The smaller weight reductions in Asian populations may also be explained by their lower baseline body weight and body mass index (BMI) compared to predominantly Western populations, which could limit the extent of weight loss observed.

The trial's strengths include its robust design, high enrollment numbers, and low dropout rate. However, limitations include a relatively short duration of 26 weeks and participant health criteria that may not represent the wider Chinese population with type 2 diabetes.

In conclusion, oral semaglutide effectively reduced HbA1c (at doses of 3 mg, 7 mg, and 14 mg) and body weight (at 7 mg and 14 mg) after 26 weeks in the trial. Its safety profile aligns with that of the GLP-1 receptor agonist class. Given the high prevalence of uncontrolled type 2 diabetes in China, exploring new treatment options is essential.

10. Comparative Renal Outcomes of Matched Cohorts of Patients with Type 2 Diabetes Receiving SGLT2 Inhibitors or GLP-1 Receptor Agonists Under Routine Care

Ref: Fadini GP, Longato E, Morieri ML, Bonora E, Consoli A, Fattor B, et al. Comparative renal outcomes of matched cohorts of patients with type 2 diabetes receiving SGLT2 inhibitors or GLP-1 receptor agonists under routine care. Diabetologia. 2024;67:2585-97.

ABSTRACT

Objectives and hypotheses: We examined the effects of glucagon-like peptide 1 receptor agonists (GLP-1 RA) and sodium-glucose cotransporter-2 inhibitors (SGLT-2i) on renal outcomes in people with type 2 diabetes, with an emphasis on alterations in estimated glomerular filtration rate (eGFR) and albuminuria.

Techniques: A multicenter retrospective observational analysis of newly prescribed diabetes drugs was conducted. Prior to and following propensity score matching, participant characteristics were evaluated. Mixed-effects models were used to analyze the primary endpoint, which was the change in eGFR. Changes in albuminuria and categorical eGFR-based outcomes were secondary objectives. To evaluate the findings' robustness, sensitivity and subgroup analyses were conducted.

Findings: Following matching, each group had 57,01 members. The majority of participants were male, aged 61, had had diabetes for 10 years, had a baseline glycated hemoglobin (HbA1c) of 64 mmol/mol (8.0%), and had a body mass index (BMI) of 33 kg/m². In 23% of patients, chronic kidney disease (CKD) was present. Over the course of the observation period, the SGLT-2i group's eGFR stayed higher than that of the GLP-1 RA group by 1.2 ml/min/1.73 m², from a baseline of 87 mL/min/1.73 m² over a median of 2.1 years. There were no discernible variations in albuminuria. Despite a smaller HbA1c decrease, the SGLT-2i group showed better improvements in blood pressure and lower rates of deteriorating CKD class than the GLP-1 RA group. In individuals without pre-existing CKD, SGLT-2i also lessened the fall in eGFR more effectively than GLP-1 RA.

Conclusions/Interpretation: SGLT-2i medication was linked to better renal function preservation in people with type 2 diabetes than GLP-1 RA administration, as seen by a slower fall in eGFR. In this patient population, these results support SGLT-2i as the recommended medication for renal protection.

CRITICAL APPRAISAL

Diabetic kidney disease (DKD) is the leading global cause of end-stage kidney disease (ESKD), posing significant societal and healthcare burdens. Sodium–glucose cotransporter-2 inhibitors (SGLT-2i) have revolutionized DKD management, with strong evidence supporting their renal benefits. Glucagon-like peptide 1 receptor agonists (GLP-1 RA) also demonstrate renoprotective effects, as shown by cardiovascular outcome trials (CVOTs) reporting reductions in nephropathy risk compared to placebo.

The renoprotective mechanisms of both drug classes involve improvements in glycemic control, blood pressure, and body weight. However, SGLT-2is are thought to exert stronger hemodynamic effects, whereas GLP-1 RAs are noted for their anti-inflammatory properties. Real-world studies yield mixed findings, with some favoring SGLT-2i for renal preservation and others suggesting similar efficacy.

To address this knowledge gap, this multicenter, retrospective observational study was conducted using real-world clinical data to compare the long-term kidney outcomes of patients who initiated SGLT-2i or GLP-1 RA under routine care.

This DARWIN-Renal study was conducted by the Italian Diabetes Society across 50 specialist care centers in Italy between January 2015 and September 2020. Eligible participants were aged 18–80 years, had been diagnosed with type 2 diabetes for at least 1 year, and had renal outcome data available. Patients with prior use of SGLT-2i or GLP-1 RA within 12 months, simultaneous initiation of both, chronic kidney disease (CKD) stage V, or dialysis were excluded.

The study's primary endpoint was the change in estimated glomerular filtration rate (eGFR), with secondary outcomes including eGFR slopes, urinary albumin–creatinine ratio (uACR), glycated hemoglobin (HbA1c), body weight, blood pressure, and renal events such as CKD progression, ESKD, and dialysis initiation. These measures were analyzed in an intention-to-treat population, censored at event occurrence or last observation.

Propensity score matching resulted in two well-balanced cohorts of 5,701 participants each. The matched populations had a mean age of 61 years, 10-year diabetes duration, body mass index (BMI) of 33 kg/m², HbA1c of 8.0%, and eGFR of 86 mL/min/1.73 m², with 23% having CKD and 15% a uACR >30 mg/g. SGLT-2i users were predominantly prescribed dapagliflozin (52.8%) or empagliflozin (38.6%). GLP-1 RA prescriptions were primarily for dulaglutide (52.3%) and liraglutide (30.8%), with fewer patients receiving exenatide (10.7%), semaglutide (3.8%), or lixisenatide (2.3%).

Over a median follow-up of 2.1 years with a median of 5 eGFR measurements per patient, SGLT-2i users showed a slower eGFR decline compared to GLP-1 RA users, with a 1.2 mL/min/1.73 m² higher eGFR and a 0.5 mL/min/1.73 m²/year less negative slope. SGLT-2i also offered superior protection against CKD progression, serum creatinine doubling, and new-onset CKD, effects were more prominent in a population with preserved baseline kidney function (mean eGFR 86 mL/min/1.73 m²). No significant differences were observed between the two groups regarding changes in albuminuria. GLP-1 RA showed slightly better glycemic control (HbA1c reduction), while SGLT-2i provided greater reductions in blood pressure and body weight.

The study supported the preferential use of SGLT-2i for renal protection in patients with type 2 diabetes, reinforcing its role in preserving kidney function.

The study's findings are largely consistent with existing research, particularly regarding the renal benefits of SGLT-2i. However, the comparison with GLP-1 RA on weight loss is an outlier compared to most previous studies, where GLP-1 RA typically results in greater weight reduction.

The study design was observational rather than a randomized trial. Despite using propensity score matching (PSM), there is a chance that some unmeasured factors, such as diet and physical activity, could have influenced the results. Baseline differences between groups, such as longer diabetes duration and worse kidney function in SGLT-2i users, as well as the lack of adherence data and incomplete GLP-1 RA dosing details, may have affected the findings. The low representation of semaglutide in the GLP-1 RA group likely reduced the observed weight-loss effects for this class.

The other limitation of the study is the inclusion of subjects with relatively preserved kidney function, which limits the results' applicability to patients with more advanced kidney disease or those in primary care. Additionally, the short follow-up period made it difficult to assess long-term outcomes such as ESKD or cardiovascular events. The lack of data on combining SGLT-2i and GLP-1 RA, which might provide better renal protection, is another limitation.

Despite the strengths of the study including large sample size and the use of PSM, due to above-mentioned limitations and the incomplete assessment of relevant outcomes (e.g., cardiovascular events and long-term renal complications) restrict the ability to draw definitive conclusions. Future randomized controlled trials, with more robust reporting of dosing, adherence, and long-term outcomes, are needed to confirm these findings.

11. Glucagon-like Peptide-1 Receptor Agonists and Risk of Thyroid Cancer: A systematic Review and Meta-analysis of Randomized Controlled Trials

Ref: Silverii GA, Monami M, Gallo M, Ragni A, Prattichizzo F, Renzelli V, et al. Glucagon-like peptide-1 receptor agonists and risk of thyroid cancer: A systematic review and meta-analysis of randomized controlled trials. Diabetes Obes Metab. 2024;26(3):891-900.

ABSTRACT

The purpose of this study is to perform a meta-analysis of randomized clinical trials (RCTs) in order to determine whether treatment with glucagon-like peptide 1 receptor agonists (GLP-1 RA) is linked to thyroid cancer.

Methods and materials: We included studies that compared a GLP-1 RA with any comparator, lasted at least 52 weeks, and reported the incidence of adverse events without regard to the population or major endpoint in this meta-analysis of RCTs. Every instance of thyroid carcinoma was compiled.

Findings: Out of the 64 trials we were able to extract, 26 of them included at least one incidence instance of thyroid cancer. The chance of developing thyroid cancer overall was significantly increased by GLP-1 RA medication [Mantel-Haenszel odds ratio (MH-OR) 1.52 (95% CI) 1.01, 2.29; $p = 0.04$, I2 = 0%), with a fragility index of 1 and a 5-year number needed to harm of 1,349. When only trials with a duration of at least 104 weeks were included, the link was still significant [MH-OR 1.76 (95% CI 1.00, 3.12); $p = 0.05$]. Neither medullary thyroid cancer [MH-OR 1.44 (95% CI 0.23, 9.16); $p = 0.55$] nor papillary thyroid cancer [MH-OR 1.54 (95% CI 0.77, 3.06); $p = 0.22$] showed any significant correlation.

Conclusion: According to our meta-analysis, GLP-1 RA therapy may be linked to a slight increase in absolute risk and a moderate increase in relative risk for thyroid cancer in clinical trials. Longer term studies are needed to evaluate this finding's clinical significance.

CRITICAL APPRAISAL

Glucagon-like peptide 1 receptor agonists (GLP-1 RAs) are increasingly used to treat type 2 diabetes and manage overweight and obesity due to their significant efficacy with cardiovascular benefits. However, some retrospective studies suggest a potential link between GLP-1 RAs and thyroid cancer, supported by reports to the FDA and the World Health Organization. This aligns with preclinical findings that show GLP-1 receptors in thyroid C cells, which can stimulate cell growth in rodent models. However, these effects appear weaker in humans, and significant evidence of GLP-1 RAs affecting the proliferation of papillary thyroid carcinoma (PTC) cells is lacking. Thus, the connection between GLP-1 RA treatment and thyroid cancer risk is not firmly established, with methodological limitations in epidemiological studies. Randomized clinical trials (RCTs) may provide clearer evidence, which is the focus of this meta-analysis assessing the association between GLP-1 RA treatment and thyroid cancer risk.

The present meta-analysis included RCTs published in Medline, Embase, Clinicaltrials.gov, and Cochrane CENTRAL Database up to 20 August 2023 with a duration of follow-up of at least 52 weeks, in which any GLP-1 RA approved by the European Medical Agency for any indication (i.e., type 2 diabetes or obesity) was compared with either placebo or active comparators. A total of 64 studies were included, overall enrolling 46,228 patients on GLP-1 RA treatment and 38,399 subjects on placebo or a comparator. GLP-1 RA treatment was found to be associated with a significant increase in the risk of overall thyroid cancer in the fixed-effect analysis [MH-OR 1.52 (95% CI 1.01, 2.29); $p = 0.04$), with no heterogeneity (I2 = 0%). The 5-year number needed to harm (NNH), which denotes the number of patients that must be treated with a drug for 5 years to observe one additional case of thyroid neoplasm, was calculated to be 1,349.

Subgroup analyses revealed no significant differences in effects based on the use of different GLP-1 RA molecules or different comparators. Results were also similar irrespective of patients' age, body mass index (BMI), or the indication of treatment (obesity or diabetes mellitus). This association of GLP-1 RA with thyroid cancer remained statistically significant when the trials lasting at least 24 weeks were included. However, upon individual analysis of the incidences of papillary thyroid cancer and medullary thyroid cancer, no significant association was identified with the utilization of GLP-1 RAs.

This is, to our knowledge, the first meta-analysis of randomized controlled trials demonstrating such results. Previous meta-analyses did not find a significant effect on thyroid cancer, likely due to insufficient statistical power. A notable strength is the low heterogeneity of results, indicating that the observed association of GLP-1 RA treatment with thyroid cancer is independent of trial characteristics and case mix.

However, the statistical power of this analysis is too low to determine whether the increase in overall thyroid cancer incidence was caused by medullary thyroid carcinoma (MTC), PTC, or both. Another thing to note is that thyroid malignancies were not a part of predefined endpoints of clinical trials, but rather recorded only if listed as serious adverse events. Hence, most of the trials might have had an insufficient duration for the assessment of their effects on the development of malignancies.

The fragility index in this study was observed to be 1, meaning that it would take only one additional case of thyroid cancer occurring in the comparator arm for the association to lose significance indicating that further trials could modify the present results. One additional limitation is the specificity of the case mix. The population enrolled in clinical trials does not fully represent those receiving treatment in routine clinical practice. In particular, the study protocols of most trials tend to exclude patients with a personal or family history of MTC or with elevated calcitonin levels, thus selecting a population at relatively low risk for this specific malignancy.

While the results are not definitive, the analysis of existing randomized trials indicates a clear safety concern, suggesting a potential link between GLP-1 RA and a moderate increase in the risk of thyroid cancer. However, the clinical significance of this association is constrained by the relatively low incidence of thyroid cancer in the general population. The estimated NNH from GLP-1 RAs is over 1,000 patients in 5 years, while the number needed to treat (NNT) to prevent major cardiovascular events in high-risk diabetes patients is much lower. For individuals with diabetes and obese patients at high cardiovascular risk, the possible risk of thyroid cancer from GLP-1 RAs is outweighed by their significant clinical benefits. However, it might not hold true for those without any comorbid conditions like cardiovascular disease.

In conclusion, the findings from randomized controlled trials indicate a possible moderate increase in the risk of thyroid cancer for patients receiving treatment with GLP-1 RAs. Nonetheless, additional data is required to validate this association, to more accurately evaluate its clinical significance, and to distinguish the effects across various types of thyroid malignancies.

12. Beneficial Effect of Oral Semaglutide for Type 2 Diabetes Mellitus in Patients with Metabolic Dysfunction-associated Steatotic Liver Disease: A Prospective, Multicentre, Observational Study

Ref: Arai T, Atsukawa M, Tsubota A, Oikawa T, Tada T, Matsuura K, et al. Beneficial effect of oral semaglutide for type 2 diabetes mellitus in patients with metabolic dysfunction-associated steatotic liver disease: A prospective, multicentre, observational study. Diabetes Obes Metab. 2024;26(11):4958-65.

ABSTRACT

Objectives: To assess oral semaglutide's safety and effectiveness in treating type 2 diabetes mellitus (T2DM) in individuals with metabolic dysfunction-associated steatotic liver disease (MASLD).

Materials and procedures: This was a prospective, multicenter, single-arm trial. An effectiveness analysis was conducted on 70 of the 80 consecutive patients with MASLD and T2DM who received oral semaglutide for the first time and finished the 48-week course of treatment as planned. Each doctor adjusted the dosage of oral semaglutide while keeping an eye on side effects and effectiveness.

Findings: At 48 weeks, there were notable changes in body weight, lipid profile, liver enzymes, and glycemic control when compared to baseline values (all $p < 0.01$). Between baseline and 48 weeks, the values of the controlled attenuation parameters dropped significantly ($p < 0.01$). Body weight variations were substantially connected with changes in alanine aminotransferase concentrations ($r = 0.37$, $p < 0.01$) and controlled attenuation parameter values ($r = 0.44$, $p < 0.01$). From baseline to 48 weeks, there was a substantial decrease in liver fibrosis markers, including type IV collagen 7S, Wisteria floribunda agglutinin-positive Mac-2-binding protein, fibrosis-4 index, and liver stiffness measurement (all $p < 0.01$). Grades 1–2 transitory gastrointestinal symptoms, including nausea (23 patients, 28.8%), dyspepsia (12, 15.0%), and appetite loss (4, 5.0%), were the most frequent side events.

Conclusion: Patients with MASLD who get oral semaglutide treatment for type 2 diabetes see improvements in their lipid profile, diabetic status, liver steatosis and damage, and surrogate indicators of fibrosis. They also lose weight.

CRITICAL APPRAISAL

Metabolic dysfunction-associated steatotic liver disease (MASLD), formerly known as nonalcoholic fatty liver disease, is a common liver condition linked to metabolic syndromes such as obesity and diabetes. Very few approved specific drugs are available for MASLD and most of the current treatments primarily rely on lifestyle modifications and managing extrahepatic comorbidities. Given the growing prevalence of both type 2 diabetes mellitus (T2DM) and MASLD, the use of glucagon-like peptide 1 receptor agonists (GLP-1 RAs) like semaglutide holds potential for improving both liver health and metabolic parameters. Previous studies have demonstrated the benefits of GLP-1 RAs in addressing liver steatosis and fibrosis in patients with MASLD, but the focus has mostly been on injectable forms of the medication. The need to evaluate the oral formulation of semaglutide is crucial for increasing treatment adherence and providing an alternative to patients who may be averse to injections.

This was a single-arm, multicenter, prospective study. A total of 80 patients with MASLD and T2DM were enrolled and treated with oral semaglutide for 48 weeks. Out of these, 70 patients completed the study, with the remaining discontinuing due to adverse events or other personal reasons. The treatment regimen began with a 3 mg daily dose, which was adjusted according to patient response and tolerability. A comprehensive set of clinical and laboratory data was collected at baseline and every 12 weeks, including body weight, liver enzyme levels, lipid profiles, glycemic control markers, and liver fibrosis markers. Noninvasive tests, such as controlled attenuation parameters (CAP) and liver stiffness measurement (LSM), were used to assess liver condition. The analysis included statistical methods to evaluate changes from baseline and the correlation between different variables.

At the 48-week mark, patients experienced reductions in body weight, liver enzymes [such as alanine transaminase (ALT) and aspartate transaminase (AST)], and improved lipid profiles, including lower triglyceride levels and better low-density lipoprotein (LDL) cholesterol. Furthermore, glycemic control was significantly enhanced, as evidenced by lower plasma glucose and HbA1c levels. Liver health also improved, with decreases in liver stiffness and CAPs, suggesting a reduction in liver steatosis and fibrosis. Notably, changes in liver markers were correlated with weight loss, emphasizing the role of GLP-1 RAs in addressing both metabolic and hepatic components of the disease. However, the effects were not significantly correlated with changes in HbA1c values. The treatment was well tolerated, with gastrointestinal symptoms being the most common adverse events, but most were mild-to-moderate in severity and transient in nature. Only a small proportion of patients discontinued treatment due to these side effects.

The strengths of the study include its prospective design, multicenter approach, and the use of noninvasive, reliable measures to assess liver condition and fibrosis. The study population was diverse, providing a broad understanding of the treatment's effects across different patient groups. Moreover, the study was one of the first to evaluate the effects of oral semaglutide on both T2DM and MASLD over a 48-week period, providing valuable insights into the long-term benefits of this treatment.

However, the study also has several limitations. As a single-arm, nonrandomized study, it lacks a control group, which limits the ability to directly compare the effects of oral semaglutide to other treatments or a placebo. Additionally, the study's sample size was relatively small, and the absence of liver biopsies to confirm improvements in liver histology limits the ability to draw definitive conclusions about changes in liver fibrosis. Also, because the study focused on patients with both MASLD and T2DM, it is unclear whether these results apply to patients with MASLD without diabetes, which constitutes a large proportion of the MASLD population.

In conclusion, the study provides strong evidence that oral semaglutide is an effective and well-tolerated treatment for improving both metabolic and hepatic outcomes in patients with T2DM and MASLD. The findings suggest that oral semaglutide not only helps to control blood sugar and reduce body weight but also leads to improvements in liver health, including reductions in steatosis and fibrosis markers. The treatment's safety profile was favorable, with most adverse events being mild and transient.

Future studies, especially randomized controlled trials, are needed to confirm these findings and explore the long-term impact of oral semaglutide on liver histology and fibrosis. Further research should also examine the effects of oral semaglutide in broader patient populations, including those with MASLD without T2DM. Finally, exploring the combination of oral semaglutide with other therapeutic strategies could open new avenues for treating MASLD and its associated comorbidities.

13. Fluoroquinolones and the Risk of Severe Hypoglycaemia Among Sulphonylurea Users: Population-based Cohort Study

Ref: Dimakos J, Cui Y, Platt RW, Renoux C, Filion KB, Douros A. Fluoroquinolones and the risk of severe hypoglycaemia among sulphonylurea users: Population-based cohort study. Diabetes Obes Metab. 2024;26(8):3088-98.

ABSTRACT

Goal: Although fluoroquinolone-induced hypoglycemia is uncommon, it may become clinically significant in people with high baseline hypoglycemia risk, such as sulfonylurea-using diabetic patients. Our population-based cohort study evaluated whether fluoroquinolones, as opposed to amoxicillin, are linked to a higher incidence of severe hypoglycemia in sulfonylurea-treated patients.

Materials and procedures: We created a base cohort of patients who started second-generation sulphonylureas between 1998 and 2020 using the UK's Clinical Practice Research Datalink Aurum, which is connected to hospitalization and vital statistics data. Patients starting amoxicillin or fluoroquinolones while taking sulfonylureas were included in the study cohort. We evaluated the 30-day risk of severe hypoglycemia (hospitalization or mortality due to hypoglycemia) linked to fluoroquinolones versus amoxicillin using an intent-to-treat exposure definition.

Hazard ratios (HRs) with 95% CIs of severe hypoglycemia were calculated using Cox models following a 1:5 match based on propensity scores and prior sulfonylurea use. Demographics and glycated hemoglobin were used to stratify secondary analyses. Overall, 143,417 individuals started using amoxicillin ($n = 130,294$) or fluoroquinolones ($n = 13,123$) while on sulfonylureas. Fluoroquinolones did not increase the incidence of severe hypoglycemia as compared to amoxicillin (HR 1.17; 95% CI 0.91–1.50). In stratified analyses, fluoroquinolones were linked to a higher risk in patients under 65 (HR 2.90; 95% CI 1.41–5.97) but not in those over 65 (HR 1.03; 95% CI 0.79–1.35). Glycated hemoglobin and sex did not appear to alter the effect.

Conclusion: When compared to amoxicillin, fluoroquinolones did not raise the risk of severe hypoglycemia in individuals on second-generation sulfonylureas. There may be a higher risk among younger adults.

CRITICAL APPRAISAL

Fluoroquinolones are highly effective in treating common bacterial infections but are linked to safety concerns, including hypoglycemia, which has led to the withdrawal of gatifloxacin and class-wide safety warnings. The underlying pharmacologic mechanism involves the inhibition of K+ channels in pancreatic beta-cells and a subsequent increase in insulin secretion. While fluoroquinolone-induced hypoglycemia is rare in the general population, it may be clinically relevant for high-risk groups, especially patients with type 2 diabetes using sulfonylureas. Previous studies suggest a sevenfold increased risk of severe hypoglycemia with fluoroquinolones and sulfonylureas, but they had methodological limitations. Given the high risk of bacterial infections among diabetic patients and the frequent use of both antibiotics and antidiabetic medications, this population-based cohort study aimed to assess the risk of severe hypoglycemia in sulfonylurea users treated with fluoroquinolones, compared to amoxicillin.

This study utilized data from the UK's Clinical Practice Research Datalink (CPRD) Aurum, linked to the Hospital Episode Statistics (HES) and Office for National Statistics (ONS) databases. The base cohort included patients prescribed second-generation sulfonylureas from 1998 to 2020, excluding those with insufficient medical history or prior use of insulin or other insulin secretagogues. From this, a study cohort was formed of patients who initiated fluoroquinolones or amoxicillin while on sulfonylureas. Amoxicillin was used as a comparator because it does not carry a hypoglycemia risk. Propensity score matching accounted for confounders such as age, comorbidities, diabetes severity, and prior medication use. The outcome of interest was severe hypoglycemia, defined as hospitalization or death due to hypoglycemia.

This study analyzed 325,549 patients who initiated sulfonylureas, with 143,417 using fluoroquinolones or amoxicillin while on sulfonylureas. Before propensity score (PS) matching, fluoroquinolone users were older and had more previous antibiotic use and hospitalizations, while amoxicillin users had more diabetic complications and comorbidities. After matching, the groups were well-balanced except for previous antibiotic use, which was adjusted for in the outcome model.

The primary analysis showed no increased risk of severe hypoglycemia with fluoroquinolones compared to amoxicillin (incidence rates 38.3 vs. 31.2 per 1,000 person-years, HR 1.17; 95% CI 0.91–1.50). There were no fatal hypoglycemia events. Stratification by sex or glycated hemoglobin did not reveal significant differences. However, an age-related effect was observed: fluoroquinolones were associated with an increased risk of severe hypoglycemia in patients under 65 years (HR 2.90; 95% CI 1.41–5.97), but not in those aged 65 or older (HR 1.03; 95% CI 0.79–1.35).

The study's findings contrast with previous studies that reported higher risks of hypoglycemia in older adults using sulfonylureas and fluoroquinolones. The mechanism behind this potential interaction involves both sulfonylureas and fluoroquinolones stimulating insulin secretion through the inhibition of pancreatic beta-cell channels. However, the study suggests the hypoglycemic effect may be limited due to the already high insulin secretion from sulfonylureas, particularly for ciprofloxacin (the most commonly used fluoroquinolone in the cohort).

Despite this, the study found an increased risk of severe hypoglycemia among younger adults. This could be due to a lack of "protective" beta-cell dysfunction seen in older adults. Sensitivity analyses also showed increased risk in those with no prior antibiotic use, which could reflect confounding by infection severity.

The study's strengths include its large sample size, use of amoxicillin as a comparator, and PS matching to reduce confounding. However, there are limitations as well. These include potential exposure misclassification due to the intention-to-treat approach, outcome misclassification despite using strict criteria, and the inability to explore infection types and severity.

The study could contribute to updated clinical guidelines on antibiotic use in diabetic patients, particularly for those using sulfonylureas, helping to refine recommendations based on age and comorbidities. Additional studies could explore the role of different infections in the interaction between fluoroquinolones and sulfonylureas, as well as investigate other potential drug-drug interactions that might affect hypoglycemia risk.

14. Denosumab, for Osteoporosis, Reduces the Incidence of Type 2 Diabetes, Risk of Foot Ulceration and All-cause Mortality in Adults, Compared with Bisphosphonates: An Analysis of Real-world, Cohort Data, with a Systematic Review and Meta-analysis

Ref: Henney AE, Riley DR, O'Connor B, Hydes TJ, Anson M, Zhao SS, et al. Denosumab, for osteoporosis, reduces the incidence of type 2 diabetes, risk of foot ulceration and all-cause mortality in adults, compared with bisphosphonates: An analysis of real-world, cohort data, with a systematic review and meta-analysis. Diabetes Obes Metab. 2024;26(9):3673-83.

ABSTRACT

Objective: The objective is to assess the effect of denosumab on (1) the incidence of type 2 diabetes (T2D) and (2) long-term health outcomes [microvascular (neuropathy, retinopathy, and nephropathy) and macrovascular (cardiovascular disease and cerebrovascular accident) complications and all-cause mortality] in patients with T2D and (3) also to integrate data from prior studies using meta-analysis.

Techniques: 331,375 people without a history of cancer or T2D who were prescribed either denosumab (treatment, $n = 45,854$) or bisphosphonates (control, $n = 285,521$) across 83 healthcare institutions had their data retrospectively analyzed in a large global federated database (TriNetX; Cambridge, MA). Confounders were matched by propensity score (1:1), yielding 45,851 in each cohort. The effect of denosumab on long-term health outcomes in T2D patients was further assessed using secondary analysis.

We also conducted a thorough review of earlier research that evaluated the relationship between denosumab and T2D. Using a random-effects meta-analysis, estimates were combined. Cochrane-endorsed instruments were used to evaluate the quality of the evidence and the risk of bias.

Findings: Compared to bisphosphonates, denosumab was linked to a decreased incidence of incident T2D over a 5-year period [hazard ratio 0.83 (95% CI 0.78–0.88)]. Significant risk reductions in foot ulcers [0.67 (0.53–0.86)] and all-cause mortality [0.79 (0.72–0.87)] were found by secondary analysis. Additionally, a meta-analysis of the pooled data from four studies (three observational and one randomized controlled trial) revealed that patients who were administered denosumab had a lower relative risk [RR (95% CI)] for incident T2D [0.83 (0.79–0.87)] (I2 = 10.76%).

Conclusion: This is the largest cohort study to demonstrate that treatment with denosumab is linked to a lower risk of incident T2D, along with a lower risk of all-cause mortality and microvascular complications. These findings could potentially impact the development of guidelines for treating osteoporosis, especially in patients who are at high risk of developing T2D.

CRITICAL APPRAISAL

The relationship between type 2 diabetes (T2D) and osteoporosis is intriguing yet controversial. Studies indicate an association between T2D and osteopenia/osteoporosis, emphasizing the need for effective diabetes prevention in these patients. Traditional osteoporosis treatments focused on bisphosphonates, but denosumab, a humanized monoclonal antibody that inhibits RANK ligand (RANKL), has gained attention for its ability to reduce bone resorption.

Current guidelines support denosumab for postmenopausal women, men, and those with glucocorticoid-induced osteoporosis. Notably, some studies suggest that denosumab may also improve glucose homeostasis, potentially reducing T2D incidence. Animal research indicates that RANKL inhibition enhances insulin sensitivity and lowers plasma glucose levels. A meta-analysis suggests denosumab may reduce fasting glucose and insulin resistance, especially in those with impaired glucose tolerance.

However, results on T2D incidence in denosumab-treated patients are mixed. A posthoc analysis of a randomized controlled trial (RCT) found no significant effect on diabetes risk, likely due to limited power and few incident events. Conversely, observational studies from Taiwan and the UK reported lower T2D incidence in patients prescribed denosumab. Despite these findings, differences in study design create challenges in interpretation.

Hence, this study was conducted to understand the impact of denosumab on T2D incidence, and its influence on long-term complications associated with T2D.

The study was a retrospective analysis of data in a large global federated database (TriNetX; Cambridge, MA) taken across 83 healthcare organizations. The primary analysis included patients without T2D and prescribed either denosumab ($n = 45,851$) or bisphosphonates ($n = 285,521$). Secondary analysis further evaluated the impact of denosumab (vs bisphosphonates) on long-term health outcomes in another cohort of patients with T2D. All the participants in each cohort were followed up for next 8 years after the treatment initiation.

Treatment with denosumab significantly reduced the risk of incident T2D by 17%. When stratified, this effect was significant regardless of ethnic background but varied based on age and body mass index (BMI) status.

In BMI-stratified analysis, denosumab treatment was linked to a significantly lower risk of T2D specifically in overweight or obese patients, not in those of normal weight. This association is expected, given the higher prevalence of T2D in these groups.

Additionally, age-stratified analysis supports previous findings that denosumab may be more beneficial for older adults. This result suggests the study findings are particularly relevant in this vulnerable population of older people living with overweight/obesity, from any ethnic background.

In patients with T2D, treatment with denosumab reduced all-cause mortality and lowered the risk of incident foot ulceration.

However, denosumab did not significantly reduce risks for retinopathy, peripheral neuropathy, or amputations. Notably, it increased the risk of nephropathy. Denosumab did not impact the risk of cardiovascular diseases or cerebrovascular accidents.

Overall, this is the largest cohort study to date showing that patients prescribed denosumab, compared with bisphosphonates, have a 17% lower risk of developing T2D over a 5-year follow-up period. Additionally, this is the first study to show that patients with T2D, who are prescribed denosumab, have a survival benefit with a 21% reduced risk of all-cause mortality and a 33% reduced risk of foot ulceration.

However, the study got certain limitations as well. First, the data are real-world, not from RCTs, so causation cannot be established. Second, since the data come from electronic health records, there may be issues with completeness, such as missing information or unanalyzed free text. We were unable to determine whether patients in the comparator arm received oral or intravenous bisphosphonates, nor could we accurately assess whether patients switched agents within the bisphosphonate drug class.

In conclusion, denosumab may effectively prevent the progression to T2D in high-risk osteoporosis patients compared to bisphosphonates. In those with both osteoporosis and established T2D, denosumab may lower all-cause mortality and the risk of foot ulcers, though it might increase nephropathy risk. These findings could help guide the design of future RCTs to confirm or challenge the conclusions.

15. The Use of Composite Endpoints in Cardiovascular Outcome Trials for Diabetes: A Review of 22 Randomized Clinical Trials Published Since 2008

Ref: Kafai Yahyavi S, Kristensen PL, Hjorthøj C, Hansen KB, Krogh J. The use of composite endpoints in cardiovascular outcome trials for diabetes: A review of 22 randomized clinical trials published since 2008. Diabetes Obes Metab. 2024;26(12):5537-45.

ABSTRACT

Objective: To explain the application of composite endpoints (CEs) in type 2 diabetes cardiovascular outcome trials (CVOTs) and assess the importance of the different outcomes that are part of these CEs from the viewpoints of patients and physicians. Estimating the gradient of treatment effects and events across outcomes was one of the secondary goals.

Materials and procedures: Randomized controlled trials evaluating the cardiovascular outcomes of diabetic individuals from 2008 onward were considered eligible studies. The Diabetes and CV Disease EASD (European Association for the Study of Diabetes) Study Group's CVOT Summit papers were searched in order to find trials. The CE's individual outcomes were compared for differences in effect size, proportion of events, and importance for patients and physicians.

Results: A total of 8,098 patients were randomly assigned to either an active intervention or a comparison group for an average of 33 months (standard deviation 16) across 22 studies. All primary outcomes were CEs, and in 22 of 22 (100%) CEs, there was no gradient of relevance across outcomes from the standpoint of the patient, but in 22 of 22 (100%) CEs, the gradient was minimal from the standpoint of the clinician. While evaluation of events was available in 15 of 22 studies (68%), three of 15 (20%) exhibited a gradient of effect of >5% points between included outcomes. 9 of 18 (50%) reporting studies had a gradient of effect that was moderate to substantial. 10 out of 22 study reports (45%) had unclear outcomes.

Conclusion: Clinical professionals and regulatory bodies should exercise caution when evaluating trial results, of which CEs are the primary outcome, to prevent misunderstandings.

CRITICAL APPRAISAL

A growing trend of using composite endpoints (CEs) in cardiovascular outcome trials (CVOTs) has been observed, particularly since 2008, following the US Food and Drug Administration's (FDA's) guidance to evaluate cardiovascular risks associated with new glucose-lowering therapies for type 2 diabetes mellitus (T2DM). CEs combine several outcomes, such as heart attacks, strokes, and deaths, into a single measure to make it easier to evaluate treatments. While this approach saves time and resources, it assumes that all these outcomes are equally important to patients and doctors, which may not always be true. The interpretation of CEs may further be compromised if the overall number of events in a trial is largely represented by events of less important outcomes or that each individual outcome is not presented in the trial report. Various studies have reported the variability in the perceptions of patients and clinicians regarding the severity of various outcomes. Furthermore, in a previous study of CEs in CV trials, more than half of the included trials consisted of outcomes with both major and little importance to patients.

No prior studies have systematically addressed whether the components of CEs reflect equal importance for patients and clinicians in this context. To address the issue, this study was conducted with a primary objective to evaluate the significance and gradient (variability) of individual outcomes within CEs in CVOTs for diabetes from both patient and clinician perspectives. Secondary objectives included examining the variability in treatment effects and event distributions across outcomes, as well as assessing the quality of CE reporting.

The study reviewed 22 CVOTs conducted since 2008. Randomized controlled trials (RCTs), were included, comparing a treatment (like a new diabetes drug) with a placebo or another treatment. All included trials used CEs as primary endpoints, with the majority employing three components, such as cardiovascular mortality, nonfatal myocardial infarction, and stroke. Data were extracted from primary trial reports, focusing on CEs used as primary and secondary outcomes. The authors assessed the adequacy of reporting and discussed potential limitations. Gradients of importance, effect, and events were analyzed based on predefined criteria: For importance, they referred to surveys of patients and doctors who ranked various health outcomes based on how critical they felt they were. For effects, they looked at how much the treatment reduced the risk of each individual outcome (e.g., percentage reduction in heart attacks versus strokes). For events, they counted how often each outcome occurred in the study population and compared the numbers.

From a patient perspective, outcomes were deemed equally important in most cases, while clinicians perceived small gradients of importance, particularly favoring mortality over nonfatal events. Moderate to large gradients of effect were observed in about half of the studies, indicating significant variability in the impact of interventions on different outcomes. A lack of clarity and consistency in CE reporting was evident, with many trials failing to detail individual outcome effects, mechanisms, or event distributions adequately.

The findings reveal a general lack of quality in CE reporting across studies, particularly concerning gradients of importance, effect, and events. CEs provide a practical approach to summarizing trial outcomes, but their validity is compromised if individual components vary significantly in importance or treatment effect. The study underscores the need for transparent reporting and careful interpretation of CEs to avoid misrepresenting trial results. Clinicians should prioritize comprehensive data on individual outcomes to enhance decision-making and patient care.

The study's strengths lie in its systematic approach and inclusion of all relevant CVOTs for diabetes. However, reliance on patient and clinician surveys introduces subjectivity.

The authors propose that future studies prioritize the transparency of CE composition and reporting. Engaging patients in the design phase could refine endpoint selection and align it with patient-centered care goals. Regulatory bodies and clinicians must critically evaluate CE-based results to ensure they reflect clinically significant benefits.

16. Efficacy, Adherence and Persistence of Various Glucagon-like Peptide-1 Agonists: Nationwide Real-life Data

Ref: Kassem S, Khalaila B, Stein N, Saliba W, Zaina A. Efficacy, adherence and persistence of various glucagon-like peptide-1 agonists: nationwide real-life data. Diabetes Obes Metab. 2024;26(10):4646-52.

ABSTRACT

Goal: Since the advent of glucagon-like peptide 1 receptor agonists (GLP-1 RAs) 20 years ago, type 2 diabetes mellitus treatment has improved. However, improving glycemic control may be hampered by a number of circumstances. This study assessed the variations in efficacy, adherence, and persistence among different GLP-1 RAs.

Materials and procedures: We used Clalit Health Services' computerized medical database to do a retrospective cohort analysis. Included were those with type 2 diabetes mellitus who bought any GLP-1 RA from 2009 to 2021. The date of any GLP-1 RA's initial purchase was designated as the Index Date. Following the start of GLP-1 RAs, we assessed adherence, persistence, and glycemic control. Glycemic controls at baseline and after treatment were examined.

Findings: There were 70,654 patients in all. 51% of the population were female, and the mean age was 11.7 ± 60.4. All patients who took GLP-1 RAs showed a significant decrease in their glycated hemoglobin (HbA1c). Nonetheless, weekly GLP-1 RA initiators had a greater percentage of HbA1c changes than daily initiators (14.6% vs. 10.2%, $p < 0.001$). The once-weekly dose had a higher percentage of individuals with any decrease in HbA1c than the daily dose (82.4% vs. 74.7%), and the majority of patients started on semaglutide or dulaglutide, which had reductions of 16.0% and 14.7%, respectively. The weekly group odds ratio = 1.25 (95% CI 1.21–1.28) had a substantially greater frequency of good adherence (the percentage of days covered $\geq$ 80%). Good adherence was noted among those who were older, female, Jewish, and high socio-economic status ($p < 0.001$).

Conclusion: Those who started weekly GLP-1 RAs showed greater adherence, persistence, and glycemic control. Epidemiological factors may contribute to this objective.

CRITICAL APPRAISAL

Type 2 diabetes mellitus (T2DM) is a chronic disease that requires medication for long-term glycemic control, yet optimal control rates remain low. The US National Health and Nutrition Examination Survey (NHANES) found that between 1999 and 2018, good glycemic control was achieved by only 50–60% of patients. Factors affecting glucose control include low treatment adherence, persistence issues, disease progression, and inadequate treatment intensification. Over the past 20 years, diabetes management has advanced with the introduction of new antidiabetic medications, such as glucagon-like peptide 1 receptor agonists (GLP-1 RAs). GLP-1 RAs vary in structure and dosing; some are taken daily, like liraglutide, while others are weekly, such as dulaglutide and semaglutide.

While RCTs show promising benefits of GLP-1 RAs in terms of not only glycemic control but cardio-renal benefits as well, real-world (RW) studies reveal a significant gap in outcomes, primarily due to poor medication adherence. RCT participants are often more motivated and healthier than those in the general population.

To date, only a few RW studies have examined the efficacy, adherence, and persistence of different GLP-1 RAs in T2DM patients. This study aimed to assess these factors in users of daily versus weekly GLP-1 RAs and explore how socioeconomic status influences adherence and persistence.

This retrospective study analyzed data from Clalit Health Services (2009–2021) to evaluate the effectiveness and adherence of GLP-1 RAs in adults with T2DM. The study included 70,654 participants, split into two groups: those receiving once-daily GLP-1 RAs (exenatide, liraglutide, and lixisenatide) and those on once-weekly GLP-1 RAs (exenatide ER, dulaglutide, and semaglutide). The index day (ID) marked the first purchase of a GLP-1 RA, with adherence and persistence tracked over the following year.

Participants had a mean age of 60.4 years, with weekly users tending to be older, more likely male, Arab, of lower socioeconomic status, and with lower baseline HbA1c levels. Across all treatments, mean HbA1c levels dropped significantly ($p < 0.001$). Weekly regimens achieved a greater reduction (14.6%) than daily ones (10.2%) ($p < 0.001$). Among weekly users, semaglutide had the most substantial reduction (16.0%), while liraglutide was the most effective among daily users (10.7%).

Discontinuation rates were higher in the daily group (50.1% vs. 44.1%, $p < 0.001$). Adherence, defined as a proportion of days covered (PDC ≥ 80%), was better for weekly regimens (51.4% vs. 46%, $p < 0.001$), with semaglutide users showing the highest adherence (54%). Factors such as age over 60, female gender, Jewish ethnicity, and higher socioeconomic status were associated with better adherence. The HbA1c reductions observed were consistent with previous trials, though slightly lower than those reported in randomized controlled trials (1.7% vs. 1.2% in the once-weekly group and 1.3% vs. 0.8% in the once-daily group).

This discrepancy is likely due to the differences between the patient populations in RCTs and those in RW settings. Patients in RCTs are typically highly selected, with fewer comorbidities, and higher motivation levels. These factors can significantly influence HbA1c levels, adherence, and persistence with therapy. In contrast, semaglutide demonstrated the most significant reduction in HbA1c among GLP-1 RAs in both RCT and RW studies.

The study also confirmed that adherence was higher among patients using weekly dosing (51.4%) compared to daily dosing (46%). Notably, good adherence rates were similar between semaglutide and dulaglutide, which may be attributed to the convenience of their delivery devices. When assuming similar efficacy, patients preferred the once-weekly dosing regimen with a single-use pen or autoinjector over the once-daily regimen. This preference is likely because the weekly schedule may lead to fewer missed doses, resulting in higher adherence rates.

Additionally, the study evaluated the relationship between adherence to GLP-1 RAs and patients' demographic characteristics. Adherence was more among older patients, females, those with high and middle socioeconomic status, and individuals of Jewish ethnicity. The differences between ethnicities might be linked to variations in purchasing power or health practices.

In conclusion, patients initiating weekly GLP-1 RA therapy were more adherent and persistent and achieved better glycemic control than those starting with daily GLP-1 RAs. Various demographic factors, particularly socioeconomic status, age, and gender, may play a crucial role in achieving these outcomes. Further studies are needed to better understand the advantages and disadvantages of each GLP-1 RA in RW settings.

17. Association of Iron Status with All-cause and Cause-specific Mortality in Individuals with Diabetes

Ref: Shen C, Yuan M, Zhao S, Chen Y, Xu M, Zhang Y, et al. Association of iron status with all-cause and cause-specific mortality in individuals with diabetes. Diabetes Res Clin Pract. 2024;207:111058.

ABSTRACT

Goals: There is currently little data on the relationship between iron status and mortality risk in diabetic individuals. The purpose of this study was to assess the relationship between iron indices and the risk of death from all causes as well as from particular causes in diabetic patients.

Methods: This analysis included 2,080 persons with diabetes from NHANES 1999–2018 (with ferritin data), 1,974 (with transferrin saturation (Tsat) data), and 1,106 (with soluble transferrin receptor (sTfR) data). Through December 31, 2019, death outcomes were derived from the National Death Index. Hazard ratios and 95% confidence intervals for mortality were computed using Cox proportional hazards models.

Findings: It was shown that the relationship with all-cause mortality was linear for sTfR ($P_{linearity}$ < 0.01), U-shaped for Tsat ($P_{nonlinearity}$ < 0.01), and J-shaped for serum ferritin ($P_{nonlinearity}$ < 0.01). The risk of all-cause mortality was lower for ferritin 300–500 ng/mL than for ferritin < 100 ng/mL, 100–300 ng/mL, and > 500 ng/mL. The risk of all-cause mortality was protected by Tsat 25–32% as opposed to Tsat ≤ 20%, 20–25%, and >32%. The risk of all-cause death was lower for those with sTfR < 4 mg/L than for those with higher sTfR.

Conclusion: Serum ferritin (300–500 ng/mL), Tsat (25–32%), and sTfR (< 4 mg/L) were found to be moderately elevated.

CRITICAL APPRAISAL

Diabetes has reached epidemic levels globally, with over 536 million cases reported, posing significant risks for cardiovascular disease (CVD), cancer, and premature mortality. Identifying modifiable factors to delay complications is crucial. Iron, a key micronutrient, is vital for cellular metabolism but is prone to dysregulation in diabetes. Excessive iron accumulates in organs such as the pancreas and liver, impairing their function, while deficiency is a primary cause of anemia, exacerbating mortality risks. The dual challenges of iron overload and deficiency are particularly relevant in diabetes, where both conditions influence complications such as insulin resistance, impaired insulin secretion, and cardiovascular dysfunction. Given the pivotal role of iron metabolism in developing diabetes and its associated complications, it is essential to examine the potential relationship between iron indices and the mortality of individuals with diabetes.

Iron indices typically incorporate ferritin, transferrin saturation (Tsat) and soluble transferrin receptor (sTfR). Studies exploring the association between ferritin, sTfR, and mortality risk in individuals with diabetes are rare and limited to individuals with diabetes accompanied with specific comorbidities. Additionally, the available studies yield conflicting results. Hence, this study aimed to fill this gap, examining the dose-response relationship between these markers and mortality outcomes.

The analysis included 2,080 adults for ferritin data, 1,974 for Tsat, and 1,106 for sTfR, drawn from NHANES data collected between 1999 and 2018. Those with pregnancy, cancer, or absolute iron deficiency were excluded. Mortality data, spanning all-cause, CVD, and cancer deaths, were extracted from the National Death Index through 2019.

Iron markers were assessed through standardized laboratory instruments, adjusted for consistency across NHANES cycles. The study employed Cox proportional hazard models to estimate hazard ratios (HRs) for mortality while adjusting for confounders, including age, sex, body mass index (BMI), diabetes duration, HbA1c, and kidney function. Stratified and sensitivity analyses were performed to ensure robustness.

The study identified distinct patterns linking iron markers to mortality risk. Ferritin exhibited a J-shaped relationship with all-cause mortality. Moderate ferritin levels (300–500 ng/mL) were associated with the lowest risk, while both low (<100 ng/mL) and high (>500 ng/mL) levels increased mortality. This pattern was more pronounced for CVD-related deaths, highlighting ferritin's role in cardiovascular health. Tsat displayed a U-shaped relationship with all-cause mortality. Tsat levels between 25% and 32% were associated with the lowest risk, while lower (≤20%) or higher (>32%) levels increased risk. Tsat's association with cancer mortality was stronger than with CVD mortality, suggesting distinct mechanisms linking iron levels to different causes of death. sTfR demonstrated a linear relationship with mortality, where sTfR < 4 mg/L had significantly reduced mortality risks compared to those with higher levels. These findings were consistent across sensitivity analyses underscoring the robustness of the associations.

The study establishes that both iron deficiency and overload contribute to increased mortality risk in diabetes. Moderate ferritin levels (300–500 ng/mL) were identified as protective, supporting iron's central role in oxygen transport, energy metabolism, and inflammation modulation. Low ferritin levels reflect functional iron deficiency, impairing oxygen delivery and cellular respiration, while excessive ferritin is linked to organ dysfunction, oxidative stress, and arterial stiffness.

For Tsat, the U-shaped relationship highlights the dual risks of iron deficiency and oxidative stress caused by iron overload. High Tsat levels, associated with increased oxidative stress, predominantly influenced cancer mortality, while ferritin had a stronger link to CVD mortality. This divergence suggests different pathways for iron's impact on chronic diseases.

The linear association of sTfR with mortality reinforces its role as a sensitive indicator of functional iron deficiency, reflecting intracellular iron demand. Unlike ferritin and Tsat, sTfR showed no nonlinearity, suggesting that even modest increases in sTfR signal significant mortality risks.

The study also emphasizes the independence of these associations from anemia, highlighting the broader implications of iron metabolism beyond hemoglobin levels. This aligns with findings in other chronic conditions, such as heart failure, where iron supplementation improved outcomes irrespective of anemia status.

A key strength of this study is its use of a nationally representative sample, which enhances the generalizability of the findings to US adults with diabetes. Comprehensive adjustments for confounders and robust sensitivity analyses strengthen the reliability of the results. However, the observational nature of the study limits causal inference. Additionally, sample sizes for cause-specific mortality analyses, particularly cancer deaths, were limited, warranting cautious interpretation.

This study underscores the importance of monitoring iron markers in diabetes management. Establishing optimal ranges for ferritin (300–500 ng/mL), Tsat (25–32%), and sTfR (<4 mg/L) could guide interventions to reduce mortality risk. Further research, including randomized controlled trials, is needed to confirm these thresholds and evaluate the efficacy of targeted iron therapies in diabetic populations. Integrating iron metabolism into diabetes care may provide a novel approach to improving long-term outcomes.

18. Fair Allocation of GLP-1 and Dual GLP-1–GIP Receptor Agonists

Ref: Emanuel EJ, Dellgren JL, McCoy MS, Persad G. Fair Allocation of GLP-1 and Dual GLP-1-GIP Receptor Agonists. N Engl J Med. 2024;390(20):1839-42.

ABSTRACT

Context: Glucagon-like peptide 1 (GLP-1) receptor agonists and dual GLP-1–GIP receptor agonists have demonstrated significant efficacy in treating obesity and diabetes. However, worldwide shortages of these drugs require the creation of fair distribution systems to tackle racial, ethnic, and socioeconomic inequities in availability.

Objective: To suggest an ethical and pragmatic approach for the equitable distribution of GLP-1 and dual GLP-1–GIP receptor agonists, with an emphasis on optimizing health outcomes, minimizing disparities, and combating early mortality.

Approach: The researchers devised a stratified allocation system based on four ethical tenets: maximizing benefits and reducing harm, ensuring equal ethical consideration, giving priority to disadvantaged groups, and recognizing social contributions. The system ranks patients according to the intensity of obesity or diabetes and potential years of life lost (PYLL), utilizing body mass index (BMI) and glycated hemoglobin measurements as clinical indicators.

Findings: The proposed system classifies patients into four levels: The highest priority is given to individuals with class III obesity (BMI ≥ 40) or severe, unmanaged diabetes (glycated hemoglobin > 8%) that has not responded to other treatments. Subsequent levels address patients with progressively milder BMI and diabetes severity, with a focus on younger patients to reduce premature mortality.

The system discourages allocation for nonmedical or aesthetic purposes and supports continued access for current users unless ethical redistribution is necessary.

Summary: Implementing this system can guide fair distribution during shortages, lessen health inequities, and prevent early deaths. While the fragmented US healthcare system presents obstacles, applying this approach could inform both national and international policies for managing limited medical resources.

CRITICAL APPRAISAL

Obesity and type 2 diabetes have reached critical levels globally. These conditions significantly increase risks for cardiovascular diseases, cancer, and premature death. Medications such as glucagon-like peptide 1 (GLP-1) receptor agonists (e.g., semaglutide) and dual GLP-1-GIP receptor agonists (e.g., tirzepatide) are highly effective in managing obesity and diabetes, leading to weight loss and reduced cardiovascular risks. However, a global shortage of these drugs has created significant inequities in access, primarily favoring individuals with higher financial means or better insurance coverage. While some countries, such as Belgium and the UK, have implemented policies to prioritize diabetes management over weight loss, the United States lacks centralized guidance. As a result, access to these medications is often determined on a first-come, first-served basis, exacerbating racial, ethnic, and socioeconomic disparities.

The article proposed a fair and ethical framework for the allocation of these scarce medications, aiming to maximize their impact while addressing systemic inequities. The framework is grounded in four core ethical values—benefiting people and minimizing harm, ensuring equal moral concern for all individuals, prioritizing disadvantaged populations, and rewarding social contribution where relevant. Using these principles, the authors developed a tiered allocation system based on clinical severity and the potential years of life lost (PYLL) metric. This system considers factors such as body mass index (BMI), glycated hemoglobin levels, and age. Younger patients within each tier are prioritized to address their greater risk of premature death, reflecting the principle of equal moral concern and the ethical goal of maximizing life-years saved.

The proposed allocation system stratifies patients into four tiers, beginning with those at the highest risk of premature death or severe complications. Tier 1 includes individuals with class III obesity (BMI ≥ 40) or severe, uncontrolled diabetes (glycated hemoglobin > 8%) that has not responded to other treatments. Subsequent tiers gradually include individuals with lower levels of obesity or diabetes severity. Tier 4, the lowest priority, includes patients with overweight (BMI 25–29.9) or mild diabetes. Within each severity tier, younger patients (<50 years of age) are prioritized because of the distinctive risk of premature death they face. The framework deprioritizes use of these medications for cosmetic purposes, emphasizing the need to reserve them for patients who face the greatest clinical risks.

The article underscores the importance of adopting an equitable approach to allocating GLP-1 receptor agonists and dual GLP-1–GIP receptor agonists. By prioritizing individuals with severe disease and younger patients with a higher risk of premature death, the framework aims to maximize societal benefit while addressing existing health inequities. The authors highlight that current practices in the United States, which often favor those with greater financial resources, are ethically problematic and perpetuate disparities. The proposed framework also considers practical challenges, such as the need to continue treatment for existing users to prevent harm from weight regain or worsening diabetes. The inclusion of metrics such as BMI and glycated hemoglobin levels ensures that allocation decisions are based on objective clinical criteria.

One limitation of the framework is its reliance on BMI as a primary metric, which may not fully capture the metabolic risks associated with obesity in diverse populations. Additionally, implementing this system in the fragmented US healthcare environment poses significant logistical challenges, particularly given the lack of centralized oversight and variations in insurance coverage. The framework's exclusion of patient preferences, such as the choice between oral and injectable formulations, may also raise concerns among patients and providers.

To conclude, adopting this framework could significantly reduce disparities in access to GLP-1 and dual GLP-1–GIP receptor agonists, leading to better health outcomes and fewer premature deaths. Policymakers could use it as a basis for developing national or global allocation guidelines, particularly in resource-constrained settings. Future research should explore alternative metrics to BMI and evaluate the long-term outcomes of implementing such a framework in diverse healthcare systems.

19. Intensive Blood-pressure Control in Patients with Type 2 Diabetes

Ref: Bi Y, Li M, Liu Y, Li T, Lu J, Duan P, et al. Intensive Blood-Pressure Control in Patients with Type 2 Diabetes. N Engl J Med November 16, 2024. DOI: 10.1056/NEJMoa2412006.

ABSTRACT

Background: It is unclear what the best targets are for controlling systolic blood pressure in patients with type 2 diabetes.

Methods: At 145 clinical sites throughout China, we recruited individuals aged 50 and above who had type 2 diabetes, high systolic blood pressure, and a higher risk of cardiovascular disease. Intensive treatment aimed at achieving a systolic blood pressure of <120 mm Hg or regular treatment aimed at achieving a systolic blood pressure of <140 mm Hg for a maximum of 5 years were given to patients at random. A composite of nonfatal myocardial infarction, nonfatal stroke, heart failure therapy or hospitalization, or cardiovascular death was the main outcome. Assuming that the data were missing, multiple imputation was applied to the missing outcome data.

Results: 5,803 (45.3%) of the 12,821 patients (6,414 in the intensive-treatment group and 6,407 in the standard-treatment group) who were enrolled between February 2019 and December 2021 were female; the patients' mean (±SD) age was 63.8 ± 7.5 years. The mean systolic blood pressure at 1 year of follow-up was 133.2 mm Hg (median, 135.0 mm Hg) in the standard-treatment group and 121.6 mm Hg (median, 118.3 mm Hg) in the intensive-treatment group. Primary-outcome events occurred in 492 patients (2.09 events per 100 person-years) in the standard-treatment group and 393 patients (1.65 events per 100 person-years) in the intensive-treatment group over a median follow-up of 4.2 years (hazard ratio 0.79; 95% CI 0.69–0.90; $p < 0.001$). Serious adverse event rates were comparable across treatment groups. However, compared to the conventional therapy group, the intensive treatment group experienced symptomatic hypotension and hyperkalemia more frequently.

Conclusion: In patients with type 2 diabetes, intensive treatment aimed at a systolic blood pressure of fewer than 120 mm Hg was associated with a considerably reduced incidence of severe cardiovascular events than standard care, which aimed for a systolic blood pressure of <140 mm Hg (Funded by the Ministry of Science and Technology of China's National Key Research and Development Program and others; BPROAD ClinicalTrials.gov number, NCT03808311).

CRITICAL APPRAISAL

Type 2 diabetes is often accompanied by elevated systolic blood pressure (SBP), a key modifiable risk factor for cardiovascular disease (CVD). While lowering blood pressure has well-documented benefits in reducing cardiovascular events, optimal SBP targets for patients with type 2 diabetes remain contentious. The ACCORD trial, a notable predecessor, compared intensive (<120 mm Hg) and standard (<140 mm Hg) SBP targets but found no significant difference in cardiovascular outcomes, partly due to limited statistical power and design complexities. Other studies, such as the SPRINT trial, showed the benefits of intensive SBP control but excluded diabetic patients. Against this backdrop, this Blood Pressure Control Target in Diabetes (BPROAD) trial was designed to directly investigate whether intensive SBP treatment improves cardiovascular outcomes in patients with type 2 diabetes.

The BPROAD trial was a multicenter, randomized controlled study involving 12,821 patients aged 50 or older with type 2 diabetes and high cardiovascular risk across 145 clinical sites in China. Key inclusion criteria included an SBP of 130–180 mm Hg for those on antihypertensive medications or ≥140 mm Hg for untreated patients, along with one or more cardiovascular risk factors. Participants were assigned to either an intensive treatment group, targeting an SBP of <120 mm Hg, or a standard treatment group, aiming for <140 mm Hg. Treatment adjustments were made monthly for the first 3 months and quarterly thereafter, following a standardized protocol. The primary outcome was a composite of nonfatal stroke, nonfatal myocardial infarction, heart failure treatment or hospitalization, and cardiovascular death, with secondary outcomes including individual components of the primary outcome, all-cause mortality and chronic kidney disease (CKD) progression.

After a median follow-up of 4.2 years, the intensive treatment group achieved a mean SBP of 121.6 mm Hg, significantly reducing primary outcome events (hazard ratio 0.79; $p < 0.001$), with 1.65 events per 100 person-years compared to 2.09 in the standard group. Stroke risk was notably lower in the intensive group (hazard ratio 0.79). While adverse events were comparable, the intensive group had slightly higher rates of symptomatic hypotension and hyperkalemia. There was no significant difference in all-cause mortality between the two groups.

To conclude, BPROAD trial demonstrated that intensive SBP control (<120 mm Hg) significantly reduces major cardiovascular events in patients with type 2 diabetes compared to standard control (<140 mm Hg). These findings support the adoption of stricter SBP targets in clinical guidelines for diabetic populations, emphasizing the importance of personalized antihypertensive strategies. However, the potential for adverse effects such as hypotension and hyperkalemia necessitates careful monitoring, particularly during treatment initiation and dose adjustments.

The strengths of the study include its large sample size, diverse patient population, and robust statistical design, which provided sufficient power to detect clinically meaningful differences between treatment groups. The trial's multicenter design enhances the generalizability of findings to real-world settings, particularly in populations with similar demographics and cardiovascular risk profiles.

However, several limitations warrant consideration. First, the open-label design meant that patients and physicians were aware of treatment assignments, which could influence treatment adherence and patient-reported outcomes. However, outcome assessors and statisticians were blinded, reducing potential bias in outcome evaluation. Second, despite intensive treatment, only 60% of patients in the intensive group achieved the target SBP after 1 year, potentially diluting the observed treatment effect. Third, the trial's results may not be directly applicable to non-Chinese populations or those with different healthcare infrastructures. Additionally, the study relied on home blood pressure monitoring during the COVID-19 pandemic, which may introduce variability in measurements.

Overall, This trial paves the way for further research into optimizing hypertension management in diabetes. Future studies could explore the long-term effects of intensive SBP control on mortality, quality of life, and healthcare costs. Additionally, investigations into the interplay between SBP targets, glycemic control, and other cardiovascular risk factors may yield a more integrated approach to managing complex diabetic populations.

20. Type 2 Diabetes in Patients with G6PD Deficiency

Ref: Israel A, Raz I, Vinker S, Magen E, Green I, Golan-Cohen A, et al. Type 2 diabetes in patients with G6PD deficiency. N Engl J Med. 2024;391(6):568-9.

ABSTRACT

Objective: This research examined how glucose-6-phosphate dehydrogenase (G6PD) deficiency affects the diagnosis, management, and complications of type 2 diabetes (T2D).

Methods: A retrospective cohort analysis was performed using Leumit Health Services data from 2003 to 2023. The study included 3,913 G6PD-deficient patients and 19,565 matched controls. Researchers compared fasting glucose and glycated hemoglobin (HbA1c) levels between groups. They also assessed the cumulative likelihood of receiving key diabetes medications, such as glucagon-like peptide 1 (GLP-1) receptor agonists and sodium-glucose cotransporter-2 (SGLT-2) inhibitors, and evaluated the occurrence of diabetes-related complications, including severe kidney disease, ischemic heart disease, and neuropathy.

Findings: G6PD-deficient patients exhibited significantly lower HbA1c levels compared to controls (4.79% vs. 5.50%, $p < 0.001$), despite comparable fasting glucose levels. These patients were less likely to receive diabetes medications, with hazard ratios of 0.77 for GLP-1 receptor agonists and 0.78 for SGLT-2 inhibitors. They also showed higher rates of complications, including severe kidney disease (hazard ratio 1.51), ischemic heart disease (1.33), and neuropathy (1.33).

Conclusion: The research highlights the necessity for alternative diagnostic tools and customized treatment strategies for managing diabetes in G6PD-deficient individuals. The unreliability of HbA1c in this population calls for updated guidelines to prevent delayed treatment and reduce complications. Implementing equitable healthcare approaches is crucial to enhance outcomes for this high-risk group.

CRITICAL APPRAISAL

Type 2 diabetes (T2D) and glucose-6-phosphate dehydrogenase (G6PD) deficiency are both significant public health concerns. G6PD deficiency, an X-linked enzymatic disorder, impairs redox balance and is prevalent in individuals of African and Mediterranean ancestry. It has been associated with increased oxidative stress, which can exacerbate metabolic disorders such as diabetes. Glycated hemoglobin (HbA1c) is widely used to diagnose and monitor diabetes, but its reliability in G6PD-deficient individuals is questionable due to altered hemoglobin glycation rates.

While prior studies have examined the physiological effects of G6PD deficiency, little is known about its influence on diabetes management, including the accuracy of HbA1c as a diagnostic tool, medication use, and complication rates.

Hence, this study was conducted to investigate the impact of G6PD deficiency on the diagnosis, treatment, and complications of T2D. The research explored how G6PD deficiency affects HbA1c levels, diabetes medication use, and the incidence of complications, highlighting challenges in managing this vulnerable population.

This was a large-scale cohort study conducted within Leumit Health Services, a national healthcare provider. From 2003 to 2023, the study included 3,913 patients with G6PD deficiency and 19,565 matched controls. The groups were matched for demographic characteristics, including age (mean 47 years) and sex (60.5% male). The primary objective was to compare HbA1c levels, diabetes treatment patterns, and complications between the two groups.

Patients with G6PD deficiency had significantly lower HbA1c levels than controls (4.79% vs. 5.50%, $p < 0.001$), despite similar fasting glucose levels. Regression analyses showed that HbA1c underestimated glycemic control in these patients; for example, a fasting glucose of 168 mg/dL corresponded to an HbA1c of 6.5%, compared to 126 mg/dL in the general population. Diabetes medications were prescribed less frequently to patients with G6PD deficiency, leading to delays in treatment. The likelihood of receiving modern oxidative-stress-targeting medications such as glucagon-like peptide 1 (GLP-1) receptor agonists and sodium–glucose cotransporter 2 (SGLT2) inhibitors was significantly lower in this group, with adjusted hazard ratios of 0.77 and 0.78, respectively.

Additionally, G6PD-deficient patients with diabetes experienced higher incidences of severe complications—kidney disease (adjusted HR 1.51), ischemic heart disease (adjusted HR 1.33), and neuropathy (adjusted HR 1.33).

The study highlighted certain challenges in diabetes management in G6PD patients. HbA1c, a standard marker for diagnosing and monitoring diabetes, is unreliable in patients with G6PD deficiency due to reduced hemoglobin glycation. This can lead to delayed diagnoses and inadequate glycemic management. The underprescription of GLP-1 receptor agonists and SGLT-2 inhibitors in these patients indicates disparities in care, possibly due to diagnostic challenges or clinicians' unfamiliarity with this subgroup. These medications are crucial as they help counter oxidative stress, which is particularly concerning for G6PD-deficient individuals. G6PD deficiency is associated with a higher incidence of severe diabetes complications, revealing the need for early interventions and tailored management.

Strengths of the study include the large sample size which increases the robustness of the findings. However, the absence of direct measurement of oxidative stress markers limits the study's conclusions. Additionally, coexisting conditions and medication adherence were not fully explored in the study.

In conclusion, alternative diagnostic tools are essential for accurately diagnosing DM in patients with G6PD deficiency. Future studies should investigate how G6PD deficiency contributes to diabetes complications, particularly through chronic oxidative stress, which may lead to new treatments such as antioxidants. Further, longitudinal studies are needed to understand the progression of these complications, refining risk stratification, and preventive strategies. Guidelines that consider the specific metabolic and oxidative stress profiles of G6PD-deficient patients could enhance treatment effectiveness. Additionally, identifying genetic and metabolic factors that influence diabetes outcomes in this group could inform personalized treatment plans. Finally, educating healthcare providers about the implications of G6PD deficiency in diabetes management is crucial for improving diagnostics and interventions.

REFERENCES (Others)

1. Hemmingsen B, Gimenez-Perez G, Mauricio D, Roque I, Figuls M, Metzendorf MI, et al. Diet, physical activity or both for prevention or delay of type 2 diabetes mellitus and its associated complications in people at increased risk of developing type 2 diabetes mellitus. Cochrane Database Syst Rev. 2017;12:CD003054.
2. Hou L, Wang Q, Pan B, Li R, Li Y, He J, et al. Exercise modalities for type 2 diabetes: a systematic review and network meta-analysis of randomized trials. Diabetes Metab Res Rev. 2023;39:e3591.
3. American College of Sports Medicine. ACSM's Guidelines for Exercise Testing and Prescription. Philadelphia: Lippincott Williams &Wilkins; 2013. pp. 456.
4. Bull FC, Al-Ansari SS, Biddle S, Li R, Li Y, He J, et al. World Health Organization 2020 guidelines on physical activity and sedentary behaviour. Br J Sports Med. 2020;54: 1451-62.
5. Erickson JD, Patterson JM, Wall M, Neumark-Sztainer D. Risk behaviors and emotional wellbeing in youth with chronic health conditions. Child Health Care. 2005;34:181-92.

6. Hanberger L, Samuelsson U, Lindblad B; Swedish Childhood Diabetes Registry SWEDIABKIDS. A1C in children and adolescents with diabetes in relation to certain clinical parameters: the Swedish Childhood Diabetes Registry SWEDIABKIDS. Diabetes Care. 2008;31:927-9.
7. Amed S, Nuernberger K, McCrea P, Reimer K, Krueger H, Aydede SK, et al. Adherence to clinical practice guidelines in the management of children, youth, and young adults with type 1 diabetes–a prospective population cohort study. J Pediatr. 2013;163:543-8.
8. Bryden KS, Peveler RC, Stein A, Neil A, Mayou RA, Dunger DB. Clinical and psychological course of diabetes from adolescence to young adulthood: A longitudinal cohort study. Diabetes Care. 2001;24:1536-40.
9. Wang B, An X, Shi X, Zhang JA. Management of endocrine disease: suicide risk in patients with diabetes: a systematic review and meta-analysis. Eur J Endocrinol. 2017;177:R169-81.
10. Pompili M, Forte A, Lester D, Erbuto D, Rovedi F, Innamorati M, et al. Suicide risk in type 1 diabetes mellitus: A systematic review. J Psychosom Res. 2014;76:352-60.
11. Wexler DJ, Krause-Steinrauf H, Crandall JP, Florez HJ, Hox SH, Kuhn A, et al; GRADE Research Group. Baseline characteristics of randomized participants in the Glycemia Reduction Approaches in Diabetes: A Comparative Effectiveness Study (GRADE). Diabetes Care. 2019;42:2098-107.
12. Kim YG, Hahn S, Oh TJ, Kwak SH, Park KS, Cho YM. Differences in the glucose-lowering efficacy of dipeptidyl peptidase-4 inhibitors between Asians and non-Asians: a systematic review and meta-analysis. Diabetologia. 2013;56:696-708
13. Curran J, Saloner B, Winkelman TNA, Alexander GC. Estimated use of prescription medications among individuals incarcerated in jails and state prisons in the US. JAMA Health Forum 2023;4:e230482.
14. Mayer-Davis EJ, Lawrence JM, Dabelea D, Divers J, Isom S, Dolan L, et al.; SEARCH for Diabetes in Youth Study. Incidence trends of type 1 and type 2 diabetes among youths, 2002-2012. N Engl J Med. 2017;376:1419-29.
15. Carson EA. Prisoners in 2019.Washington, DC: Bureau of Justice Statistics, U.S. Department of Justice; 2020.
16. U.S. Department of Health and Human Services, Centers for Disease Control and Prevention. (2020) National Diabetes Statistics Report 2020. [online] Available from https://www.cdc.gov/diabetes/pdfs/data/statistics/national-diabetesstatistics-report.pdf [Last accessed January, 2025].
17. Kouidrat Y, Pizzol D, Cosco T, Thompson T, Carnaghi M, Bertoldo A, et al. High prevalence of erectile dysfunction in diabetes: a systematic review and meta-analysis of 145 studies. Diabet Med. 2017;34(9):1185-92.
18. Defeudis G, Mazzilli R, Tenuta M, Rossini G, Zamponi V, Olana S, et al. Erectile dysfunction and diabetes: a melting pot of circumstances and treatments. Diabetes Metab Res Rev. 2022;38(2):e3494.
19. Foresta C, Ferlin A, Lenzi A, Montorsi P; Italian Study Group on Cardiometabolic Andrology. The great opportunity of the andrological patient: cardiovascular and metabolic risk assessment and prevention. Andrology. 2017;5(3):408-13.
20. Assaly R, Gorny D, Compagnie S, Mayoux E, Bernabe J, Alexandre L, et al. The favorable effect of empagliflozin on erectile function in an experimental model of type 2 diabetes. J Sex Med. 2018;15(9):1224-34.
21. Armstrong DG, Boulton AJM, Bus SA. Diabetic foot ulcers and their recurrence. New Eng J Med. 2017;376:2367-75.
22. Jupiter DC, Thorud JC, Buckley CJ, Shibuya N. The impact of foot ulceration and amputation on mortality in diabetic patients. I: from ulceration to death, a systematic review. Int Wound J. 2016;13(5):892-903.
23. Chen L, Sun S, Gao Y, Ran X. Global mortality of diabetic foot ulcer: a systematic review and meta-analysis of observational studies. Diabetes Obes Metab. 2023;25(1):36-45.
24. IWGDF. (2023). Guidelines on the prevention of foot ulcers in persons with diabetes–IWGDF 2023 update. [online] Available from https://iwgdfguidelines.org/wp-content/uploads/2023/07/IWGDF-2023-02-Prevention-Guideline.pdf [Last accessed January, 2025].
25. Bus SA, Valk GD, van Deursen RW, Armstrong DG, Caravaggi C, Hlaváček P, et al. The effectiveness of footwear and offloading interventions to prevent and heal foot ulcers and reduce plantar pressure in diabetes: a systematic review. DMRR. 2008;24(S1):S162-80.
26. Bus SA, van Deursen RW, Armstrong DG, Lewis JEA, Caravaggi CF, Cavanagh PR. Footwear and offloading interventions to prevent and heal foot ulcers and reduce plantar pressure in patients with diabetes: a systematic review. DMRR. 2015;32(Suppl 1):99-118.
27. Emerging Risk Factors Collaboration; Di Angelantonio E, Kaptoge S, Wormser D, Willeit P, Butterworth AS, Bansal N, et al. Association of cardiometabolic multimorbidity with mortality. JAMA. 2015;314(1):52-60.
28. Zinman B, Wanner C, Lachin JM, Fitchett D, Bluhmki E, Hantel S, et al. Empagliflozin, cardiovascular outcomes, and mortality in type 2 diabetes. N Engl J Med. 2015;373(22):2117-28.
29. Anker SD, Butler J, Filippatos G, Ferreira JP, Bocchi E, Böhm M, et al. Empagliflozin in heart failure with a preserved ejection fraction. N Engl J Med. 2021;385(16):1451-61.
30. Nyström T, Toresson Grip E, Gunnarsson J, Casajust P, Karlsdotter K, Skogsberg J, et al; EMPRISE Study Group. Empagliflozin mortality in Sweden compared to dipeptidyl peptidase-4 inhibitors: Real world evidence from the Nordic EMPRISE study. Diabetes Obes Metab. 2023;25(1):261-71.
31. Karasik A, Lanzinger S, Chia-Hui Tan E, Yabe D, Kim DJ, Sheu WH, et al. Empagliflozin cardiovascular and renal effectiveness and safety compared to dipeptidyl peptidase-4 inhibitors across 11 countries in Europe and Asia: results from the EMPagliflozin compaRative effectIveness and SafEty (EMPRISE) study. Diabetes Metab. 2023;49(2):101418.

32. Htoo PT, Tesfaye H, Schneeweiss S, Wexler DJ, Everett BM, Glynn RJ, et al. Comparative effectiveness of empagliflozin vs liraglutide or sitagliptin in older adults with diverse patient characteristics. JAMA Netw Open. 2022;5(10):e2237606.
33. Desai RJ, Glynn RJ, Everett BM, Schneeweiss S, Wexler DJ, Bessette LG, et al. Comparative effectiveness of Empagliflozin in reducing the burden of recurrent cardiovascular hospitalizations among older adults with diabetes in routine clinical care. Am Heart J. 2022;254: 203-15.
34. Patorno E, Pawar A, Franklin JM, Najafzadeh M, Déruaz-Luyet A, Brodovicz KG, et al. Empagliflozin and the risk of heart failure hospitalization in routine clinical care. Circulation. 2019;139(25):2822-30.
35. Patorno E, Pawar A, Wexler DJ, Glynn RJ, Bessette LG, Paik JM, et al. Effectiveness and safety of empagliflozin in routine care patients: results from the EMPagliflozin compaRative effectIveness and SafEty (EMPRISE) study. Diabetes Obes Metab. 2022;24(3):442-54.
36. Owen MR, Doran E, Halestrap AP. Evidence that metformin exerts its anti-diabetic effects through inhibition of complex 1 of the mitochondrial respiratory chain. Biochem J. 2000;348:607-14.
37. Miller RA, Chu Q, Xie J, Foretz M, Viollet B, Birnbaum MJ. Biguanides suppress hepatic glucagon signalling by decreasing production of cyclic AMP. Nature. 2013;494(7436):256-60.
38. Borg MJ, Bound M, Grivell J, Sun Z, Jones KL, Horowitz M, et al. Comparative effects of proximal and distal small intestinal administration of metformin on plasma glucose and glucagon-like peptide-1, and gastric emptying after oral glucose, in type 2 diabetes. Diabetes Obes Metab. 2019;21(3):640-7.
39. Carter D, Howlett HC, Wiernsperger NF, Bailey CJ. Differential effects of metformin on bile salt absorption from the jejunum and ileum. Diabetes Obes Metab. 2003;5(2):120-5.
40. Wu H, Esteve E, Tremaroli V, Khan MT, Caesar R, Manneråars-Holm L, et al. Metformin alters the gut microbiome of individuals with treatment-naive type 2 diabetes, contributing to the therapeutic effects of the drug. Nat Med. 2017;23(7):850-8.
41. Nauck MA, Homberger E, Siegel EG, Allen RC, Eaton RP, Ebert R, et al. Incretin effects of increasing glucose loads in man calculated from venous insulin and C-peptide responses. J Clin Endocrinol Metab. 1986;63(2):492-8.
42. Little TJ, Pilichiewicz AN, Russo A, Phillips L, Jones KL, Nauck MA, et al. Effects of intravenous glucagon-like peptide-1 on gastric emptying and intragastric distribution in healthy subjects: relationships with postprandial glycemic and insulinemic responses. J Clin Endocrinol Metab. 2006;91(5):1916-23.
43. Hashimoto Y, Tanaka M, Okada H, Mistuhashi K, Kimura T, Kitagawa N, et al. Postprandial hyperglycemia was ameliorated by taking metformin 30 min before a meal than taking metformin with a meal; a randomized, open-label, crossover pilot study. Endocrine. 2016;52(2):271-6.
44. Sun H, Saeedi P, Karuranga S, Pinkepank M, Ogurtsova K, Duncan BB, et al. IDF diabetes atlas: global, regional and country-level diabetes prevalence estimates for 2021 and projections for 2045. Diabetes Res Clin Pract. 2022;183:109119.
45. Davies MJ, Aroda VR, Collins BS, Gabbay RA, Green J, Maruthur NM, et al. Management of hyperglycemia in type 2 diabetes, 2022. A consensus report by the American Diabetes Association (ADA) and the European Association for the Study of Diabetes (EASD). Diabetologia. 2022;65:1925-66.
46. Chinese Diabetes Society. Guideline for the prevention and treatment of type 2 diabetes mellitus in China (2020 edition). Chin J Diabetes Mellitus. 2021;13(4):315-409.
47. Li C, Guo S, Huo J, Gao Y, Yan Y, Zhao Z. Real-world national trends and socio-economic factors preference of sodium-glucose cotransporter-2 inhibitors and glucagon-like peptide-1 receptor agonists in China. Front Endocrinol (Lausanne). 2022;13:987081.
48. Aroda VR, Rosenstock J, Terauchi Y, Altuntas Y, Lalic NM, Morales Villegas EC, et al. PIONEER 1:randomized clinical trial of the efficacy and safety of oral semaglutide monotherapy in comparison with placebo in patients with type 2 diabetes. Diabetes Care. 2019;42(9):1724-32.
49. Yamada Y, Katagiri H, Hamamoto Y, Deenadayalan S, Navarria A, Nishijima K, et al. Dose-response, efficacy, and safety of oral semaglutide monotherapy in Japanese patients with type 2 diabetes (PIONEER 9): A 52-week, phase 2/3a, randomised, controlled trial. Lancet Diabetes Endocrinol. 2020;8(5):377-91.
50. Mosenzon O, Wiviott SD, Cahn A, Rozenberg A, Yanuv I, Goodrich EL, et al Effects of dapagliflozin on development and progression of kidney disease in patients with type 2 diabetes: an analysis from the DECLARETIMI 58 randomised trial. Lancet Diabetes Endocrinol. 2019;7(8):606-17.
51. Neal B, Perkovic V, Mahaffey KW, de Zeeuw D, Fulcher G, Erondu N, et al. Canagliflozin and cardiovascular and renal events in type 2 diabetes. N Engl J Med. 2017;377(7):644-57.
52. Sattar N, Lee MMY, Kristensen SL, Branch KRH, Del Prato S, Khurmi NS, et al. Cardiovascular, mortality, and kidney outcomes with GLP-1 receptor agonists in patients with type 2 diabetes: a systematic review and meta-analysis of randomised trials. Lancet Diabetes Endocrinol. 2021;9(10):653-62.
53. Zhang Y, Jiang L, Wang J, Wang T, Chien C, Huang W, et al. Network meta-analysis on the effects of finerenone versus SGLT2 inhibitors and GLP-1 receptor agonists on cardiovascular and renal outcomes in patients with type 2 diabetes mellitus and chronic kidney disease. Cardiovasc Diabetol. 2022;21(1):232.
54. Suzuki Y, Kaneko H, Nagasawa H, Okada A, Fujiu K, Jo T, et al. Comparison of estimated glomerular filtration rate change with sodium-glucose cotransporter-2 inhibitors versus glucagon-like peptide-1 receptor agonists among people with diabetes: a propensity-score matching study. Diabetes Obes Metab. 2024;26:2422-30.

55. Lugner M, Sattar N, Miftaraj M, Ekelund J, Franzén S, Svensson AM, et al. Cardiorenal and other diabetes related outcomes with SGLT-2 inhibitors compared to GLP-1 receptor agonists in type 2 diabetes: Nationwide observational study. Cardiovasc Diabetol. 2021;20(1):67.
56. Davies MJ, Aroda VR, Collins BS, Gabbay RA, Green J, Maruthur NM, et al. A consensus report by the American Diabetes Association (ADA) and the European Association for the Study of Diabetes (EASD). Diabetes Care. 2022;45(11):2753-86.
57. ElSayed NA, Aleppo G, Aroda VR, Bannuru RR, Brown FM, Bruemmer D, et al. 9. Pharmacologic approaches to glycemic treatment: standards of care in diabetes—2023. Diabetes Care. 2023;46:S140-57.
58. Wang J, Kim CH. Differential risk of cancer associated with glucagonlike Peptide-1 receptor agonists: analysis of real-world databases. Endocr Res. 2022;47(1):18-25.
59. Yang Z, Lv Y, Yu M, Mei M, Xiang L, Zhao S, et al. GLP-1 receptor agonist-associated tumor adverse events: a real-world study from 2004 to 2021 based on FAERS. Front Pharmacol. 2022;13:925377.
60. Vigibase. (2024). Uppsala Monitoring Centre. [online] Available from https://who-umc.org/vigibase/ [Last accessed January, 2024].
61. Bjerre Knudsen L, Madsen LW, Andersen S, Almholt K, de Boer AS, Drucker DJ, et al. Glucagon-like peptide-1 receptor agonists activate rodent thyroid C-cells causing calcitonin release and C-cell proliferation. Endocrinology. 2010;151(4):1473-86.
62. He L, Zhang S, Zhang X, Liu R, Guan H, Zhang H. Effects of insulin analogs and glucagon-like peptide-1 receptor agonists on proliferation and cellular energy metabolism in papillary thyroid cancer. Onco Targets Ther. 2017;10:5621-31.
63. Younossi Z, Anstee QM, Marietti M, Hardy T, Henry L, Eslam M, et al. Global burden of NAFLD and NASH: trends, predictions, risk factors and prevention. Nat Rev Gastroenterol Hepatol. 2018;15:11-20.
64. Vernon G, Baranova A, Younossi ZM. Systematic review: the epidemiology and natural history of non-alcoholic fatty liver disease and nonalcoholic steatohepatitis in adults. Aliment Pharmacol Ther. 2011;34:274-85.
65. Rinella ME, Neuschwander-Tetri BA, Siddiqui MS, Abdelmalek MF, Caldwell S, Barb D, et al. AASLD practice guidance on the clinical assessment and management of nonalcoholic fatty liver disease. Hepatology. 2023;77:1797-835.
66. European Association for the Study of the Liver (EASL); European Association for the Study of Diabetes (EASD); European Association for the Study of Obesity (EASO). EASL-EASD-EASO clinical practice guidelines for the management of non-alcoholic fatty liver disease. J Hepatol. 2016;64:1388-402.
67. Tokushige K, Ikejima K, Ono M, Eguchi Y, Kamada Y, Itoh Y, Akuta N, et al. Evidence-based clinical practice guidelines for nonalcoholic fatty liver disease/nonalcoholic steatohepatitis 2020. Hepatol Res. 2021;51:1013-25.
68. Armstrong MJ, Gaunt P, Aithal GP, Barton D, Hull D, Parker R, et al. Liraglutide safety and efficacy in patients with non-alcoholic steatohepatitis (LEAN): a multicentre, double-blind, randomised, placebo-controlled phase 2 study. Lancet. 2016;387:679-90.
69. Newsome PN, Buchholtz K, Cusi K, Linder M, Okanoue T, Ratziu V, et al. A placebo-controlled trial of subcutaneous Semaglutide in nonalcoholic steatohepatitis. N Engl J Med. 2021;384:1113-24.
70. Park-Wyllie LY, Juurlink DN, Kopp A, Shah BR, Stukel TA, Stumpo C, et al. Outpatient gatifloxacin therapy and dysglycemia in older adults. N Engl J Med. 2006;354(13):1352-61.
71. Center for Drug Evaluation and Research. (2021). Serious Low Blood Sugar, New Mental Health Effects with Fluoroquinolon. U.S. Food and Drug Administration. [online] Available from https://www.fda.gov/drugs/drug-safety-and-availability/fda-reinforcessafety-information-about-serious-low-blood-sugar-levels-and-mentalhealth-side [Last accessed January, 2025].
72. Zünkler BJ, Claassen S, Wos-Maganga M, Rustenbeck I, Holzgrabe U. Effects of fluoroquinolones on HERG channels and on pancreatic betacell ATP-sensitive K+ channels. Toxicology. 2006;228(2–3):239-48.
73. Maeda N, Tamagawa T, Niki I, Miura H, Ozawa K, Watanabe G, et al. Increase in insulin release from rat pancreatic islets by quinolone antibiotics. Br J Pharmacol. 1996;117(2):372-6.
74. Wang YC, Chen YT, Kuo SC, Chen TL, Chang FY. Rapid hypoglycemia onset associated with antimicrobial use in patients with diabetes: A nationwide population-based case-crossover study. Eur J Intern Med. 2016;34:e14-5.
75. Lee S, Ock M, Kim HS, Kim H. Effects of Co-administration of sulfonylureas and antimicrobial drugs on hypoglycemia in patients with type 2 diabetes using a case-crossover design. Pharmacotherapy. 2020;40(9):902-12.
76. Schelleman H, Bilker WB, Brensinger CM, Wan F, Hennessy S. Anti-infectives and the risk of severe hypoglycemia in users of glipizide or glyburide. Clin Pharmacol Ther. 2010;88(2):214-22.
77. Lin HH, Hsu HY, Tsai MC, Hsu LY, Chien KL, Yeh TL. Association between type 2 diabetes and osteoporosis risk: a representative cohort study in Taiwan. PLoS One. 2021;16(7):e0254451.
78. Rasgado E, Pérez-Fuentes R, Gonzalez-Mejia ME. Denosumab improves glucose parameters in patients with impaired glucose tolerance: a systematic review and meta-analysis. J Drug Assess. 2021;10(1):97-105.
79. Kiechl S, Wittmann J, Giaccari A, Knoflach M, Willeit P, Bozec A, et al. Blockade of receptor activator of nuclear factor-κB (RANKL) signaling improves hepatic insulin resistance and prevents development of diabetes mellitus. Nat Med. 2013;19(3):358-63.
80. Huang HK, Chuang AT, Liao TC, Shao SC, Liu PP, Tu YK, et al. Denosumab and the risk of diabetes in patients treated for osteoporosis. JAMA Netw Open. 2024;7(2):e2354734.
81. Schwartz AV, Schafer AL, Grey A, Vittinghoff E, Palermo L, Lui LY, et al. Effects of antiresorptive therapies on glucose metabolism: results from the FIT, HORIZON-PFT, and FREEDOM trials. J Bone Miner Res. 2013;28(6):1348-54.
82. Houchen L, Sizheng Steven Z, Licheng Z, Wei J, Li X, Li H, et al. Denosumab and incidence of type 2 diabetes among

83. Cefalu WT, Kaul S, Gerstein HC, Holman RR, Zinman B, Skyler JS, et al. Cardiovascular outcomes trials in type 2 diabetes: where do we go from here? Reflections from a diabetes care Editors' expert forum. Diabetes Care. 2018;41(1):14-31.
84. Federal Register; The U.S. Food and Drug Administration (FDA). (2008). Guidance for Industry Diabetes Mellitus- Evaluating Cardiovascular Risk in New Antidiabetic Therapies to Treat Type 2 Diabetes. [online] Available from https://www.federalregister.gov/documents/2008/12/19/E8-30086/guidance-for-industry-on-diabetes-mellitus-evaluating-cardiovascular-risk-in-new-antidiabetic [Last accessed January, 2025].
85. U.S. Department of Health and Human Services, Food and Drug Administration. (2017). Multiple Endpoints in Clinical Trials Guidance for Industry. [online] Available from http://www.fda.gov/Drugs/GuidanceComplianceRegulatoryInformation/Guidances/default.htm [Last accessed January, 2025].
86. EUnetHTA—European network for Health Technology Assessment. Endpoints Used for Relative Effectiveness Assessment of Pharmaceuticals Composite Endpoints Final Version. EUnetHTA; 2013.
87. Yahyavi SK, Kristensen PL, Nagras ZG, Hjorthøj C, Krogh J. Rating the importance of outcomes from diabetes trials. A survey of patients' and doctors' opinions. J Diabetes Metab Disord. 2021;21:51-59.
88. Ferreira-González I, Busse JW, Heels-Ansdell D, Montori VM, Akl EA, Bryant DM, et al. Problems with use of composite end points in cardiovascular trials: systematic review of randomised controlled trials. Br Med J. 2007;334(7597):786-8.
89. Fang M, Wang D, Coresh J, Selvin E. Trends in diabetes treatment and control in US adults, 1999-2018. N Engl J Med. 2021;384:2219-28.
90. Almigbal TH, Alzahra SA, Aljanoubi FA, Alhafez NA, Aldawsari MR, Alghadeer ZY, et al. Clinical inertia in the management of type 2 diabetes mellitus: a systematic review. Medicina. 2023;59(1):182.
91. Giorgino F, Benroubi M, Sun JH, Zimmermann AG, Pechtner V. Efficacy and safety of once-weekly dulaglutide versus insulin glargine in patients with type 2 diabetes on metformin and glimepiride (AWARD-2). Diabetes Care. 2015;38(12):2241-9.
92. Marso SP, Daniels GH, Brown-Frandsen K, Kristensen P, Mann JF, Nauck MA, et al. Liraglutide and cardiovascular outcomes in type 2 diabetes. N Engl J Med. 2016;375(4):311-22.
93. Yao H, Zhang A, Li D, Wu Y, Wang CZ, Wan JY, et al. Comparative effectiveness of GLP-1 receptor agonists on glycaemic control, body weight, and lipid profile for type 2 diabetes: systematic review and network meta-analysis. BMJ. 2024;384:e076410.
94. Carls GS, Tuttle E, Tan RD, Huynh J, Yee J, Edelman SV, et al. Understanding the gap between efficacy in randomized controlled trials and effectiveness in real-world use of GLP-1 RA and DPP-4 therapies in patients with type 2 diabetes. Diabetes Care. 2017;40(11):1469-78.
95. Alatorre C, Fernández Landó L, Yu M, Brown K, Montejano L, Juneau P, et al. Treatment patterns in patients with type 2 diabetes mellitus treated with glucagon-like peptide-1 receptor agonists: higher adherence and persistence with dulaglutide compared with once-weekly exenatide and liraglutide. Diabetes Obes Metab. 2017;19(7):953-61.
96. Walter PB, Knutson MD, Paler-Martinez A, Lee S, Xu Y, Viteri FE, et al. Iron deficiency and iron excess damage mitochondria and mitochondrial DNA in rats. PNAS. 2002;99:2264-9.
97. Franke GN, Kubasch AS, Cross M, Vucinic V, Platzbecker U. Iron overload and its impact on outcome of patients with hematological diseases. Mol Aspects Med. 2020;75:100868.
98. Harrison AV, Lorenzo FR, McClain DA. Iron and the pathophysiology of diabetes. Annu Rev Physiol. 2023;85:339-62.
99. Ponikowska B, Suchocki T, Paleczny B, Olesinska M, Powierza S, Borodulin-Nadzieja L, et al. Iron status and survival in diabetic patients with coronary artery disease. Diabetes Care. 2013;36:4147-56.
100. Asmar J, Chelala D, El Hajj CR, Azar H, Finianos S, Aoun M. Anemia biomarkers and mortality in hemodialysis patients with or without diabetes: A 10-year follow-up study. PLoS One. 2023;18:e0280871.
101. Ellervik C, Andersen HU, Tybjærg-Hansen A, Frandsen M, Birgens H, Nordestgaard BG, et al. Total mortality by elevated transferrin saturation in patients with diabetes. Diabetes Care. 2013;36:2646-54.
102. Ellervik C, Mandrup-Poulsen T, Tybjærg-Hansen A, Nordestgaard BG. Total and cause-specific mortality by elevated transferrin saturation and hemochromatosis genotype in individuals with diabetes: two general population studies. Diabetes Care. 2014;37:444-52.
103. Jordan AS, McSharry DG, Malhotra A. Adult obstructive sleep apnoea. Lancet. 2014;383:736-47.
104. Young T, Peppard PE, Taheri S. Excess weight and sleep disordered breathing. J Appl Physiol (1985). 2005;99:1592-9.
105. McEvoy RD, Antic NA, Heeley E, Luo Y, Ou Q, Zhang X, et al. CPAP for prevention of cardiovascular events in obstructive sleep apnea. N Engl J Med. 2016;375:919-31.
106. Peker Y, Glantz H, Eulenburg C, Wegscheider K, Herlitz J, Thunström E. Effect of positive airway pressure on cardiovascular outcomes in coronary artery disease patients with nonsleepy obstructive sleep apnea: the RICCADSA randomized controlled trial. Am J Respir Crit Care Med. 2016;194:613-20.
107. Morgenthaler TI, Kapen S, Lee-Chiong T, Alessi C, Boehlecke B, Brown T, et al. Practice parameters for the medical therapy of obstructive sleep apnea. Sleep. 2006;29:1031-5.
108. Jastreboff AM, Aronne LJ, Ahmad NN, Wharton S, Connery L, Alves B, et al. Tirzepatide once weekly for the treatment of obesity. N Engl J Med. 2022;387:205-16.
109. Wilson JM, Lin Y, Luo MJ, Considine G, Cox AL, Bowsman LM, et al. The dual glucose-dependent insulinotropic polypeptide and glucagon-like peptide-1 receptor agonist tirzepatide improves cardiovascular risk biomarkers in

patients with type 2 diabetes: a post hoc analysis. Diabetes Obes Metab. 2022;24:148-53.
110. Eberly LA, Yang L, Essien UR, Eneanya ND, Julien HM, Luo J, et al. Racial, ethnic, and socioeconomic inequities in glucagon-like peptide-1 receptor agonist use among patients with diabetes in the US. JAMA Health Forum. 2021;2(12):e214182.
111. Emanuel EJ, Persad G. The shared ethical framework to allocate scarce medical resources: a lesson from COVID-19. Lancet. 2023;401:1892-902.
112. Emerging Risk Factors Collaboration. Life expectancy associated with different ages at diagnosis of type 2 diabetes in highincome countries: 23 million person-years of observation. Lancet Diabetes Endocrinol. 2023;11:731-42.
113. Ferrannini E, Cushman WC. Diabetes and hypertension: The bad companions. Lancet. 2012;380:601-10.
114. GBD 2019 Risk Factors Collaborators. Global burden of 87 risk factors in 204 countries and territories, 1990-2019: a systematic analysis for the Global Burden of Disease Study 2019. Lancet. 2020;396:1223-49.
115. Adler AI, Stratton IM, Neil HA, Yudkin JS, Matthews DR, Cull CA, et al. Association of systolic blood pressure with macrovascular and microvascular complications of type 2 diabetes (UKPDS 36): prospective observational study. BMJ. 2000;321:412-9.
116. The ACCORD Study Group. Effects of intensive blood-pressure control in type 2 diabetes mellitus. N Engl J Med. 2010;362:1575-85.
117. The SPRINT Research Group. A randomized trial of intensive versus standard blood-pressure control. N Engl J Med. 2015;373:2103-16.
118. Harris MI, Eastman RC, Cowie CC, Flegal KM, Eberhardt MS. Racial and ethnic differences in glycemic control of adults with type 2 diabetes. Diabetes Care. 1999;22:403-8.
119. Cowie CC, Port FK, Wolfe RA, Savage PJ, Moll PP, Hawthorne VM. Disparities in incidence of diabetic end-stage renal disease according to race and type of diabetes. N Engl J Med. 1989;321:1074-9.
120. Cappellini MD, Fiorelli G. Glucose-6-phosphate dehydrogenase deficiency. Lancet. 2008;371:64-74.
121. Yang HC, Wu YH, Yen WC, Liu HY, Hwang TL, Stern A, et al. The redox role of G6PD in cell growth, cell death, and cancer. Cells 2019;8:1055.

Index

A

Acetyl tartaric acid esters 47
Acute myocardial infarction 65, 83
Adapter protein-2-associated kinase 1 155
Adiposity 33
Advanced hybrid closed loop therapy 144, 145, 200
Alanine
 aminotransferase 165
 transaminase 224
Aliskiren trial 63
Alkaline phosphatase 5
American College of Sports Medicine 201
American Diabetes Association 17, 18, 81, 87, 95, 101, 140, 161, 201, 207
 statement of 207
American Heart Association guidelines 51
Amputations, risk of 85
Angiogenesis 5
Angiotensin receptor blocker 151
Angiotensin-converting enzyme inhibitor 151
Antithymocyte globulin 116
 low-dose 116
Aspartate
 aminotransferase 165
 transaminase 104, 224
Aspirin
 comparative effectiveness of 51
 daily low-dose 41
 efficacy of 87
Assisted reproductive technology 141
Atherosclerotic cardiovascular disease 51, 62, 87, 213
Autoantibodies 125
Autoimmune diseases 127

Automated insulin delivery systems 120, 194, 198-200

B

Bariatric surgery 57
Basal insulins 185
Bisphosphonates 227
Bleeding risk 88
Blindness 97
Blood
 glucose
  monitoring 196
  self-monitoring of 163, 196
 pressure 56, 97, 154, 175
  control target 237
 samples 216
Body mass index 4, 10, 13, 16, 17, 20, 25, 27, 32, 35, 43, 44, 54, 79, 94, 129, 140-142, 147, 151, 160, 166, 172, 173, 206, 210, 219, 221, 222, 228, 234, 236
Body weight 148
Bone marrow 5
 mesenchymal stem cells 5, 6

C

Canagliflozin 83
 cardiovascular assessment study program 63, 150
 impact of 150
Cancer 28, 36, 214, 233
 subsequent incidence of 15
Cardiometabolic disease spectrum 107
Cardiorenal endpoints 63
Cardiovascular death 90, 107
Cardiovascular disease 34, 36, 37, 51, 52, 60, 62, 67, 76, 87, 129, 151, 209, 233, 237
 prevalence of 67
 regardless of 67
Cardiovascular events 59, 84

Cardiovascular outcome 55, 64, 80, 150
 trials 53, 220, 229, 230
Cardiovascular properties 177
Carrageenan gum 47
Central nervous system 16
Cerebrovascular accidents 129
Chinese Diabetes Society 218
Chronic kidney disease 1, 60, 70, 73, 74, 80, 92, 98, 100, 105, 106, 150, 220, 238
 prediction consortium 1
 progression of 69
Closed-loop insulin delivery systems 194
Cohort-specific hazard ratios 49
Continuous glucose monitoring 113, 121, 144, 163, 181, 182, 188-192, 195-197, 199, 207
 efficacy of 189
 safety of 189
Controlled attenuation parameters 224
Coronavirus disease 2019 (COVID-19) 32
 pandemic 33, 114, 133, 165, 196, 238

D

Dapagliflozin 83, 209
De novo lipogenesis 12
Denosumab 227
Depression 204
Diabetes Exercise Initiative Pediatric Study 118
Diabetes mellitus 26, 28, 51, 65, 67, 76, 91, 98, 138, 148, 157, 165, 189, 214, 233
 control and complications trial 130
 diagnosis 15
 different phenotypes of 142
 gestational 138, 139, 141, 145, 146

management 207
remission clinical trial 6, 7, 31, 32
risk, development of 54
study of 218
type 1 3, 10, 68, 96, 113, 114, 116, 118, 120, 121, 123, 126, 128, 130-132, 136, 142, 144, 162, 163, 192, 198, 203, 204
type 2 8, 12, 15, 17, 32, 34, 36, 41-43, 48, 52, 57, 58, 60, 63, 64, 67, 68, 78, 80-83, 87-89, 96, 105, 138, 148, 150, 155-161, 164, 166, 170-172, 175, 179, 181, 186, 189, 190, 192, 193, 195, 196, 201, 209, 215, 217, 219, 223, 224, 227, 228, 230, 231, 237, 239
Diabetic foot ulcer 6, 211
Diabetic ketoacidosis 207, 214
Diabetic kidney disease 23, 60, 61, 98-100, 151, 220
Diabetic macular oedema 78
Diabetic microvascular complications 22, 23
Diabetic nephropathy 128
Diabetic neuropathy 23
Diabetic peripheral neuropathy 128, 155
Diabetic retinopathy 23, 78, 91, 128
 incidence of 90
 progression of 90
 risk of 78
Dipeptidyl peptidase-4 inhibitor 156, 171, 214
Dual energy X-ray absorptiometry 33, 35, 169
Dynamic light scattering 5
Dyslipidemia 92

E

Electronic health records 24
Empagliflozin 83, 213, 214
 effectiveness of 213
 effects of 64, 69, 73
 impact of 65
 safety of 213
 therapies 64
End-diastolic velocity 210
Erectile dysfunction 209
Estimated glomerular filtration rate 20-22, 70, 74, 79, 81, 94, 95, 99, 105, 106, 150, 219
European Food Safety Authority 47
Extracellular vehicles 6

F

Fasting blood glucose 16
Fasting plasma glucose 42
Fatty acid
 diglycerides of 47
 nonesterified 12, 13, 175
Fatty liver disease, nonalcoholic 58, 59, 103, 104, 157, 159, 162
Fibrosis 102
Fluoroquinolones 225, 226
Food additives 46
Foot ulceration
 diabetes-related 211
 risk of 227
Framingham risk score 77

G

Gallbladder cancers 16
Gamma-glutamyl transferase 105
Gastrointestinal adverse events, occurrence of 151
Gastrointestinal bleeding 51
Gastrointestinal problems 104
Gastrointestinal symptoms 152
Gegludec 186
Genetic risk score 4
Genome-wide association studies 9
Gestational diabetes mellitus 138, 139, 141, 145, 146
 earlier detection of 139, 140
 risk factors, prevalence of 141
Glargine 206
Glimepiride 206
Glucagon 176
 receptor, dual agonism of 102
Glucagon-like peptide 1 100, 102, 215, 216, 235, 239
 receptor 69, 78, 151, 159
 agonists 20, 26, 52, 53, 55, 56, 58, 59, 78, 80, 81, 90, 95, 149, 158, 168, 170, 172, 183, 220-222, 231
Glucose control 89
Glucose-6-phosphate dehydrogenase deficiency 239
Glucose-dependent insulinotropic peptide 161
 polypeptide 103, 104, 154
 receptor 159
Glucose-lowering drugs 156
Glucose-responsive insulin complex 13

Glutamic acid decarboxylase 11
Glycemia
 reduction approaches 76
 analysis of 148
 estimating 190
 progression of 54
 regression of 54
 reduction approaches in diabetes mellitus 19, 20, 76, 148, 205, 206
Glycemic control 88, 148, 193, 201
Glycemic index 36-39
Glycemic load 36, 38, 39
Glycemic outcomes 19, 121
Glycemic risk index 200
Glycemic status, impact of 64
Guar gum 47
Gum arabic 47

H

Heart disease, ischemic 92
Heart failure 65, 67, 90, 213, 214
 new-onset 63
 obesity-related 68
 outcomes 107
 risk of 67
Hemoglobin
 A1c 33, 77, 190
 glycated 65, 73, 89, 202
Hepatic steatosis 11
Hepatocellular carcinoma 157
High-density lipoprotein 60, 61
 cholesterol 35
HOMA-IR and Matsuda index 10
Hospital episode statistics 226
Human umbilical vein endothelial cells 6
Hybrid closed-loop 119
Hypertension 92
Hypoglycemia 13, 148, 181, 192, 206, 207
 fluoroquinolone-induced 225
 sensor-detected 192
 severe 214

I

Impaired glucose tolerance 17, 18
Inclisiran 173
Incorrectly fitting footwear 211
Inhaled insulin 120
Insulin
 efsitora 186
 formulations 13
 lispro 162
Insulin-like growth factor 1 80

Insulinogenic index 10, 11
Intense glucose management 89
Intensive blood pressure control 237
Intermittently scanned continuous glucose monitoring 121, 189
International Association of Diabetes and Pregnancy Study Groups 140
International Classification of Diseases 92
International Index of Erectile Function 5-Item 209
International Working Group on Diabetic Foot 211
Intracytoplasmic sperm injection 142
Intraduodenal glucose infusion 215
Iron status 233
Islet autoantibody frequency 3
Islet-after-kidney transplantation 134
Isolated impaired fasting glucose 17, 18

K

Kidney
  disease 76, 81, 95, 101
    chronic 1, 60, 70, 73, 74, 80, 81, 92, 98, 100, 105, 106, 150, 220, 238
    diabetic 23, 60, 61, 98-100, 151, 220
    end-stage 97, 214, 220
    non-diabetic 98
    primary 73
  injury, acute 214
  transplant recipients 134

L

Lactococcus lactis 124
Large for gestational age 142
Laser photocoagulation 78
Lipid-lowering therapies 174
Liver
  fibrosis 103
  related outcomes 156
  stiffness measurement 224
Lotiglipron 164
Low-density lipoprotein 7, 56, 61, 167, 173
  cholesterol 173, 219, 224

Lower urinary tract symptoms, mild 209
Lower-limb amputation 214

M

Macrovascular outcomes 88
Major adverse cardiovascular events 52, 55, 56, 58, 64, 89, 106, 177, 213
Malignancies 214
Markov model 18
Mass spectrometry 7
Maternally inherited diabetes and deafness 2, 3
Matsuda index 10
Mean arterial pressure 97
Medical therapy, metabolomic fingerprints of 57
Medullary thyroid carcinoma 223
Mesenchymal stem cell 5
Metabolic dysfunction 103, 223
Metabolic health 33
Metabolic surgery 57
Metabolic syndrome 12
Metformin 59, 138, 151, 205, 216
  administration 215
  therapy 138
Microvascular outcomes 88
Mixed meal tolerance test 163, 165
Monotherapy 123
Mortality rate 76
Multicentre randomised controlled trial 196, 198
Multiple daily insulin injections 196
Myocardial infarction 38, 61, 64, 65, 83, 90, 97, 214

N

National Death Index 234
National Diabetes Audit 44
National Health Insurance Fund Administration 29
National Health Insurance Research Database 92
National Health Service 32, 43, 44
Neonatal intensive care unit 138
Nephrosclerosis 98, 99
Nitric oxide 209
Non-high-density lipoprotein 174
Nonsteroidal mineralocorticoid receptor antagonists 101, 107
Noradrenaline 176

Normoalbuminuria 93
Normoglycemia 13
Nuclear magnetic resonance 7
NutriNet-Santé Prospective Cohort Study 46

O

Obesity 26, 54, 55, 57, 68, 71, 164, 166, 173, 235
Oral antidiabetic drugs 149
Oral glucagon-like peptide-1 receptor agonist 171
Oral glucose tolerance test 18, 146
Oral semaglutide
  beneficial effect of 223
  monotherapy
    efficacy of 217
    safety of 217
Osteoporosis 227
Overweight 54, 55

P

Pain, diabetic peripheral neuropathic 155
Pancreas volume, longitudinal assessment of 114
Peak systolic velocity 210
Peripheral artery disease 85, 86, 92
Peripheral vascular disease 97
Phenylboronic acid 13
Pioglitazone 175
Polycystic ovary syndrome 30, 142
Polygenic risk score 1
Polypyrimidine tract 11
Postexercise glycemia 118
Postprandial glucose 163
  control 162
  excursion 120
Prediabetes 71, 72
Premature mortality 233
Proliferative diabetic retinopathy 97
Propensity score weighting 28
Proteinuria, effect of 98

R

Randomized controlled trials 7, 44, 52, 61, 62, 80, 85, 86, 90, 95, 106, 121, 122, 145, 152, 183, 184, 195-199, 228
  meta-analysis of 193, 221

Randomized second-line therapy, comparative effects of 148
Rapid kidney function 98
Rapid-acting analog insulin 120
Real-time continuous glucose monitoring 121, 122, 195
Red blood cell 191
Renal disease, end-stage 150
Renal function 71
Renin-angiotensin system inhibitor 101
Roux-en-Y gastric bypass 57, 58

S

Self-injury 26
Semaglutide 55, 68, 71, 160, 169, 179
 effect of 54, 55, 105
 flows 100
Sensor-augmented pump 199
Serum alanine transaminase 104
Serum ketone bodies 175
Severe hypoglycemia 214
 risk of 225
Shanghai Municipal Center for Disease Control and Prevention 16
Shanghai Standardized Diabetes Management System 16
Single nucleotide polymorphisms 136
Sleeve gastrectomy 57
Small for gestational age 138, 140
Sodium citrate 47
Sodium-glucose cotransporter-2 59, 63, 64, 71
 inhibitors 27, 52, 59, 61, 69, 70, 74, 77-80, 82, 84, 85, 90, 91, 95, 106, 108, 150, 156, 175, 213, 219, 220, 239
 effect of 61, 107
 efficacy of 183
 safety of 183
 uric acid-lowering effects of 84

Standard insulin therapy 144
Steatohepatitis 103
 metabolic dysfunction-associated 103, 104
 nonalcoholic 159
Steatotic liver disease 223
 metabolic dysfunction-associated 12, 224
Stroke, ischemic 82, 92
Structured weight maintenance support 32
Sugar-sweetened beverages 24
Suicidal
 attempts 203, 204
 deaths 203
 ideation 26, 203, 204
Sulfonylureas 177, 225
Survodutide, phase 2 randomized trial of 102

T

Teplizumab 123, 132
 efficacy of 130
 safety of 130
Thiazolidinediones 77, 156, 157
Thyroid cancer, risk of 221
Tirzepatide 103, 160, 179
 effect of 166
 treatment 153
Total cholesterol 219
Total diet replacement 32, 43, 44
Transmission electron microscopy 5
Triglyceride-rich lipoproteins 60
Triglycerides 167, 219
Tripotassium phosphate 47
Tumor necrosis factor alpha 210
Type 1 diabetes mellitus 3, 10, 68, 96, 113, 114, 116, 118, 120, 121, 123, 126, 128, 130-132, 136, 142, 144, 162, 163, 192, 198, 203, 204
 progression of 125
 treatment of 130
 young-onset 96

Type 2 diabetes mellitus 8, 12, 15, 17, 32, 36, 41-43, 48, 52, 58, 63, 67, 68, 78, 80-83, 87-89, 96, 105, 138, 148, 150, 155-161, 166, 170-172, 181, 189, 193, 196, 201, 209, 217, 219, 223, 227, 231, 237, 239
 cardiovascular outcomes trials 52
 diagnosis 3
 duration 150
 early-onset 153, 154
 management of 20, 169, 189
 natural history of 17
 non-obese 175
 prevalence of 66
 risk of 38, 46
 treatment of 96, 97, 179, 205
 young-onset 96, 142

U

Ultra-rapid lispro 162, 163
Uric acid 84
Urinary albumin 93, 101
 abnormal 93
 to-creatinine ratio 93, 101

V

Valencia Health System Integrated Database 27
Vascular endothelial growth factor 78
Visceral adipose tissue 166

W

Weight loss
 maintenance 31
 metabolomic signature of 6
Western blot analysis 5
World Health Organization 201
Wound healing 5

X

Xanthan gum 47

Z

Zinc 11